UNDERSTANDING
TYPE 2 DIABETES

UNDERSTANDING TYPE 2 DIABETES

Fewer highs, fewer lows, better health

PROFESSOR MERLIN THOMAS

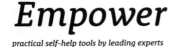

Empower

practical self-help tools by leading experts

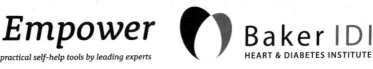

Baker IDI

HEART & DIABETES INSTITUTE

Professor Merlin Thomas is a clinician scientist from Melbourne, Australia. He works extensively with patients with diabetes and their doctors, as well as performing research in experimental models of diabetes and its complications. His research aims to identify new targets and advance new treatments to prevent, reverse and retard the development and progression of diabetic complications. His work on diabetic complications has received both local and international recognition. He has written over two hundred and seventy papers, book chapters and books on diabetes management. He is also a consummate storyteller, speaker and communicator on the diagnosis, prevention and treatment of all aspects of preventive health.

'*Understanding Type 2 Diabetes* is a terrific addition to your library if you have Type 2 and want to gain a deeper knowledge of it, or if you have just been diagnosed and don't know where to start.'

Diabetes Diet Choices, May 2014

'Written by Professor Merlin Thomas from the world-renowned Baker IDI Heart and Diabetes Institute, *Understanding Type 2 Diabetes* offers clear and effective guidance on how to manage all aspects of diabetes.'

Diabetes Matters, April 2013

'This book is a clear guide for any diabetic sufferer on how to manage all aspects of the disease. The text covers what diabetes is and how it comes about, what is the right diet for someone with diabetes and how to achieve it and how exercise can improve and maintain health. The medical aspects of diabetes care, such as the best ways to control your waistline, blood glucose, blood sugar and cholesterol, as well as how to prevent major complications, are all covered in the book.'

Australian Nurses Journal, April 2013

'This book aims to help those living with diabetes manage the condition, giving you the knowledge you need to choose the right diet, exercise and medication, and prevent complications.'

Good Health Magazine, May 2013

First published 2013. This edition published 2017.

Exisle Publishing Pty Ltd
'Moonrising', Narone Creek Road, Wollombi,
NSW 2325, Australia
P.O. Box 60–490, Titirangi, Auckland 0642,
New Zealand
www.exislepublishing.com

A CiP record for this book is available from the
National Library of Australia.

ISBN 978-1-925335-55-2

Designed by Tracey Gibbs
Typeset in Miller Text
Printed in China

This book uses paper sourced under ISO 14001
guidelines from well-managed forests and other
controlled sources.

10 9 8 7 6 5 4 3 2 1

Disclaimer

This book is a general guide only and should never be a substitute for the skill, knowledge and experience of a qualified medical professional dealing with the facts, circumstances and symptoms of a particular case. The nutritional, medical and health information presented in this book is based on the research, training and professional experience of the author, and is true and complete to the best of their knowledge. However, this book is intended only as an informative guide; it is not intended to replace or countermand the advice given by the reader's personal physician or diabetes care team. Because each person and situation is unique, the author and the publisher urge the reader to check with a qualified healthcare professional before using any procedure where there is a question as to its appropriateness. Your diabetes practitioner or care team should be consulted before beginning any new treatment program, including diet, lifestyle and/or physical activity. The author, publisher and their distributors are not responsible for any adverse effects or consequences resulting from the use of the information in this book. It is the responsibility of the reader to consult a physician or other qualified healthcare professional regarding their personal care. This book contains references to products and procedures that may not be available everywhere. The intent of the information provided is to be helpful; however, there is no guarantee of results associated with the information provided. Use of drug brand names is for educational purposes only and does not imply endorsement.

CONTENTS

INTRODUCTION

In ancient times there lived a king called Sisyphus. Because of his past excesses and hubris he was cursed by the Gods. His penance was to push an immense boulder up a steep hill, only to have it roll back down and the task to start all over again. Having diabetes often feels like this, the ripened fruit of our actions or inattention. Equally, the treatment regime for managing diabetes often feels like an appropriate punishment: boring ritualized repetition and relentless austerity to make up for our previous bad behaviour. But it's really not like that at all.

First, your goals of understanding and managing your diabetes are achievable. With the application of good diabetes care, healthy nutrition and regular physical activity, most people with type 2 diabetes lead full and healthy lives. Your effort is never futile.

Second, managing diabetes is not as hard as it sounds. What might appear on the surface to be an enormous or complex undertaking can become quite effortless with practice and application.

Third, diabetes management is not a punishment. It is easy to fall into the trap of believing that some suffering is the price of good health, like the distasteful medicine you must swallow to get well. But dieting is not punishment for the nutritionally wicked, nor is exercise the castigation of the couch potato. These are positive steps that have their own rewards.

Fourth, diabetes management requires a careful coordination of physical activity, diet and medication. But this does not mean you have to do the same things every day or eat the same restrictive diet, trapped in a tedious and repetitive cycle of care. In fact, diabetes management can be very flexible, matching individual requirements and capabilities with diet, exercise or medications.

Finally, you are not alone with your burden. Diabetes management will harness the support of your doctor, diabetes educator, dietician, podiatrist and many other professionals that comprise your diabetes care team. Each person will help you manage your diabetes and make the task of managing diabetes not only feasible but also revitalising.

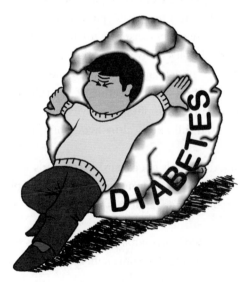

Diabetes can sometimes feel like a curse to a lifetime of futile repetition. But it is not like this at all!

This book is your guide to diabetes and outlines the many opportunities you have to make a positive difference to your health. It begins by examining what diabetes is and how it comes about. It then goes on to describe the many practical changes you can make to your diet, and the potential strengths as well as weaknesses of these changes. It also looks at physical activity and the different ways exercise can be used to both maintain and improve your health. The book also explores the medical aspects of diabetes care, including practical ways to achieve control of your waistline, blood glucose, blood pressure and cholesterol levels, as well as the best means to avoid major complications.

You can do this. It is nothing like pushing a rock up a hill.

1

WHAT IS DIABETES?

Understand

- The human body runs on fuel, like the petrol in your car. Glucose is chiefly used to fuel chemical reactions inside the body.
- To keep the brain and body healthy, blood glucose levels are normally kept within a narrow range, balanced by the actions of insulin and other hormones.
- Insulin is made and released by the beta-cells of the pancreas to coordinate the body's response to rising glucose levels.

- Diabetes occurs when there is not enough insulin (or its functions) to keep glucose levels under control.
- High glucose levels usually start out as a silent problem. Most people diagnosed with type 2 diabetes are completely unaware they have it, and have probably had it for many years.

Manage
- Recognize what your own symptoms of high glucose levels are and how they might be affecting your health and wellbeing.
- Frequently assess how well your glucose levels are being controlled with the help of your diabetes care team.
- Work with your diabetes care team to define the most appropriate targets for the intensity of your own glucose control.
- Learn to monitor your own glucose levels using a blood glucose meter.

- Follow and learn what different foods or activities do to your glucose levels, and use this information to develop diet and lifestyle plans that best meet your individual needs.

The name **glucose** comes from the Greek word *glukus*, meaning 'sweet'. Glucose is a sweet sugar. It is also the major sugar that circulates inside your blood, so the terms 'glucose' and 'sugar' are often used interchangeably when managing diabetes. But glucose is not the same thing as the white sugar used in cooking or in your coffee.

The human body runs on fuel, like the petrol in your car. Glucose is chiefly used to fuel chemical reactions inside your body. This is known as **metabolism**. Metabolism provides the vital energy for every cell to do what needs to be done. Every cell needs fuel for its metabolism. Most cells will eat anything that is available. But your brain is a very picky eater — it will only eat glucose.

However, the problem is that your brain has little stored glucose of its own. It can't make glucose itself and won't use any other fuel if glucose runs out. Instead, it must rely on the glucose dissolved in your blood being present all of the time to maintain continuous supply and continuous functioning. From the brain's point of view, blood sugar is as important as the oxygen in the air you breathe: it can only function for a few minutes without either before it stops working altogether.

To guarantee your brain keeps running night and day, the body must ensure that glucose is always present in your blood in roughly the same concentration. To achieve this level of control is not easy. Some days you might eat a few pieces of cake, a sandwich or even a huge bowl of pasta. Other times you might eat hardly anything at all. Yet through it all, glucose levels will normally fluctuate only very slightly:

- between 4–6 mmol/L (72–108 mg/dL) when you are not eating and
- between 4–7 mmol/L (72–126 mg/dL) after a meal.

This amazing level of control is achieved thanks to an elaborate system of checks and balances that carefully regulates how much glucose is going into the blood and how much is going out.

In essence, diabetes is the state in which this balance fails and glucose levels rise.

Every time you eat or drink something that contains any **carbohydrate** (also known as **carbs**) your body gets a dose of sugar. Whether you are eating chocolate cake or spaghetti or drinking a Coke, the carbs contained in each product are broken down by your digestion into simple sugars, one of which is glucose.

As these sugars are digested and absorbed, they trigger the release of hormones, the most important of which is **insulin**. Hormones are chemical signals that communicate a message from one part of the body to another, usually via the bloodstream. Insulin is made and released by the **beta-cells of the pancreas**. The message insulin sends coordinates the body's response to rising blood glucose levels. This message tells the cells of the liver, muscles and fat to take away glucose from the blood (and store it for later use). It also tells the liver to stop making and releasing any extra glucose, which is rendered unnecessary by having just had a sugary meal.

This is a proportional response. The greater the amount of

sugar contained in a product and the faster it hits your system, the greater the amount of insulin that is released. This keeps glucose levels from rising too fast or too high. In contrast, a meal that is low in sugar or contains sugars that are only slowly digested will need to trigger a proportionally smaller insulin response to make sure glucose levels don't drop too rapidly.

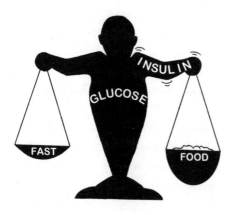

Diabetes occurs when there is not enough insulin (or its functions) to keep glucose levels balanced.

The net result of this finely balanced system is that, in people without diabetes, glucose levels in the blood only rise slightly and very briefly following a meal, regardless of what they eat.

When you are not eating, such as at night, your brain still needs glucose to keep functioning. So to keep up with the brain's unceasing demands, the liver slowly releases its glucose stores and also manufactures new glucose, which it releases into the blood like a kind of controlled drip feed for your hungry brain.

To make this happen before glucose levels in the blood start to fall, the pancreas immediately stops releasing insulin and starts making other hormones such as **glucagon**. These hormones send a different message. They say that any unnecessary uptake of glucose must now stop, leaving any glucose for your fussy brain. Also, the brakes that insulin has placed on the liver's glucose production should be removed, to start the drip feed.

Again, the rate at which glucose is released into the blood is finely balanced to match the rate at which the body (and in particular the brain) uses glucose. So glucose levels in the blood don't fall very much, if at all, between meals in people who do not have diabetes. Even if you skip a meal, or wish to fast for several days, glucose levels always remain sufficient for the brain to keep working.

So in people without diabetes, day and night, feeding or fasting, the levels of glucose in their blood do not rise or fall much at all, balanced by the actions of insulin and other hormones.

Diabetes only occurs when there is not enough insulin to keep this balance and maintain glucose levels under tight control.

How and why this happens is complicated. Many different factors can contribute to the decline and loss of insulin's functions, leading ultimately to the development of type 2 diabetes. These are discussed in detail in Chapter 2.

DIABETES AND GLUCOSE CONTROL

Not having enough insulin has major consequences for glucose control.

In diabetes, glucose levels in the blood can rise excessively after a meal

The job of insulin is chiefly to coordinate your body to deal with the sugars in your meal. So one of the first signs that insulin is not doing this job is a rise in your glucose level after a meal, especially one rich in carbohydrate. This is when you need to make the greatest amount of insulin to cope with the extra glucose entering your blood, so this is also when any limited capacity for insulin production is first challenged.

One simple way to test for type 2 diabetes is an **oral glucose tolerance test (OGTT)**. This test involves drinking a large amount of glucose and then determining how quickly it is cleared from your blood and glucose balance is restored. It is essentially a 'road test' of your pancreas to see if it can rev up and handle the (sugar) hills. An OGTT is usually performed in the morning after having not eaten anything overnight. Drinking water beforehand is allowed, but no coffee, tea or juice, which can upset the results. At the start of the OGTT a blood sample is drawn. You are then given a sweet solution (containing 75g of glucose) to drink within 5 minutes. A further blood sample is drawn 2 hours later and the glucose level is measured.

In healthy people, the glucose level in their blood 2 hours after drinking this big wallop of glucose will be below 7.8 mmol/L (140mg/dL). This means they quickly made enough insulin to efficiently put all this sugar away.

If your glucose level is above 11 mmol/L (198 mg/dL) 2 hours after drinking the glucose, insulin has not done its job. This indicates a diagnosis of diabetes.

If glucose levels are modestly elevated (between 7.8 and 11 mmol/L) (140.4 and 198 mg/dL) then **impaired glucose tolerance** is said to exist. This is also known as **pre-diabetes**, as without significant changes in diet and lifestyle most people with these intermediate levels ultimately go on to develop full-blown diabetes.

In diabetes, glucose levels in the blood can stay elevated even when you are not eating

Most of the glucose in your blood does not come from your diet. It has been made and released by your liver. As detailed earlier in this chapter, in the healthy human body the production of glucose is perfectly in tune with the glucose levels in your blood and the rate at which it is used up. So glucose levels in the blood do not usually fall very much when you are not eating, because glucose production springs into action.

Equally, if glucose levels are too high or sugar is coming into the body after a meal, unnecessary glucose production by the liver should be shut down, so balancing the system. But in type 2 diabetes this shutdown does not happen very well. This is partly because there is not enough insulin (function) to stop glucose production. In addition, the signals that drive glucose production, like glucagon and free fat in the blood, fail to be adequately suppressed.

Without the right signals, your liver mistakenly believes you are hungry all the time and need more glucose in your blood, even when you have just eaten.

So diabetes is like a state of anarchy (literally out of control). Even though glucose levels may be already high in the blood, in diabetes extra glucose is still made by the anarchic liver and released into the blood. Consequently, glucose levels become and remain elevated in people with type 2 diabetes even if they are on a stringent diet or are eating almost nothing at all. Indeed, most people are first diagnosed with type 2 diabetes because they are found to have a glucose level greater than 7 mmol/L (126 mg/dL) on a routine blood test taken when they were not eating (e.g. before a meal).

THE CONSEQUENCES OF HIGH GLUCOSE

High glucose levels usually start out as a silent problem. Most people are completely unaware they have type 2 diabetes. Yet glucose levels have usually been elevated in the blood for an average of 5 to 10 years before a diagnosis of type 2 diabetes is first made.

The most common symptoms associated with type 2 diabetes are easily dismissed as a signs of getting old or other problems. These may include:

- feeling tired and weak all the time
- having difficulty concentrating
- feeling restless and uncomfortable
- not doing the things you usually do with the same skill or enthusiasm
- finding the things that were difficult now even harder to do
- trouble with your eyesight and/or dry eyes
- dry and itchy skin
- yeast infections in the feet, groin and under your breasts
- being irritable or moody
- reduced interest in (and difficulties during) sex
- general aches and pains
- passing urine more frequently during the day and especially during the night
- feeling thirsty and hungry, even though you seem to be drinking and eating more
- difficulty getting to sleep and staying asleep and/or waking up still feeling 'hung over'.

All of these symptoms are caused by having high glucose levels in your blood. They are not permanent or a sign of damage. When diabetes is treated and glucose control is restored most of these symptoms will go away. This is one reason why you and your diabetes care team will be working to keep your glucose levels as close to normal as possible.

There is no symptom here that is particularly unique to type 2 diabetes. It is very easy to simply explain these symptoms away, ignore them or misattribute them to other conditions. This is why today it is recommended that all people at risk for type 2 diabetes should have regular blood tests to look for diabetes regardless of how they feel.

GLUCOSE MONITORING USING HbA1c

The most common way to get a handle on your glucose control is for a doctor to measure your **haemoglobin A1c** (also known as HbA1c or A1c). The test for this involves having a blood sample taken and sent away to a clinical laboratory. The HbA1c shows the amount of glucose that is stuck onto a protein — haemoglobin — in your red blood cells. The higher your glucose levels have been during the previous 3 to 4 months, the more glucose will be stuck to the haemoglobin and the higher your HbA1c will be. This means that taking a blood test to measure your HbA1c is one way to confirm if you have diabetes.

In people without diabetes, their HbA1c is almost always less than 6 per cent (or 48 mmol/mol in the new units for this test now used by many doctors). By comparison, without treatment, people with type 2 diabetes usually have an HbA1c of greater than 6.5 per cent (50 mmol/mol). An HbA1c greater than 8 per cent (64 mmol/mol) suggests persistently elevated glucose levels and generally indicates your blood glucose is not well controlled and the risk of complications is increased.

Your HbA1c will be measured when you are diagnosed with type 2 diabetes and then at least twice a year thereafter. It is also common to measure your HbA1c about 3 months after starting any new treatment to lower your glucose levels, as it takes this long for its full effect to be seen on your HbA1c.

Often the first step in diabetes management will be to set an appropriate target for your HbA1c. Usually, getting and keeping the HbA1c to less than 7 per cent (53 mmol/mol) is the goal. This is not quite as good as people without diabetes, who normally run an HbA1c less than 6 per cent. However, achieving an HbA1c of less than 7 per cent (53 mmol/mol) will eliminate most of the symptoms caused by high glucose levels in people with diabetes. In addition, improving glucose control beyond this level does not appreciably reduce your risk from the complications of diabetes detailed later in this book, while exposing you to the burden of additional treatment.

However, sometimes even aiming for this level of glucose control is not the right thing for you to do. The right target for your HbA1c should take into account your age, lifestyle, work practices, the treatment you are receiving and its side effects, and a host of other factors. This kind of careful individualised assessment of the adequacy of your current level of glucose control, and the value and safety of going lower, will be made almost every time you see your physician or diabetes care team.

MONITORING USING BLOOD GLUCOSE LEVELS

Another way to come to grips with your glucose control is to directly measure and monitor your own blood glucose levels using a **blood glucose meter**. This is known as **self-monitoring**. Most good hospitals and many diabetes practices have educator nurses who will teach you this technique. The glucose test involves pricking your finger to release a drop of blood. (It is not very painful or particularly complicated to do.) The drop of blood is then applied to a plastic strip and placed in a small machine that measures the glucose level in the blood.

When glucose levels are under good control, most of the results from self-monitoring will be between:

- 6–8 mmol/L (108–144 mg/dL) when not eating and before meals, and
- 6–10 mmol/L (108–180 mg/dL) after a meal.

Testing your own blood glucose levels is a practical way to make sure that your diabetes management is on track. Self-monitoring also enables you to find out how different foods and activities affect your own individual blood glucose levels, and makes it easier to develop and modify diet and lifestyle plans that best suit your individual needs. In addition, self-monitoring provides valuable and prompt feedback about anything you might be doing to improve your glucose control, such as changes in your medication, physical activity, diet or lifestyle. Blood glucose monitoring can also be a useful way to reduce the risk of hypoglycaemia (see Chapter 5).

It is not essential to monitor your own glucose levels. However, most people with type 2 diabetes are encouraged to monitor when there are adequate resources, support and assessment.

A strategic plan for blood glucose monitoring will usually be developed in conjunction with your physician or diabetes care team. The frequency of self-monitoring will always need to be different for different people and different situations. For example, people with very stable glucose control may need to monitor less often than those starting out on a new treatment regimen, or those troubled by lots of highs and/or lows. How often you need to test may range from once or twice a week to many times a day, timed to coincide with key problem periods. More testing will usually be undertaken if you are unwell, because this is commonly the time that glucose control, as well as other aspects of your health, goes awry.

A new way to monitor glucose levels has recently become more widely available. This is known as **continuous glucose monitoring** (CGM) and involves wearing a small device that is able to measure glucose levels every 5 minutes. It can be worn for up to 6 days and can track changes in your glucose levels throughout the day and night. Some devices also have alarms for glucose highs and lows. These devices can provide a very accurate picture of your daily fluctuations in blood glucose control and help find the best approach to tackling your own individual glucose control problems.

At present, CGM devices are mostly used only for brief periods, and give a brief snapshot of glucose control over a few days. However, some people are starting to use this technology every day. It is likely that the future management of diabetes will increasingly involve continuous blood glucose monitoring.

2

WHY DID IT HAPPEN TO ME?

Understand

- Many different factors can contribute to the decline and loss of insulin's functions, leading ultimately to the development of type 2 diabetes.
- By the time type 2 diabetes is diagnosed it may be that over half of the insulin-producing beta-cells in the pancreas have been lost.
- Beta-cells may become progressively exhausted because of the demands of an unhealthy diet or having to work against insulin resistance to keep your metabolism under control.

- Most people develop type 2 diabetes because they cannot safely contain the excess energy from their diet and a 'toxic waist' starts to accumulate.
- To develop type 2 diabetes, you also need to be susceptible either to developing ectopic fat or your beta-cells must be susceptible to exhaustion, which can be the result of genes, ethnicity or acquired during your development or as you age.

Manage
- Unburden your pancreas from too much work by reducing the carbs and calories you eat, and slowing their delivery using low GI, high fibre substitutes.
- Measure your waist circumference and compare it to what it should be in someone of your gender and ethnic background. Set targets to make it smaller.
- Increase your level of physical activity to achieve a negative energy balance

    that will help to remove ectopic fat
    from your body.
- Restrict the amount of energy you get
  from your food and drink by improving
  your dietary choices or adhering to a
  diet.

Diabetes is a simple disease. It occurs when there is not enough insulin (or not enough of its functions) to keep your glucose levels under control. Insulin is a hormone made and released by the beta-cells of the pancreas. Its job is to coordinate the body's response to rising blood glucose levels in the blood. Diabetes develops only when it can't do this anymore. But while diabetes is a simple problem, the reasons diabetes comes about are much more complex.

Many different factors can contribute to the decline and loss of insulin's functions, leading ultimately to the development of diabetes.

In some people, the immune system can inadvertently destroy the insulin-producing beta-cells of the pancreas. This is called **type 1 diabetes**. Type 1 diabetes accounts for around 8 to 10 per cent of all people with diabetes. It can occur at any age, not just in children and adolescents. Type 1 diabetes used to be known as insulin-dependent diabetes because the ability to make insulin is completely lost and insulin injections are always needed to survive. However, people with other forms of diabetes may also need insulin to control their glucose levels, so this name has become largely obsolete.

The most common form of diabetes is **type 2 diabetes**, which accounts for over 90 per cent of all diabetes in adults and is the sole topic of this book. In type 2 diabetes, the capacity to produce enough insulin to adequately control your glucose levels is progressively exhausted over many years (probably at least 20 years). By the time type 2 diabetes is finally diagnosed it may be that over half of the insulin-producing beta-cells in the pancreas have been lost.

WHAT CAUSES TYPE 2 DIABETES?

Broadly, there are three key factors that combine to prevent the beta-cells of the pancreas doing their job to make enough insulin to keep blood glucose levels under control. These act to a greater or lesser extent in different people, but collectively mean that the capacity for insulin production eventually fails to keep up with demands, and glucose levels start to rise.

Too much work can be exhausting for the pancreas

The beta-cells of the pancreas make insulin in proportion to the amount of sugar in a meal and how quickly it is digested and absorbed (known as the **glycaemic load** or **GL** — see Chapter 3). If you regularly eat a diet rich in sugars, especially those that are rapidly digested, your pancreas will have to make more insulin more quickly. And these demands to make more and more insulin eventually take their toll. People who habitually eat this kind of unhealthy sugar-rich diet have a higher risk of developing type 2 diabetes.

The pancreas will also have to work harder if the cells of the body become less sensitive to insulin (known as **insulin resistance**).

Resistance to the actions of insulin is a common early finding in people who ultimately develop type 2 diabetes. If there is resistance to insulin's actions, much more insulin must be made and released every time sugar is eaten to compensate and keep glucose under control. So insulin levels in type 2 diabetes initially run higher than normal. For a while this is possible, but not forever.

Insulin resistance is like driving your car with the handbrake still partly on. You can still get to your destination but it takes much more effort. Eventually, all that revving damages your engine and the car can no longer make it down the street. In the same way, type 2 diabetes occurs when you reach a point that your pancreas simply can no longer make enough insulin to overcome the resistance.

The most common cause of insulin resistance is being overweight or inactive, and especially both. But these are not the only causes. In every pregnancy, hormones and other factors normally cause resistance to the actions of insulin. This means that insulin production in pregnant women needs to be almost doubled to keep glucose levels under control. Most women's bodies can capably do this. However, some women do not have the kind of extra capacity to double their insulin production, especially older and/or overweight women. And when there is not enough insulin (function) to keep metabolism under control, glucose levels will inevitably rise. When this happens during pregnancy it is known as **gestational diabetes**.

Although glucose levels usually return to normal after giving birth, women with gestational diabetes are four times more likely to eventually develop type 2 diabetes as they age when compared to those who have a diabetes-free pregnancy. Many people think of a 9-month pregnancy as a kind of road test of your pancreas, for what might happen in the future should you remain overweight or inactive over much longer periods.

Another condition associated with type 2 diabetes is **polycystic ovarian syndrome**, or **PCOS**. PCOS affects between 5 and 10 per cent of all women. It can cause women to experience irregular periods, acne, and excessive facial hair and weight gain. Having PCOS also makes you more likely to develop type 2 diabetes, which may affect up to 40 per cent of women with PCOS by the time they are 40 years old. This is partly because those women with PCOS also have greater resistance to the (glucose-lowering) actions of insulin.

Some medicines used in the treatment of other diseases may also cause type 2 diabetes in some people through making the body more resistant to the effects of insulin. These include steroid pills (especially in high doses), some diuretics and antipsychotics used in the treatment of mental illness.

Too much fat in all the wrong places

Most people develop type 2 diabetes because they cannot safely contain the excess energy from their diet and a toxic waist starts to accumulate.

Most of the excess energy from your diet is stored as fat. The equation is simple: if you eat it and you'll don't burn it in your metabolism or physical activities, then you store it. Energy is too precious a thing for the body to waste.

Your fat normally turns over about 10 per cent of its energy stores every day. This means it always has plenty in reserve in case of extra requirements, such as if you miss a meal or need to be more active than usual.

The body initially stores its fat mostly under the skin, in the thighs, buttocks and breasts (known as **peripheral fat**). These depots are very efficient at impounding fat and keeping it safe until its energy is needed. This is partly because peripheral fat is sensitive to the signals that regulate metabolism, the most important of which is insulin, which promotes fat storage.

Peripheral fat is not unhealthy. If you remove all this fat from under your skin (e.g. by liposuction) you do not become any healthier or reduce your chances of developing type 2 diabetes. In fact, it is thought that having this kind of healthy fat might prevent the dangerous spill-over of fat into other tissues. Transplanting peripheral fat into people who have an abnormal deficiency of fat tissue (known as lipodystrophy) can actually improve their health.

However, the problem comes when these peripheral fat stores are filled up or stop listening to insulin. If they can no longer act as an efficient energy reservoir, what do you do with all the extra energy now? You can't afford to waste it. So you need to build additional storage capacity outside of where fat is normally stored. This is known as **ectopic fat**. Most of these new 'dump sites' are around the internal organs (also known as **visceral fat**) or inside them (known as **steatosis**).

The easiest way to determine whether you have any of this ectopic fat is to place a tape measure around your waist, two finger breadths above the top of your hip bone.

In people of a European, white, Caucasian background, a healthy waist circumference is considered to be

- **for men: less than 94 cm (37 in)**
- **for women: less than 80 cm (31½ in)**

In people of an Asian, Indian or Middle Eastern background, a healthy waist circumference is considered to be

- **for men: less than 78 cm (30½ in)**
- **for women: less than 72 cm (28½ in).**

Few people with a waist circumference persistently in the healthy reference range will develop type 2 diabetes. But as your waistline increases beyond these levels, the chances that you might develop type 2 diabetes will significantly increase. Today, over half of all adults exceed these measurements. Some by quite a bit. This is the dominant reason type 2 diabetes is increasing exponentially around the world.

Today, at least three out of four people with type 2 diabetes have abdominal obesity, defined by a waist circumference that is:

- greater than 102 cm (40 in) in men (Asian men: greater than 90 cm/35½ in)
- greater than 88 cm (34½ in) women (Asian women: greater than 80 cm/31½ in).

Diabetes is not inevitable if you have a waist of this size, but it does become more likely. For example, when compared to people with a healthy waist circumference, developing diabetes in the next 5 years is four times more likely if you have abdominal obesity.

Most people develop type 2 diabetes because they cannot safely store the excess energy from their diet and a 'toxic waist' starts to accumulate.

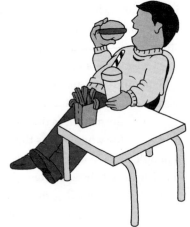

This girth implies that there is probably a large amount of ectopic fat in the body and it is definitely worth doing something about it. In fact, if you specifically measure the amount of (ectopic) fat in the liver (known as **fatty liver** or hepatic steatosis) you find the same sort of numbers — that is, at least three out of four people with type 2 diabetes also have too much fat in their liver.

The problem with ectopic fat is that it is not very good at its job. It is really a makeshift solution to the 'problem of fat storage' when all other options are exhausted. And in not doing its job very well, a number of things can go wrong.

In particular, unlike healthy fat, ectopic fat is far less efficient at safekeeping its fat stores. It tries really hard to compensate and is much more metabolically active than peripheral fat, but it is just not very good at it. So instead of being efficiently stored, free fat leaches out into the tissues and the blood, particularly after a meal, when fat levels should normally be going down.

These free floating fats and their by-products are directly toxic in many parts of the body, including the beta-cells of the pancreas. Free fat is only supposed to be a drip feed, released into the blood in carefully regulated amounts when you are not eating, in order to spare the glucose for the brain. But if your fat is not safely stored, and levels are high in the blood, it is a free meal for cells, which get fatter themselves as a result. So cells like the beta-cells of the pancreas accumulate ectopic fat in great globules that ultimately distort the way they function. Cells that are eating fat also don't need glucose for fuel, so glucose utilization falls.

This excessive flux of free fat through a cell's metabolism also causes problems, as toxic by-products are generated through inefficiency. The best known of these by-products are **free**

radicals (also known as reactive oxygen species), which react with and damage anything they come into contact with.

Cells that are stuffed full of fat also don't respond well to insulin. This is particularly the case when ectopic fat accumulates in the cells of the liver. As detailed above, insulin resistance in the liver forces the pancreas to have to make much more insulin to bring glucose production by the liver back under control. And this means more work for the beta-cells of the pancreas, which are already feeling the strain.

Finally, fat is not a lifeless lump of lard. In fact, it is a dynamic regulator of health and wellbeing. All fat, but especially ectopic fat, is able to produce a range of chemicals (known as **adipokines**) that railroad healthy functioning. In fact, fat tissue is the largest producer of hormones in the human body. People with type 2 diabetes often have high levels of adipokines in their blood, chiefly because they also have high levels of ectopic fat.

You also need to be susceptible

There are a great many people who are overweight, some of them extremely so. But only some develop type 2 diabetes. This is because you also often need a third factor to be present for type 2 diabetes to occur.

To develop type 2 diabetes, you also need to be susceptible either to developing ectopic fat or your beta-cells must be susceptible to exhaustion.

Some people are better than others at safely setting aside any excess energy from their diet as healthy peripheral fat. This might be because they have a bigger storage capacity or are more able to expand it when needed, rather than dumping fat inappropriately around their organs. What determines when the peripheral fat store reaches its capacity (in essence its size and expandability) may be different in different people depending on their age, gender, race, genes and a host of other factors.

For example, people of Indian or Asian descent are generally more prone to lay down fat around their internal organs if they eat too much or are inactive. This is because Asian people have an inherently smaller storage capacity in their peripheral fat. This is one reason why type 2 diabetes seems to occur in much thinner people from Asia than it does in the West. However, if you look on the inside those with diabetes are just as likely to have excess fat whether they are of Indian, Asian or European heritage.

Diabetes also doesn't affect everyone who has resistance to the effects of insulin or affect everyone who is eating a bad diet. This appears to be because some people remain quite capable of making enough insulin to control their glucose levels even though they may need to make very large amounts of insulin in the face of stiff insulin resistance or dietary excesses. By contrast, other people simply can't sustain this extra workload for long and eventually there is not enough insulin (function) to keep glucose levels under control, and type 2 diabetes develops.

There are a number of different factors that make your pancreas susceptible to the effects of too much work or too much fat.

In the family

Type 2 diabetes tends to run in families. One in every three people with type 2 diabetes also has a close family member with type 2 diabetes. If either of your parents, your brother or your sister has type 2 diabetes, you are five to six times more likely to develop type 2 diabetes yourself. If three family members have type 2 diabetes, you are over fifteen times more likely to develop type 2 diabetes yourself than someone without a family history. The reason that type 2 diabetes runs in families is partly due to similar diet, lifestyle habits and exposure to environmental factors. It may also be partly determined by your genes.

Genes are the basic instructions encoded in your DNA that are used to determine how your body works. These gene instructions are passed down from parents to their children, who all share similar genes. In some cases, the genes you inherit may increase your risk of type 2 diabetes. Most of these genes appear to influence how well beta-cells handle the stress of having to make more insulin. But while genes are important in some families, overall they explain only a small fraction of why most people develop type 2 diabetes.

During early development

Susceptibility to type 2 diabetes may also be acquired during your life, particularly during your early development in your mother's womb. For example, babies very small for their age have an increased risk of developing type 2 diabetes when they grow up. This is probably because the same thing that restricts the growth of a baby also restricts the development of the pancreas and ultimately its capacity to take the strain of controlling glucose levels during adulthood. A mother's high glucose levels during pregnancy can also increase the risk of type 2 diabetes in her children, partly because their beta-cells become more susceptible to damage.

Increased susceptibility with ageing

Some people develop type 2 diabetes only when they are very old, without having been very overweight or inactive during their life. This is probably because the regenerative capacity of the pancreas is not limitless, and the ability to make insulin slowly declines with time in everyone. But ageing just brings you closer to the edge — usually something else is also required to push you over. Whether 'getting old' will result in type 2 diabetes is determined by how great the demands are for insulin production and how great this capacity has already been reduced by other factors. Of those people who develop type 2 diabetes in their eighties, it is often suggested that it was probably always going to happen no matter what, given enough time. But if these same people had been overweight and inactive during their lives, it would probably have happened much earlier.

TYPE 2 DIABETES: THREE STRIKES AND YOU'RE OUT

Type 2 diabetes will affect at least one in every three people at some point during their lifetime. But it will not affect everyone.

There are many people who are overweight who don't get diabetes. There are many who have a poor diet or the wrong genes, and they don't get diabetes either. To get type 2 diabetes you need all three things to happen.

- You need the beta-cells of the pancreas to be overworked.
- You need too much fat in the wrong places.
- You need to be susceptible (such that your ability to compensate for overwork of your beta-cells and too much fat in your body ultimately fails).

Type 2 diabetes is made more likely if any one of these factors is increased. For example, an unhealthy diet will increase the work of the pancreas and increase the risk of diabetes. Similarly, being overweight can increase your risk of diabetes even without a strong family history. Equally, some people have a strong family history of diabetes so it doesn't take much extra work or being very overweight for diabetes to occur. Of course, if more than one of these factors is increased, your risk will multiply and diabetes will become both more likely and more likely to occur at an earlier age.

At the same time, the best ways to prevent and treat diabetes will target these important areas. For example, changes in the amount and types of sugar and fibre in your diet can reduce the strain on your pancreas to produce large amounts of insulin (see Chapter 3). Getting rid of any extra fat in your body through diet (Chapter 4) and increased physical activity (Chapter 5) will reduce its limiting effects on your metabolism and reduce insulin resistance. Some medicines will also help to protect the beta-cells and make them more able to compensate for the demands of glucose control.

In its early stages, diabetes is reversible. For example, gastric bypass surgery dramatically reduces food intake and causes a great decline in the amount of ectopic fat in your body (see Chapter 4). This is able to 'cure' type 2 diabetes such that many people having this procedure can keep control of their glucose levels without the need for any medications. It requires complicated, invasive major surgery that is not an answer for the over 430 million people worldwide with type 2 diabetes. But it does illustrate that once you understand some of the factors involved in the development of diabetes (like ectopic fat), and target them early enough, anything is possible.

3

A SPOON LESS OF SUGAR

Understand

- Reducing the demands on your pancreas to make insulin can be achieved by reducing the amount of carbohydrates you eat and/or changing the type of carbohydrates you eat.

- You can reduce the amount of carbs you eat by following a diet or meal plan that is low in carbs (low carb diet) or by restricting the amount of carbs you eat through carb counting.

- Sugar substitutes and sweeteners can safely reduce the carbs in your diet, as between 10 and 15 per cent of the energy in carbs probably comes from added sugars.

- Some foods have greater and faster effects on your glucose control than others. This can be estimated as their glycaemic index or GI.
- Dietary fibre plays an important role in good glucose control, even though it is not digested by your body.

Manage

- Incorporate a serve of fruit and vegetables into every meal.
- Explore the nutritional information guide on the foods you currently eat, or download a program for your phone to help you do this on the fly. Look at the content of carbs, fibre and GI where available.
- Experiment with different recipes that use sugar substitutes and find a product that works for your taste buds as well as your glucose control.
- Find new ways to put fibre into

your diet by substituting wholegrain alternatives, bran or fruit, or using fibre supplements.

- Monitor your glucose control, as improvements that come from changes in the amount or type of carbohydrate in your diet can reduce your requirements for certain glucose-lowering medications.

A hundred years ago, the only rational treatment for type 2 diabetes was to avoid all sugar in your diet. It is still widely thought that having type 2 diabetes only means you have to avoid sugar and any sweet foods and drinks that contain it. While this is not strictly true, managing your sugar intake is one important strategy for achieving and maintaining good glucose control.

A typical diet consists of foods that are rich in sugars (also known as **carbohydrate** or **carbs**). Some of the carbohydrate in your diet is in the form of simple sugars, like sucrose (the white 'table sugar') and fructose (in fruit and honey). Your taste buds are able to detect the presence of simple sugars in food or drink, which is why such things taste sweet. Simple sugars occur naturally in sweet foods or may be added in food processing or by consumers (e.g. into your coffee) for extra sweetness. On average, between 10 and 15 per cent of the total energy (calories) in your diet comes from these added sugars, but in some people's diets this can exceed 25 per cent.

Most carbohydrate in your diet is in the form of complex chains of hundreds to thousands of glucose molecules.

This is known as **starch**. Starch is the major store of energy in plants and is found in many plant-based foods, from bread and cereal to potatoes, pasta and rice. It does not taste sweet as its sugars are locked up into these complex chains. However, starch is rapidly digested in your intestines, where its sugars are released and subsequently absorbed into the bloodstream in precisely the same way as table sugar.

As any sugar is digested and absorbed, it triggers the release of hormones. The most important of these is **insulin**, which coordinates the body's response to ensure the levels of glucose in your blood rise only slightly after a meal, if at all. This is a proportionate response: the greater the amount of carbohydrate/ sugar in a meal and the faster it is digested and absorbed, the more insulin needs to be made to keep your glucose levels from rising dangerously. The combined effects of these two components — the quantity and quality of carbohydrate in a meal — is known as the **glycaemic load** (GL). Essentially, GL is an estimate of the demand placed on your pancreas to make insulin by any particular meal.

Of course, what happens in type 2 diabetes is that there is not always enough insulin to keep glucose under control, especially after meals.

So one way to make sure that your limited capacity for insulin production will still be enough to keep control is to reduce the glycaemic load imparted by your diet.

This can be done in essentially two different ways:

- by reducing the amount of carbs you eat (e.g. following a low carb diet, carb counting or using sugar substitutes)
- by slowing the absorption of carbs from your diet by selecting the carbs you eat (by their GI index),

mixing meals and/or by substituting more soluble fibre into your meals.

This chapter will look in detail at these two common ways to manage diabetes and their role in helping to improve your glucose control. Although discussed separately, there is no reason some or all of these interventions can't be combined for even better glucose control. In addition, changes in your diet have a far greater role in managing diabetes than just making your glucose levels easier to control. A good diet will improve waist management, the control of lipids and blood pressure levels as well as the prevention of complications. These facets are discussed in specific chapters dedicated to these topics found elsewhere in this book. However, this chapter will just look at how you can reduce the rise in glucose levels after a meal by making changes to your diet.

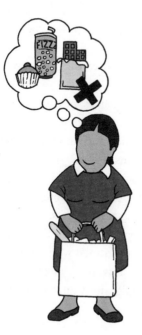

One way to make sure your limited capacity to produce insulin is still enough to keep glucose under control is to slow the absorption of sugars from your diet.

LOW CARBOHYDRATE DIETS

Low carb diets have become very popular for the management of type 2 diabetes. In theory, by reducing the amount or proportion of carbohydrate you are eating you can also reduce the demands on your pancreas to make insulin. So if you have only a limited capacity to make insulin, as occurs in people with type 2 diabetes, reducing the carbohydrate component in your diet can make it more likely your limited capacity will be sufficient to keep control of your glucose levels.

Typically, half of the energy in a standard diet comes from carbohydrates. In fact, because of the push from modern consumers to reduce the amount of fat in their diets, people in the 21st century are eating more carbohydrates than ever before. Diabetes may be one of the consequences.

Carbohydrates are found in high proportions in many common foods, including:

- breads, buns, muffins, cakes, pastry, cookies, crackers and tortillas
- pasta, noodles, rice and cereal grains (such as oats and barley)
- starchy vegetables such as potatoes, yams, beets, corn, pumpkin (squash), plantain, beans and peas
- milk and milk products such as cheeses and yoghurt
- fruits, juices and jams (jellies)
- sugar-sweetened soda, sports drinks and alcoholic beverages (e.g. beer, cider and wine)
- candy, frosting, icing and desserts.

In low carb diets, these common foods that are high in carbohydrates are limited or substituted with foods containing more proteins and/or more fats (e.g. meat, poultry, fish, shellfish, and eggs). For example, substitute rice with a low-fat meat. Alternatively, some low carb diets simply replace common carb-rich products with other foods that are essentially low in carbohydrates (e.g. non-starchy vegetables like okra and eggplant/aubergine for potatoes or rice). Generally, low carb diets mean you eat differently rather than eating less.

Perhaps the best known example of a low carb diet is the Atkins Diet. However, there are a range of other diets that share roughly the same principles with respect to carbs but vary in their relative amounts of other nutrients (e.g. how much fat or protein you eat). These are all discussed in more detail in Chapter 4.

CARB COUNTING

Limiting your carbohydrate intake is also relatively easy to achieve by yourself, simply by estimating how many carbs are contained in different products then planning your meal and how much of it you will eat to match your chosen limit. This practice is known as **carbohydrate counting** or counting carbs and is widely recommended for people with type 2 diabetes as a means to control their blood glucose levels.

Some information about the carbs in your food can be obtained simply by reading the 'nutritional information panel' present on the labels of most processed foods. Look first at the serving size section. All the information below it will be about what you will get when you eat this amount of this product. If you eat more than this, which is usually the case with most of these products, all the nutrients you will be getting will increase proportionally, including the carbs.

On the label, total carbohydrates are measured in grams (g), for instance, one serve is said to be equal to 15g of carbohydrate.

When counting carbs it is common to subtract half the amount of fibre from the total amount of carbohydrate to determine what is known as the effective carbs or **net carbs.** For example, if a product contains 23g of carbohydrate (total) and 6g of fibre, then its net carbs will be around 20g per serve. This figure approximates the amount of carbohydrate in a product that will impact insulin production and potentially your blood glucose levels. It is also another good reason to choose high fibre products which have their own benefits (detailed below).

Most of the food we commonly eat has no labels at all. But there are many recipe books, websites and phone apps now available that provide useful information about how many carbs are contained in most kinds of food and drinks, which can help in planning your meals.

There is approximately 15g of net carbohydrate in:
- one slice of bread
- one tablespoon of syrup, jam, jelly, sugar or honey
- one apple, orange, pear or banana
- twenty grapes
- one tub of natural or diet yoghurt
- half a tub of flavoured yoghurt
- half a cup of baked beans
- two to three biscuits/cookies
- one muffin
- one scoop of ice-cream
- half a cup of pasta or rice
- half of cup of cereal or one and half Weetabix
- one baked potato or medium corn cob
- six squares of milk chocolate
- half a can of soft drink (soda).

A typical low carb diet will aim to limit carbs to only five to ten serves a day. A good place to start is to limit your carbohydrate intake to no more than three to four serves (45–60g) of carbs in each meal, or no more than ten serves (150g) of carbs each day.

The maths involved in calculating carbs is not as hard as it sounds and becomes easier as you go. A dietician or diabetes educator can help to get you started with meal plans based on fixed serves of carbohydrate spread throughout the day. This also makes it easier to control your glucose levels after meals, as when you know what's coming you also know what it will do to your glucose levels.

Low carb diets and type 2 diabetes

A number of studies have consistently shown that low carb diets and carb counting are able to improve glucose control in people with type 2 diabetes. This may be partly because these strategies can also cause weight loss, which is often achieved quite rapidly much to the delight of anyone starting out on a diet (see Chapter 4). However, even in those people who don't achieve much in the way of weight loss with a low carb diet, there can still be a useful improvement in glucose levels and/or a reduced requirement for medications to control them.

Low carb diets are not without their problems in people with type 2 diabetes, the most important of which may be the increased intake of fat that can sometimes occur when trying to avoid carbs, which can have unwanted effects on your lipid levels (see Chapter 8).

Some people can find that elimination of carbohydrate-rich foods from their diet also reduces or removes many of their favourite (staple) dishes, such as rice, bread and pasta. This can lead to them feeling overly restricted with a low carb diet, especially when sharing a meal with their family. It may also be particularly difficult for vegetarians and vegans, for whom finding low carbohydrate alternatives can be difficult (though not impossible). Such restrictions can also lead to many eventually breaking their diet and falling back into old habits.

Some people with diabetes are worried that a low carb diet will increase their risk of experiencing dangerously low glucose levels (known as **hypoglycaemia** — see Chapter 7). This is seldom the case as much of the sugar in the body is made by the body, so there usually is little chance of running out. However, the improvements in glucose control and weight loss that are achieved through changes in your diet can sometimes mean that if you are taking glucose-lowering medications that can sometimes cause hypoglycaemia, such as sulphonylureas or insulin, these may need to be reduced or stopped to prevent hypos. It could be said that a spoon less of sugar really does helps the medicine go down.

SWEETENERS AND SUGAR SUBSTITUTES

Another popular way to reduce the total amount of sugar in your diet is to choose foods and beverages that substitute any sugar with a **sweetener**. Sweeteners can provide the sweet taste of sugar but have less or no effect on your glucose levels or the amount of energy you are getting from your food. This is the principle of many 'diet' drinks and low-energy products now on the market. These 'diet' products can be quite effective for people who get a lot of their dietary carbs from sweet foods or drinks.

The most commonly used sugar substitutes are **artificial sweeteners**, such as saccharin, aspartame and Acesulfame K. These have a very intense sweet taste when compared to table sugar, so can be used in very small amounts while producing a similar sweetness. Artificial sweeteners have minimal or no effect on blood glucose levels. In addition, the energy (calories) contained in diet products containing sweeteners can also be much less than that in regular products made with added sugars. And less energy in your diet means less fat will accumulate in your body. Importantly, when used in recommended amounts, artificial sweeteners appear to have no adverse effects on human health.

However sweet, though, the taste of artificial sweeteners is not quite the same as sugar. Sugar also contributes to the thickness or 'syrupiness' of a product, particularly a drink, so products with artificial sweeteners can sometimes feel 'thinner' in the mouth when compared to the usual sugar-laden products. To solve these dual problems of taste and bulk, many diet products are now made up of complex mixtures of artificial sweeteners and bulking agents, and achieve a reasonable approximation of a natural sweet sensation. This is harder to do on your own, so simply replacing table sugar in your house with artificial sweeteners may not be as practical or as tasty as it sounds. Also some of these artificial sweeteners break down when heated, so they can't be used in baking.

Another group of so-called 'natural sweeteners' has more recently emerged as a low calorie alternative to sugar, including sucralose (also known as Splenda®) and **stevia**. Some formulations of these products are stable when heated and can therefore be used for cooking and baking.

Sucralose is just ordinary table sugar (sucrose) that has been chlorinated. This makes it over 500 times as sweet as sugar, so you need 500 times less to achieve the same sweetness. Only 15 per cent of it is absorbed into the body (compared with nearly

100 per cent of sucrose) so its footprint on your glucose control is also very small.

Extracts of *Stevia rebaudiana*, a South American herb plant, are also increasingly used as natural sweeteners. Stevia is over 300 times as sweet as sugar, again meaning you need to use very little to get a sweet fix, and it contains no sugar and no food energy (calories).

Some recent studies have questioned the benefits of sweeteners, arguing that they might have adverse effects on the functions of insulin or on the composition of bacteria in the gut. However, the consensus is that they are safe, and realistically are much safer than drinking large amounts of sugar and calorie-laden beverages and foods.

THE GLYCAEMIC INDEX

It used to be believed that eating too many sweet things was the main reason for glucose levels to rise in people with diabetes. Consequently, the management of diabetes was all about not eating sweet things. Certainly, sweet foods and drinks often contain large amounts of simple sugars that are rapidly digested and absorbed. But many other foods also have the potential to release their sugars very quickly and cause your glucose levels to rise if enough insulin is not also quickly made and released.

Another approach to lower the load of glucose on the pancreas is simply to target just the right kind of carbohydrate in your food. This is because the carbs contained in some foods have greater and faster effects on your glucose control than others. This effect can be measured as a food's glycaemic index or **GI** for short.

The glycaemic index scores different foods on how quickly and how much their carbs raise glucose levels when compared with eating the same amount of glucose. For example, a meal with a GI of 50 will raise the glucose levels by half as much as eating the same amount of glucose.

By convention, low GI foods have a GI of less than 55 (which means 55 per cent of the effect on glucose levels of eating an equivalent amount of glucose). Low GI products deliver their carbohydrate load slowly, so the demands on the pancreas to produce insulin are not so steep. This is why these low GI foods are sometimes called **slow carbs**.

Foods that have a GI greater than 70 are called high GI. The carbohydrate contained in these foods is digested and absorbed quickly. This causes a rapid surge of glucose into the blood and the requirement for an equally rapid surge in insulin production in response, to prevent blood glucose levels from rising. Interestingly, table sugar (sucrose) has a GI of around 60. Many sweet foods containing lots of table sugar have a lower GI than ordinary white bread or standard breakfast cereals. This means that they have less effect on your glucose levels. From the low GI standpoint, avoiding table sugar and foods that contain it may therefore be less important for your glucose control than tackling the high GI starches in a slice of bread or a bowl of pasta or rice.

The GI was originally developed to help people with diabetes improve their blood glucose control. In people with type 2 diabetes, producing large amounts of insulin rapidly is exactly what their pancreas can't do very well. This is one of the reasons glucose levels rise more rapidly in people with diabetes after eating high GI foods, and why finding a low GI alternative is a good idea for glucose control in people with type 2 diabetes.

Low GI diets

Many people with type 2 diabetes are now recommended to go on a low GI diet, which simply aims to substitute any high GI products in your diet with low GI alternatives so that the carbs you do eat are mostly slow carbs. Again, this can be achieved in one of two ways. You can follow a low GI meal, recipe or menu plan in which the authors have already made sure the foods you will be eating are low GI. Alternatively, you can make a low GI diet yourself by finding out the GI of the foods you currently eat and then finding alternatives that have a slower glucose profile. At least initially, this may require you to check tables, books, websites and phone apps. These can give you an estimate of the GI of most foods and help you to choose the lowest GI alternative. Some products also display their GI proudly on their label. An example of some of the simple carb swaps you can consider include:

Common high GI food	Lower GI alternative
Puffed and flaked breakfast cereals	Unrefined cereals (e.g. bran)
White bread, bagels, buns	Wholegrain breads, sourdough, fruit loaf
Potato (especially baked, boiled or mashed)	Legumes, sweet potatoes, yam, sweet corn
White rice	Basmati rice, pearled barley, quinoa, pasta
White bread sandwich	Sushi (the stickiness means low GI)
Plain biscuits or crackers	Fruit

The reason one product is low GI and another is high GI is complex and hard to predict. Low GI foods are not simply those with high fibre (although many are). For example, puffed wheat is high in fibre but also high GI. Equally, high GI foods are not all starchy or sweet (although many are).

The GI of food is influenced not only by the type of carbohydrate it contains but also its content of fat, protein, fibre and water. For example, protein and fat in foods can lower its GI by slowing its passage through the stomach and subsequent digestion. This means that some potato chips that are also high in fat can have a lower GI than baked potatoes.

The GI can also vary significantly between foods that look and taste the same. For example, some potatoes have a low GI while others have a GI greater than 100 (i.e. worse than eating straight glucose). This is why tables, books, phone apps etc. are so essential for making the most of a low GI diet. With practice you will come to know which foods increase your glucose levels and which ones don't, and can then make your choices accordingly.

But while each of these can be a good guide, the GI of any food is not static. The preparation and processing of a food (cooking method and time, amount of heat or moisture used, etc.) can change its GI. For example, although pasta falls into the low GI category, the more it is cooked the higher its GI becomes. For this and other reasons it is best to eat pasta al dente and not out of a tin. Drinking small amounts of alcohol with meals can also lower your meal's GI by slowing the emptying of your stomach. The GI for a piece of fruit can also change as the fruit ripens or with prolonged storage.

The other important feature of GI is that only foods containing carbohydrate are given a score, and GI only ranks food on their effect on glucose levels. It doesn't rank them based on how healthy they are for other things, such as fat or calories. For example, sausages are low GI but are often high in fat.

These reservations aside, a low GI diet is a practical and potentially useful tool for the management of type 2 diabetes. It is relatively easily to achieve, perhaps more so than any other dietary intervention for the management of diabetes. It is not particularly restrictive, as it does not require you to avoid any category of food, or change your menu (only substitute foods within it). It doesn't require you to reduce the volume of what you eat or count carbs or calories (but you can as well if you want to lose weight). It also means that you don't end up eating more fat, which may be a problem for people with type 2 diabetes on a strict low carb diet.

There is also now good data to show that adherence to a low GI diet is able to improve glucose control in people with type 2 diabetes. Indeed, results have suggested that, in people with type 2 diabetes, the effect on glucose levels of sticking to a low GI diet is approximately equivalent to adding medications that specifically target blood glucose levels after meals. Low GI diets may also have beneficial effects on lipids, blood pressure and weight control.

Importantly, while glucose levels may fall if you go on a low GI diet, the risk of hypoglycaemia is not increased. In fact, it may be reduced as the slower delivery of glucose from low GI foods acts to maintain glucose levels for longer after meals, when glucose levels are usually at their lowest. By contrast, the rapid rise in glucose induced by high GI foods not only leads to high swings in glucose levels but can also lead to rebound lows as increased insulin released in response causes a much steeper fall in glucose levels.

HIGH FIBRE DIETS

Another way to target carbohydrates is to focus on the amount of fibre in your diet. Fibre is only found in plants and their products. There is no fibre in meat, even if it is chewy. Fibre is the indigestible part of plant material (also known as roughage). Chemically, fibre is mostly made up of long chains (polymers) of sugars joined together so that they won't come apart when you eat them. This is why eating fibre has little or no effect on your glucose levels.

There are two types of dietary fibre: soluble and insoluble. Some fibre is able to dissolve in water. This is called soluble fibre. This kind of fibre is found in almost all plant foods. The highest amounts are found in legumes, such as lentils, beans and peas. Other excellent sources of soluble fibre include wholegrains (such as wheat, rye, oats, barley and brown rice), nuts and popcorn.

Some fibre tends to absorb water but does not dissolve in it. This is called **insoluble fibre**. This kind of fibre is most abundant in wholegrains. The highest levels are found in the outer husk of the grain, which is called the bran. Significant but lower levels of insoluble fibre are also found in nuts and seeds and refined cereals. Insoluble fibre is also found in the skins of vegetables and fruits, such as strawberries, prunes, tomatoes, apples, potatoes and onions.

The presence of soluble fibre in food slows its digestion and the subsequent absorption of glucose. Think about eating an apple compared to drinking apple juice. Of course, the same amount of juice will cause a greater rise in your glucose levels than just eating the apple. This is because soluble fibre transforms what you have just eaten into a sticky gel that releases its nutrients only gradually, making it less of a challenge for your insulin-producing capacity.

By holding food in your intestine for longer, a meal rich in fibre can also make you feel satisfied for longer when compared to an identical product devoid of its fibre. This means you may be less likely to feel hungry or need to snack between meals. A high fibre diet can also reduce the levels of harmful cholesterol in your blood (see Chapter 9).

In addition, fibre is also good for the health of your bowels and helps to prevent constipation, which is a common problem for people with type 2 diabetes. Fibre will act to absorb water, which makes your stool softer and more bulky. This makes it much easier for your bowels to push. However, if you increase the amount of fibre in your diet too quickly, or don't drink enough, fibre can actually cause constipation. If you double your fibre intake, you should generally also double your water intake.

All fibre is resistant to human digestion. But some fibre is digested by the bacteria of your large intestine, which releases gas. If you add fibre into your diet too quickly it can make you feel bloated and flatulent. This appears to be its only major drawback. So when ramping up the amount of fibre in your diet or using fibre supplements it is important to start slowly to allow your bowels and their bacteria to adjust to the change. Increasing your fibre intake gradually over a month until you reach your target should be sufficient.

Increasing the amount of fibre in your diet

All people with type 2 diabetes should aim for around 30g of fibre each day in their diet. Most adults eat less than half this amount. There are a number of simple ways in which you can increase your intake of fibre.

Many processed foods, such as bread and breakfast cereals, list their fibre content on the 'nutritional information panel'. In general, an excellent source of fibre will contain at least 5g per serve. A good source of fibre will contain more than 2.5g per serve. A product that claims to have added fibre will have at least 2.5g more per serve than if it wasn't added.

If you also want to go low carb (i.e. five to ten serves of carbs a day), you must ensure that almost all your carbs are coming from good or excellent sources of fibre to reach the recommended daily target of 30g.

Another way to increase the intake of fibre in your diet is to substitute products that use refined grains with **wholegrain alternatives**. These products retain either intact grains, flaked or 'cracked' grain kernels, coarsely ground kernels or use flour that is made from wholegrains (known as wholemeal flour). Milling or the refining of grains removes the germ and the bran (which contain most of the fibre) leaving behind only the inner starchy (high GI) part of the grain. For example, the amount of fibre in standard white flour is ten times lower than that of wholemeal flour.

Some simple ways to increase the amount of fibre in your diet include:

- Eat a breakfast cereal that lists 'wholegrain' or bran as the main (first) ingredient instead of one that contains just wheat. You should be able to find one containing at least 5g of fibre per serve. Alternatively, add a few tablespoons of bran to your favourite cereal. Brans are more concentrated sources of fibre, meaning you need to eat less to get the same amount.
- Switch white bread for wholegrain or wholemeal bread. Many breads contain some or all of these components, but they may not be truly wholegrain or high in fibre unless a wholegrain is the main (first)

ingredient. Many breads are made brown because of added sugar (molasses) or are made to look healthy with a few scattered seeds. However, some products are fortified with significant amounts of added fibre. Again, most commercial breads will now list their nutritional contents on the label. So to select one that is a good source of fibre, choose one that has at least 2.5g of fibre per serve.

- For the same reasons, substitute some or all of the white 'all purpose' flour you use for your own baking with wholegrain wheat or chickpea flour. You might need more yeast and baking powder to get your baking to rise, because wholemeal flour is heavier than traditional white flour. Also throw in some bran when you bake anything, from meatloaf to muffins and biscuits/cookies.

- Replace some or all of the white rice in your diet with brown rice. To make brown rice, only the husk is removed from the rice grain. But to make white rice, the brown coloured fibre-rich layers (the bran and the germ) are removed, again leaving behind only the inner starchy (high GI) part of the grain. This allows white rice to cook faster and fluff up nicely, but it also means that white rice contains four times less fibre than brown rice. Alternatively, throw in some barley with your white rice for some added fibre and flavour.

- Different kinds of whole wheat pasta are also now available as a substitute for standard white pasta. These can take a little getting used to because of their colour, nutty taste, texture and longer cooking time, which is about twice that of regular pasta. Some products are more palatable than others. But if you are making a good sauce, especially one that contains legumes, it is hard to tell the difference. Just by replacing refined products with wholegrain equivalents, without changing anything else in your diet, you can more than double your intake of total and soluble fibre.

Other simple tricks to increase your fibre intake include:

- When making fruit juice, don't get rid of the skin and pulp. These are the good parts. Choose the whole fruit every time where possible.
- Don't peel off the skin from fruit, such as apples and pears, and vegetables such as carrots, potatoes, sweet potato and the pods of peas, as peeling them decreases their fibre content.
- For snacks, instead of processed carbs eat fruits with edible (whole) seeds, such as berries and kiwi fruit or fibre-rich fruits such as apples, pears, bananas, citrus and stone fruit. Vegetables with good soluble fibre content include cauliflower, zucchini (courgettes), broccoli, carrots, Jerusalem artichokes and celery.
- Substitute animal protein in your diet with legumes. For example, use beans, chickpeas, lentils and soybeans instead of some or all of your steak mince in your spaghetti bolognese, or in your curry instead of some or all of the meat. Again, these highly flavoured dishes mean that the taste of the meal is not substantially changed, while its fibre content is increased and fat content decreased.

A cup of red kidney beans will provide almost half your daily fibre requirements. If you don't like beans you can also try substituting other fibre-rich vegetables such as broccoli, artichoke or Brussels sprouts.

For some people with diabetes, changing to a diet with large amounts of wholegrain, bran and legumes is a major shift. Another simple way to get fibre into your day without changing what you eat too much can be to take fibre supplements. These are available in many different forms, such as tablets, capsules and powders (which can be mixed up as a drink). These supplements don't provide the extra nutrients contained in wholegrain products that may be beneficial to your health, but they give you the fibre that may be lacking in your diet. It is also important to remember that fibre supplements must be started slowly and only gradually increased to your target intake over a month. This will give your bowels a chance to adjust, in order to reduce problems with bloating, flatulence and constipation.

DIABETES AND FEASTING

Multiple festivals and festivities make feasting an integral part of everyday life. If it's not a birthday, it's Christmas, a wedding or another family gathering. These happy occasions can easily lead to excessive exposure to sugars and potentially dangerous elevations in blood sugars in those with diabetes. It is not easy, and often not appropriate, to say no to food on such occasions. You don't want to put the host to any trouble (or not be invited next time). However, with careful selection of the foods you eat, it is possible to not only join in but also to enjoy the feast.

All of the ways to limit carb intake detailed in this chapter become especially important at festive occasions. The two most important factors are moderation and selectivity. You can absolutely still enjoy a sweet or chocolate with your friends, but don't overdo it. Carefully choosing those dishes with no added sugar doesn't mean they are not sweet or delicious. Often they are laden with fruit or nuts, which is just fine.

The other trick is fibre. Lots of legumes will slow the delivery of sugars and make it easier for your body to cope with any sugar load. There is usually so much food, you just need to be picky and restrict the rice, bread, potatoes, and cakes in favour of other dishes.

Some people with diabetes will be able to adjust their medication when they are eating more. This takes a degree of expertise and should not be done without supervision and support (at least initially). Another useful technique is to increase physical activity coming up to a festive occasion and of course to join in the dancing or take a walk after the meal. It can also help to remember that the focus of these occasions should be on friends, family and observance activities rather than the food.

4

WAIST MANAGEMENT

Understand

- The most important goal of changing your diet is to reduce the amount of fat in your body.
- Most weight loss diets focus on only one key component in your diet (calories, fat, carbs or GI), which makes them simple to follow and easy to stick to.
- There is no such thing as the best diet for weight loss. On average, most diets achieve about the same amount of weight loss of around 2 to 4 kg (4½–9 lb).

- It is likely that the mere process of embracing any dietary restrictions, thinking about and coordinating the foods you eat, makes you tend to eat less (energy) and eat better.
- Successful waist management is not all about changing what you eat; it also involves changing how you eat.

Manage

- Adopt a diet. It probably doesn't matter which one, so long as you enjoy it and are able to stick with it for the long term.
- Find out what you are eating. Explore the nutritional information guides on the foods that you currently eat, or download a program for your phone to help you do this on the fly.
- Start simply with realistic goals and small changes, and slowly work your way up to life-changing things.
- Get help from your doctor, dietician or other health professionals to find a diet

that is best for you. Get help from your
family. It's always hard to do just on
your own.

The biggest health challenge of type 2 diabetes is not glucose control, but its direct antecedent, the accumulation of fat outside of where it is normally safely stored. You may not look or feel overweight. But it is your excess fat that has probably got you over the line. And losing it should be high on the agenda for managing your diabetes.

Possibly the most important goal of changing your diet is to reduce the amount of fat in your body.

Long-term waist management is not only possible in people with type 2 diabetes but is also associated with a reduced risk of many of its complications. This can be achieved in many different ways, including regular exercise, medications and surgery. But the most common way to weight loss is through changing your diet.

Many of the things that you eat and drink release energy as they are broken down and used to fuel your metabolism. Different foods will release different amounts of energy when burnt by the body, depending on their composition. For example, fats release twice as much energy for every gram you eat compared to protein or carbohydrate. The amount of 'food energy' that is released can be measured and quantified as calories or kilojoules. So products that are rich in fat will usually contain more calories or kilojoules (of food energy) than low-fat products.

The energy contained in your food is essential for life. You use its energy continuously. However, food is not always available all of the time. So if you eat but you don't need the food's energy immediately for your metabolism or physical activities, then your body will store it against times when you are not eating. The biggest and most important energy store in your body is fat.

It does not seem to matter what you are eating too much of. If you eat too many sweets or too many steaks you will get fatter. You don't need super-sized overconsumption. To grow fatter it only takes a small mismatch between the energy (calories) you get from your diet and energy used up by your metabolism and physical activity. This is known as a **positive energy balance**. Every time you run your energy balance into the positive, you get a little fatter.

Most adults will eat and drink well over 10,000kJ (2390 calories) of energy every day. However, their daily energy requirements will probably be more like 8000 to 9000kJ (1910–2150 calories). This is why so many people are getting slowly fatter as they get older and so many are getting diabetes.

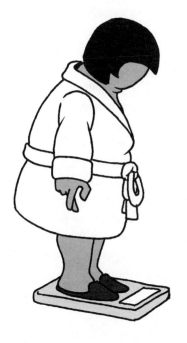

The object of changing your diet is not just to lose weight but to reduce the amount of fat in your body, especially around your waist.

The only way to get rid of the fat is to do the opposite and run a **negative energy balance**. This can be achieved by reducing the amount of energy (calories) you get from food and drink each day, burning more energy by being physically active or — best of all — by doing both. It is a very simple equation, but sadly is not as simple to implement or maintain in a modern lifestyle, full of tasty, calorie-rich things to try.

WEIGHT LOSS DIETS

Reducing the amount of energy (calories) you get from what you eat and drink can be successfully approached in any number of very different ways. There is no 'one size fits all' strategy. The most common way to try to reduce your energy intake is to go on a diet. This means regulating some or all of your entire food intake according to a plan. There are millions of diets out there. Each requires some adherence to a formula, recipe book or strategy for its success.

The media is full of inflated claims that one diet may be better than another, producing better weight loss because of a particular (magical) mix of nutrients. Whether the composition of a diet significantly affects how well it helps you to reduce the fat in your body remains controversial. On average they will all achieve about the same amount of weight loss — 2 to 4 kg (4½–9 lb). However, on an individual basis their effects may be quite variable. Some diets that work really well for some people will be unpalatable or impossible for others. The fact that there are so very many diets out there that are so very different in what they let you eat should tell you that there is no right or wrong answer. What you are eating is probably not as important as the fact that you are sticking to some sort of plan for what you eat and are eating fewer calories. It is likely that the mere process of embracing any dietary restrictions, thinking about and coordinating the foods you eat, makes you tend to eat less (energy) and eat better. No matter how well it might work, if you can't stick with it, it's never going to give you what you want.

Overall, the best outcomes are probably seen when different dietary approaches are used in combination. For example, it is often recommended that what best fits the bill in people with type 2 diabetes is to adopt a low glycaemic index, low fat diet with increased soluble fibre and protein intake together with behavioural interventions, exercise, support measures and adjustment of diabetes medications. This may sound extraordinarily complicated but it is essentially a dietician's description of a good basic, healthy diet.

Although most weight loss diets share a number of common elements, they can be divided into essentially four main categories:

- low calorie (or low energy) diets
- low fat diets
- low carbohydrate diets
- low GI diets.

Each of these different kinds of diets essentially focuses on changing only one particular component of your diet, without (directly) worrying about any of the others. This has the advantage of simplicity. As you've only got one thing to look out for, it also makes it easier to stick to.

It is beyond the scope of this book to describe any of these different diets in the detail required to make them really work for you. This information can be easily found elsewhere, in books and magazines and on the internet. However, their broad characteristics can be summarized as follows.

Low calorie diets

Low calorie diets aim to directly limit your energy (calorie) intake. As far as low calorie diets are concerned, a calorie is a calorie no matter where it comes from. You make your choices on calories alone. It doesn't really matter what you are eating so long as it adds up to fewer calories in the end.

A low calorie diet can be achieved in essentially two different ways. The first method is to estimate how much energy (calories) is contained in everything you eat, and make a plan to restrict your diet based on a set number of calories at each meal or over a day. This is known as **calorie counting** and is widely practised by people wanting to lose weight and keep it off.

The first step in calorie counting is usually to work out how much energy you actually need to be getting from your diet (known as the **daily energy requirement).** This can be estimated with a calculator using the Harris Benedict principle, which takes into account your age, gender, size and level of activity:

Women: 655.1 + (9.56 × weight in kg) + (1.85 × height in cm) – (4.68 × age in years) × activity factor × 4.12 (if you want the result in kilojoules)

Men: 664.7 + (13.75 × weight in kg) + (5 × height in cm) – (6.76 × age in years) × activity factor × 4.12 (if you want the result in kilojoules)

Note: To work out your daily energy requirement in calories, leave out the 4.12 at the end of the calculation.

The activity factor in each equation (which adjusts for how active you are) is:

- for those who do little or no exercise each day, multiply by 1.2
- for those who do light exercise one to three days a

week, multiply by 1.375

- for those who do moderate exercise three to five days a week, multiply by 1.55
- for those who do hard exercise six to seven days a week, multiply by 1.725
- for those who do daily exercise, a physical job or hard training, multiply by 1.9.

Let's say you are a 50-year-old woman who is 156 cm tall and weighs 80 kg. You're doing a little light exercise one to three days a week, but your weight is stable and doesn't want to budge. Using this equation, you can calculate that you must be eating about 8500kJ (2030 calories) of energy in your diet each day, because this is how much energy you are using up every day.

To get rid of some of your fat you need to subtract energy from your diet and run in negative balance. You could step up your exercise, let's say to do moderate exercise three to five days a week. This would mean your energy requirements would go up to 2280 calories. And if you didn't eat any more than your usual 2030 calories, you'd be running a negative balance (-250) and start losing weight.

But if you didn't have time to do more exercise and just wanted to lose weight through your diet, a good place to start is with an energy deficit of about 500kJ (120 calories) each day. So if you were calorie counting you'd plan to only eat approximately 8000kJ (1910 calories) a day. This will generally achieve a weight loss rate of approximately 0.5 kg (1 lb) per week. Using this formula you can also appreciate how combining diet and increased physical activity is the easiest way to a negative energy balance and a slimmer waistline. But more on exercise in the next chapter.

After you have determined your target calorie intake, the next step in calorie counting is to work out how many calories are actually contained in the food you are eating. Some information can be obtained by reading the 'nutritional information panel' that is present on the labels of most processed foods. Look first at the serving size section. All the information below it will be about what you will get when you eat this amount of the product. If you eat more than this, which is usually the case with most of these products, all the nutrients you will also be getting will increase proportionally, including the calories.

There are also many recipe books, websites and phone apps that are now available to provide useful information about how many calories are contained in most kinds of food and drinks, which can help in planning your meals.

Unlike the other diets detailed below, a low calorie diet can be quite flexible with what you eat. In fact it's largely your choice what you eat (e.g. whether you chose nachos or apples) so long as you stay within the limits imposed by the calorie count. The other advantage is that you quickly learn how to substitute foods that eat into your calorie count with those that eat into your waistline.

For example, the energy in a packet of corn chips is around 2000kJ (478 calories) per 100g (almost the same as butter) while most fruit and vegetables contain fewer than 400kJ (96 calories) per 100g. So if you are sticking to your new plan of 8000kJ (1910 calories) a day, you can still have your energy-rich nachos, but that's a quarter of all the energy you can have that day. And this leaves less room for other things. But if you eat an apple instead, then you have more room for something else later.

Another simple approach to limiting the energy contained in your diet is to follow a diet, meal or menu plan that swaps your intake of high calorie foods for products that carry less energy but have about the same volume and the same or more nutrients. The object is to make every mouthful contain less energy than it did before, while at the same time you get to eat the same satisfying portions. Two of the most commonly used low calorie diets are the DASH Diet and Weight Watchers.

Often the first thing a dietician will do to help you lose weight is to take a close look at what you are currently eating and find out which parts of your daily menu are providing you with energy you don't really need. Rather than causing a major shift in your diet, often only a few targeted strikes can be all it takes to successfully reduce the energy content of your diet and the fat around your middle.

For example, soft drinks (sodas) and 'juices' represent major sources of excess energy. Over one-fifth of the sugar in a typical diet comes from these unnecessary drinks. The corn syrup sugars used in most soft drinks are the same as those in concentrated apple juice used in the bulk of fruit drinks. On average the energy in a can of Coke is around 500kJ (120 calories). So substituting all soft drinks in your diet for (low calorie) water can make a big difference to your waist. Many waist-conscious drinkers have also embraced diet versions which substitute sugar with other sweet chemicals and so contain less or none of the energy of their fully sugared parents. These sugar substitutes are discussed in detail in Chapter 3.

Another important cause for the excessive amounts of calories in our diet is so-called energy-dense foods. These contain a large amount of energy (calories) for their weight and are essentially concentrated energy. Some of the most energy-dense foods are high in fat. As noted above, fat contains twice the energy (calories) per gram when compared to protein or carbohydrate. Fat also doesn't dissolve in water so fatty foods tend to be drier, meaning that calories are tightly packed. One teaspoon of butter contains almost the same amount of energy as two cups of raw broccoli. Low calorie substitutes can usually be identified as foods that are both low in fat but high in water or fibre to provide weight and volume to food, but without additional calories.

However, it's not just fat that contributes to calories. Other components in your diet may be energy dense too, including those with a high sugar content (e.g. cakes, confectionery, dried fruit and some highly processed breakfast cereals). Again, the 'nutritional information panel' will give you some idea.

Even within food groups the energy density can vary quite a lot. For example, there are 420kJ (100 calories) in a quarter of a cup of raisins. The same amount of energy is contained in two cups of grapes.

A low calorie diet might substitute:

- lean cuts for fatty chops
- reduced fat dairy for whole milk
- skinless chicken for fried chicken
- apples for apple juice
- whole fruit for dried fruit
- lentils for mince
- salads and soups for muffins
- fruit for chips or crisps.

You might think that eating low calorie foods would just make you hungry and therefore want to eat more. But this is not true. On average, if you reduce the energy-dense foods you eat by a quarter, you will reduce your energy intake by a similar amount. In fact, it has been argued that energy-dense foods make you overeat because they are less filling and this means you eat more in the long term. So reducing the energy density of every mouthful usually means that you eat less (fewer calories) and lose waist.

Low fat diets

Some of the extra energy in your diet comes from the fat you eat. Fat contributes twice the energy per gram when compared with other nutrients. Even if you are not counting calories, by assiduously avoiding fat, whatever you eat will usually contain less energy. For example, just choosing a leaner cut of meat can reduce the energy you get from your steak even if the amount you eat or the menu does not change.

So another popular way to lose weight is to focus solely on limiting the amount of fat in your diet, without worrying too much about anything else. These so-called 'low fat diets' are very popular for weight loss and are simple to follow because you only care about fat. Among the most famous are the Pritikin and Ornish diets, which can offer an effective means of weight loss for some people.

Again, you can do this quite easily yourself by seeing how much fat is contained in the food you eat (based on the 'nutritional information panel') and choosing products with the lowest fat levels. Then you can simply substitute those things that contain animal fat (meat, milk, eggs, etc.) with low fat or vegetable alternatives. This is precisely what people on a low calorie diet are also doing, although for a different reason.

The other advantage of reducing the amount of fat in your diet is that you can also improve your lipid levels (see Chapter 9) along with your waistline. Many low fat diets also tend to have a high fibre content, which also helps with glucose control.

The major problem with low fat diets is that fat is not the only source of calories. Reducing the proportion of fat in your diet will not lead to weight loss unless the total amount of energy you are getting from your diet is also reduced (and exceeded by energy expenditure). Any extra energy from carbohydrates (sugar) or protein in your diet is still going to be converted and stored as fat. So overeating will still make you fatter, even if you are following a low fat diet. In fact, most people are eating much less fat than they did 20 years ago and yet the average size of their waistlines has not improved and, if anything, has got bigger.

It has also been argued that low fat diets may not be successful because when you get rid of fat in many of these low fat diet plans you often replace it with high GI carbohydrates, which potentially makes both glucose and weight control more difficult.

Low carbohydrate (carb) diets

As discussed in Chapter 3, diets low in carbohydrates are popular for the management of type 2 diabetes because of their beneficial effects on glucose control. However, low carb diets can also help in waist management.

The sole focus of low carb diets is to reduce your carbohydrate intake. You can do this yourself by estimating how many carbs are contained in different products and planning your meal and how much of it you will eat to match your chosen limit. This practice is known as **carbohydrate counting** or **counting carbs** and is widely used by people wanting to lose weight and keep it off.

Alternatively, you can begin a low carb diet, in which any foods that are high in carbohydrates are strictly limited or substituted with foods containing more proteins and/or more fats (e.g. meat, poultry, fish, shellfish, eggs, cheese, nuts and seeds). Some low carb diets just replace common carb-rich products with other foods that are essentially low in carbohydrates (e.g. non-starchy salad vegetables for potatoes or rice).

Perhaps the best-known example of a low carb diet is the Atkins Diet. However, there are a range of other diets that share roughly the same principles with respect to carbs but vary in their relative amounts of other nutrients (e.g. how much fat or protein you eat). For example, the Atkins Diet does not restrict the fat you can eat, while the CSIRO Total Wellbeing Diet and the Zone Diet reduce both fat and carbohydrate in your diet, so the relative proportion of energy from protein goes up (which is why they are also sometimes called high protein diets). This extra protein can have the added effect of suppressing hunger and promoting your sense of fullness earlier in the meal.

Low carb diets tend to work faster than other weight loss plans. This is because the sugars stored in your body (as glycogen) are rapidly used up to make up for the carbs you are not getting from your diet. The chemical release of glycogen from its stores uses up water. So your weight quickly falls within a week, which is a great positive reinforcement. However, at the beginning you are mostly losing water rather than fat.

The other problem comes if you fall off the wagon and return to your normal diet. As you are now eating more carbs, your body is able to put away more glucose stores, which releases water. This means that your weight can very quickly rebound, even if you are not actually getting fatter. Therefore your weight can yoyo on a low carb diet more than with other strategies, as faithfulness to your diet rises and wanes.

Low GI diets

Another practical approach to waist control is to go on a **low GI diet**, which only considers how quickly a food will cause a rise in blood glucose levels (known as the **glycaemic index** or GI). It does not concern itself with the amount of carbs or calories you are eating, but rather the kind of carbs you are taking in. A low GI diet aims to substitute any high GI products in your diet with low GI alternatives that deliver their carbohydrate at a slower pace. Examples of some possible substitutions are provided in Chapter 3.

Because it is hard to predict why one product is low GI and another is high, a low GI diet relies (at least initially) on tables, recipe books, websites and apps that provide an estimate of the GI of most foods and help you to choose the lowest GI alternative. Some products also display their GI proudly on their label.

The real value of low GI diets in glucose control for people with type 2 diabetes is discussed in detail in Chapter 3. However, it is also clear that simply targeting the kind of carbohydrates you eat without doing anything else is enough to help you lose weight and keep it off. Eating predominantly low GI foods is the basis of many effective weight loss programs including the South Beach Diet and New Glucose Revolution Diet.

It is thought that high GI foods don't make you feel as full as other foods, or if they do it wears off more quickly and you're left feeling hungry again sooner. By contrast, the slow delivery of sugars from low GI foods keeps you satisfied for longer (known as satiety), which means you are less likely to want to eat again soon. This also means you tend to eat less between meals, which helps reduce your energy (calorie) intake.

MEAL REPLACEMENTS

As an alternative to organizing your own diet it is now possible to get someone else to do it for you by providing meal replacements and/or pre-packaged meals. For example, one or two of your meals each day can be effectively replaced with a low energy drink or bar that has an energy content of no more than 1000kJ (239 calories) and consists mostly of protein with a small amount of fat and carbohydrate. Some meal replacement programs provide frozen meals that you just defrost on the right day at the right time and eat. If you eat their food instead of relying on your own random habits, you are almost guaranteed to be eating less.

Meal replacement strategies have generally proved more successful for weight loss than trying to limit your calorie intake across all your meals. This has made meal replacements some of the most popular and successful (in the short term) of all commercial weight loss plans. All you need to do is not fall off the wagon.

Their key limitation is the lack of flexibility with many programs, limited food choice and predictability of diet plans. Many do not include an education component, so that when the program is completed you haven't learnt self-reliance. Waist management in type 2 diabetes is a lifelong task not a temporary fad. Ideally, diets and meal replacements should be considered a great kick-start to your weight-loss program, which sees you ultimately take control of what you eat.

CHANGING EATING BEHAVIOURS

Successful waist management is not just about changing what you eat; it also involves changing how you eat. Changing eating behaviours and assuming control over what you are eating (even if it is only one component of your diet) appears to be pivotal for the long-term struggle to keep excess fat out of your body. The desire and momentum to keep new habits in place must come from yourself.

The single most important factor in determining the success of any weight loss diet is whether you can stick with it for the long term.

To make healthy behaviours stick, it is also important to change your focus from the negative 'I can't eat that' to the positive 'I can have these'. Eating is one of life's great pleasures. When you shop, when you cook, when you eat, it is possible to get satisfaction from your diet without excess calories.

For a diet to be successful it cannot be considered a punishment that you have to endure in order to get healthy. That will never work. So the only real solution is if at first you don't succeed, try, and try again until you find something that both works and that you enjoy — then run with it.

Even if you never change what you eat, or never follow a diet as such, it is possible to reduce the amount you eat by changing the way you eat. One simple trick is to leave one in every four behind. For example, for every four spoons of cereal you would have, eat three and leave one behind. For every four potatoes you'd eat, eat three and leave one behind. On its own, this technique is challenging, as smaller portions can leave you hungry and dissatisfied. So the combination of more filling (less energy dense) foods and reduced portion sizes is better than either on its own.

Another simple trick is to use smaller plates and bowls. When presented with larger portions most people generally just eat it all up, as hunger and fullness signals are overridden by the cue to clean the plate. To stop yourself overfilling, and make it look as if you are eating more than you really are, just use a smaller plate.

One of the important reasons we often eat is simply because food is there. That is how the human brain works. So plan your environment to support waist management. But rather than having a house devoid of food, make it easier to access fruit, vegetables and salads in your home and harder to get to the carbs, sweets, biscuits/cookies and chips.

The more often you eat, the greater the chance you will take in more energy (calories). It is obvious that every calorie outside of meal times is probably a calorie in excess. However, skipping meals is not a good solution. In fact, there is good data showing that regular eating patterns help waist control. For example, breakfast gets you going and makes you feel nourished and satisfied, and less likely to overeat for the rest of the day. Missing breakfast means you have less energy and makes you hungrier for snacks or larger portions at other meals, so you are always chasing your tail when it comes to glucose control.

Snacks

It is sometimes said that snacking between meals can prevent overeating due to excessive hunger. Certainly, some diet programs allow for snacks to help manage hunger and reduce bingeing. But it is usually not necessary to snack and any means to reduce the amount you are eating is worthwhile if you have type 2 diabetes. If you just have to snack, the trick is to make sure that these snacks don't add much to your energy balance. The best example is to reach for fresh fruit or vegetables (such as carrots or broccoli) when you snack instead of a sandwich, muffin or cake.

A more practical solution is to get a handle on when you usually feel the urge to snack. Is it mid-morning, mid-afternoon or in the evening? Once you know, you can try adding in more slow carbs to the meal immediately beforehand, to try to cover this period much better and reduce your hunger cravings.

Comfort food

We eat food not just to get energy. It is also major source of pleasure in our lives and is central to the ideal of a 'good life'. This pleasure sometimes makes us want to eat even when we shouldn't be hungry. How many times have you heard people say that they have a special stomach for dessert? Equally, the reason that many diets fail is because they are less palatable, less pleasurable and less comforting than regular food.

For a weight loss diet to really work it has to be enjoyable, or even more enjoyable than your regular fare. This takes a degree of experimentation, trial and error. But the new flavourful meals you will discover can become your new best friends and bring guilt-free pleasure back into your kitchen. One way many people cope with stress in their lives is by eating. If you are depressed, anxious, strung out, angry or filled with other negative emotions, food can be a comfort, hence the term 'comfort food'. The more stress you have in your life, the more you might look to offset it by eating. And it works, but only for a moment. Eating food will reliably alter mood and emotion, typically making you less grumpy and calmer, possibly by modifying brain function and triggering the release of 'calming' hormones. What is important in stress-related eating is to deal with the stress at the same time you are trying to lose weight (see Chapter 16). This makes it more likely that both will get better.

SETTING WEIGHT LOSS GOALS

One of the most important components of a weight loss program is setting clear and achievable goals. Unrealistic expectations concerning weight loss frequently result in failure. Having a relevant and achievable target in front of you hardens your resolve and focuses your attention (not just 'I want to be thinner'). As an initial target it is recommended that those who are overweight should aim to reduce their current weight by 5 to 10 per cent (e.g. if you are 100 kg/220 lb, aim to initially reduce your weight to between 90 and 95 kg/198 and 209 lb). This might seem very small, but even this amount may be associated with improved health if it can be sustained.

It is also useful to keep a food diary or journal, recording everything you eat. You can use either a book or a phone app for this. It is not simply a good way to see how you are tracking; some studies have shown that people who keep a daily food diary lose more weight than those who don't. Again, it appears that the act of paying close attention to what you are eating, and recognizing that your choices actually matter, seems to be a key part of achieving weight loss.

Finally, waist control is not easy at the best of times. It can be even harder on your own. There are many providers out there who can offer advice and support. The most successful programs involve a strong relationship and long-term interaction between provider and consumer, be that a dietician, trainers, counsellors, motivators, a weight loss group or even your friends and family. So get some help!

OTHER OPTIONS FOR THE EXTREMELY OVERWEIGHT

In many people with type 2 diabetes, getting rid of excess fat can be achieved through keeping to a diet and increased physical activity. However, in some people who are dangerously overweight, medications and surgery are now available to make it easier to lose weight and improve health and wellbeing.

Orlistat is a medicine that reduces the absorption of fat from the diet by one-third, by inhibiting the enzymes that break down fats in the intestine. It was derived from a natural inhibitor of digestion found in bacteria. By limiting the amount of fat digested, orlistat also reduces the energy obtained from fat in your diet. In some individuals this is enough to cause a modest reduction in weight. However, many people cannot tolerate orlistat because of its side effects, including flatulence and oily, loose stools.

Phentermine and diethylpropion are **appetite suppressants** that are chemically related to amphetamines, and work by changing the balance of neurochemicals in the brain to help you feel full after meals. Again, their effects are modest at best and they may be associated with significant side effects, including behavioural changes, anxiety, increases in heart rate and blood pressure. There is also a potential for dependence so they can only be used for short-term treatment.

GLP-1 receptor agonists and SGLT-2 inhibitors that are used for the management of glucose levels can also be used to promote weight loss in some people with type 2 diabetes. These therapies are discussed in detail in Chapter 6.

A number of different complementary herbal weight loss supplements are sold in health shops and claim to promote weight loss. None of these therapies has been proven to be consistently effective and some are actually dangerous depending on what they contain and how they are used. Someone with type 2 diabetes should never take additional medications without first consulting their physician or diabetes care team for advice.

Another option for weight control is surgery (known as **bariatric surgery**). This is a very effective means to produce sustained weight loss in severely overweight individuals. In many people, the weight loss is so significant that they become free of diabetes. The most common bariatric surgery techniques are gastric banding, gastric bypass and gastric sleeve surgery. All these surgical techniques are costly and require adherence to diet and exercise regimens for the full benefits to be achieved and sustained.

Gastric banding (also known as a **lap-band**) places an adjustable band around the upper part of the stomach, creating a small pouch. This pouch is smaller than a whole stomach and means you eat much less at any one time before feeling full. In the long term this means you eat smaller portions and lose weight over time. The size of the pouch can be individually adjusted so that it prevents overeating, but not so small as to prevent adequate nutrition. Because no part of the stomach is removed, the signals for hunger sometimes remain. However, by feeling full more quickly and for a longer period of time, this can lead to significant weight loss over time in some individuals. Weight loss with lap-banding also requires adherence to dietary changes to be successful.

Gastric bypass surgery also creates a small upper pouch that reduces the amount you can eat at one time, but it also surgically connects the small intestine to the new pouch, bypassing the remainder of the old stomach which is then removed. This means less hunger and better weight loss. However, it requires more complicated invasive major surgery, but bypassing the upper intestine has more significant effects on blood glucose control, with at least three out of every four people with type 2 diabetes who undergo this procedure not needing to take glucose-lowering medication anymore.

An intermediate form of gastric surgery thins the stomach to form a tube (known as a **gastric sleeve**) rather than a restrictive pouch. The part of the stomach that regulates hunger is also removed. This kind of surgery is more effective at producing weight loss than lap-banding, but may be less effective than gastric bypass surgery in terms of its effects on 'curing' diabetes. Surgery cannot be considered a solution for the hundreds of millions with type 2 diabetes. But for those who can afford it (and can survive it) bariatric surgery can be a life-changing intervention.

5

GET PHYSICAL

Understand

- One-third of adults undertake no vigorous activity at all, or only now and then in very small/short doses. Most of their waking hours are spent sitting.
- People who sit for long periods are at greater risk of weight gain and have worse blood glucose and blood pressure control, no matter how much physical exercise they subsequently do.
- The health benefits of regular physical activity are far greater than the total amount of energy burnt, and are seen regardless of whether or not you lose weight.

- The stresses and strains that tax the body during vigorous exercise cause it to adapt. These adaptations are what is known as 'getting **fit**' and include better blood glucose, lipid and blood pressure levels.
- The same health benefits of physical activity can be achieved whether performed as a structured daily session (exercise) or as unstructured activity spread over the course of a day.

Manage

- Take all the little opportunities to be more active every day. Accumulate moderate-intensity physical activity in everyday tasks.
- Undertake a careful screening assessment of your health and fitness before commencing any new exercise program.
- Plan exercise as part of your regular daily commitments, rather than as an optional 'add on' to do 'when you have time'.

- Set yourself modest but realistic goals and keep updating them as you get fitter.
- Combine aerobic training with anaerobic exercises such as resistance training for added benefits with respect to fat burning and glucose control.
- Get help. People generally have greater success with exercise when they have supervision and encouragement from someone else, be that an exercise physiologist, trainer or a local club.

Most people don't get enough physical activity. This is not because they don't go to the gym, jog or lift weights. It is not because they are lazy. In fact, most people are far too busy — too busy, that is, to undertake any sustained vigorous activity on any regular basis. Such people are known as **sedentary**. Most of their busy waking hours are spent sitting at a desk, in a car, bus or train, sitting around the meal table or recovering from their day sitting on the couch. Think about what you did yesterday: there's a good chance you too spent at least eight to ten hours sitting down.

While it may seem innocuous enough, this sedentary lifestyle is a killer. For example, when compared to those who undertake regular physical activity, inactive people have, on average, twice the risk of heart attack. The magnitude of this effect is similar to being a smoker.

Type 2 diabetes is strongly linked to inactivity. People who engage in little physical activity are more likely to get type 2 diabetes even without an expanding waistline. Yet recognizing that one reason you're sitting in the pickle jar of diabetes is because of sitting on your backside far too often makes the potential solution all the more apparent and urgent. Having type 2 diabetes means it's time to get physical.

Of all the things that can be done to manage your diabetes, getting more physical activity is one of the most important.

You can have the best diet and take all your medication as prescribed, but if you remain inactive many of their benefits can be lost.

By contrast, the impact of diabetes and its complications can be reduced by just increasing your level of regular physical activity, often only very slightly. Engaging in regular exercise can also enhance the success of other initiatives, such as those aiming to control your blood glucose levels, your waistline, your blood pressure or lipid levels. When it comes to diabetes, if you really want to survive you need to get fitter.

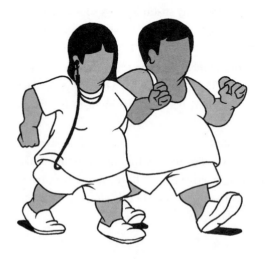

Of all the things that can be done to manage type 2 diabetes, physical activity is one of the most useful and most important.

WHY DO FIT PEOPLE SURVIVE?

There is good evidence that physical exercise has a number of direct and indirect effects on the human body that promote health and wellbeing.

Exercise burns excess energy

The most obvious reason for this is that exercise burns energy (calories) accrued from your diet that would otherwise be deposited as fat around your waistline. Consequently, alongside healthy nutrition, regular exercise is an important means to achieve and maintain weight control and to improve the body's composition. However, the health benefits of physical activity are far greater than the total amount of energy burnt, and are seen regardless of whether or not you lose weight when you exercise regularly.

Exercise offsets insulin and improves glucose control

When you are physically active, your muscles burn different kinds of fuel. The first fuel to be used is stored in the muscles themselves. Once muscle activity has burnt these limited stores, to keep going glucose is released into the bloodstream by the liver, and fat breakdown is increased so that it can also fuel the muscles. Your muscles then take up, burn and break down fats and glucose from the blood, which provides the energy for your muscles to contract and get their job done. After exercise is finished your muscles continue to take up large amounts of fat and glucose from the bloodstream to replenish their fuel stores in preparation for their next exertion. This uptake of glucose, both during and after exercise, can be very useful for people with type 2 diabetes, as it means less work for insulin and any medications to do.

Exercise triggers adaptations

The stresses and strains that tax the body during exercise cause it to adapt. These adaptations are what is known as 'getting fit' or 'the training effect'. Fitness includes adaptations in the heart, circulation, muscle, nerve and hormonal functions that vary according to the level and duration of physical activity. Precisely because it is taxing, exercise stimulates and adapts the body in ways that make you better able to cope with your next physical activity. However, these adaptations also have spin-off effects on many other aspects of your health, including those associated with diabetes and its complications. For example, muscles that are regularly used will adapt to become bigger and stronger, meaning they can do more next time with less effort and less fatigue at the end of it. At the same time, bigger muscles are also more efficient at taking up and burning glucose, which is a bonus for diabetes control.

The same sort of thing happens in your heart. Following regular exercise, the heart also becomes bigger and stronger, making it more able to provide the extra blood flow required to fuel your exertions. However, a stronger heart is a bonus for people with type 2 diabetes, who often experience reduced function of their heart. A strong heart also means a slower pulse and lower blood pressure.

Benefits from fitness are also seen in your feet. For example, type 2 diabetes can sometimes lead to reduced blood flow to your feet, which can have serious complications for your health (see Chapter 12). Regular exercise demands better blood flow to the legs to allow the muscles to work better. So the blood vessels supplying your legs progressively adapt to regular exercise to improve this blood flow. And if you have diabetes, this may be just what your feet need to stay healthy.

To trigger each of these adaptations, you have to undertake activities that tax each system. The heart must be pushed and the muscles must be tired. Not too hard, but enough to make these systems want to improve, to be better able to cope with future requirements; in essence, to get fitter.

Exercise improves risk factors for heart disease

It is still possible to improve your health as a result of increasing your physical activity levels without necessarily being bigger, stronger or faster. For example, when people with type 2 diabetes perform regular exercise they can also reduce risk factors for complications such as high cholesterol, glucose and blood pressure levels without noticeably improving traditional markers of fitness, such as strength or endurance. Nonetheless, the greatest improvements are seen in those who can also achieve and sustain level of physical fitness.

Exercise makes you feel good

Feeling well each day is an important part of diabetes management, and exercise is also good for the mind. Physical activity improves many aspects of psychological health, including self-esteem and emotional wellbeing. Exercise also lessens the impact of stress on your mood and your body, partly by modifying the synthesis or release of stress-response chemicals in the brain. It also works in preventing depression and in its treatment (see Chapter 16).

Exercise not only makes you feel better but also makes you think better. Exercise increases levels and the availability of chemicals that have protective benefits for several diseases of the brain. Exercise also directly enhances the capacity for learning and memory and slows their losses associated with age.

In addition, regular exercise improves the quality of your sleep, which is extremely beneficial for how you feel (see Chapter 17).

The problem with too much sitting

Finally, the reason couch potatoes have such poor health outcomes is not simply because they are missing out on the health benefits of exercise. While it might feel comfortable, sitting down all day every day turns out to be directly damaging to your health. This is particularly the case where sitting is unbroken for long periods (such as when on the computer, at the desk, in front of the television, etc). People who sit for long periods are at greater risk of weight gain and have worse blood glucose and blood pressure control, no matter how much physical exercise they subsequently do.

It is thought that because your muscles are inactive when sitting, more of the burden of metabolising the food you eat is placed on the pancreas (which in the setting of diabetes is having a hard time coping anyway!). So more of the energy (calories) in the diet of inactive couch potatoes ends up in the fat around their waistlines, instead of being burnt while moving your muscles. By contrast, staying on your feet at every opportunity, and breaking up long periods of sitting by getting up frequently, may be as important as engaging in a structured exercise such as going to the gym. For example, people who sit for fewer than 4 hours per day but don't exercise, appear to be at least as healthy as those who exercise at least 5 hours per week but spend most of their day sitting down.

INCREASING YOUR DAILY ACTIVITY

There are many different ways to lead a more active life. The same health benefits of physical activity can be achieved whether you are doing a structured daily session (exercise or training) or just making it up over the course of your day, as part of your life or your job.

The important part is simply being active on a regular basis, and to stop being a couch potato.

Many people can 'accumulate' the moderate-intensity physical activity they need in everyday tasks, such as:

- walking the kids to school
- walking or cycling to work
- taking the stairs instead of the lift or elevator
- getting off the bus one stop earlier and walking home
- parking a little further away and walking the difference
- speaking to colleagues in person rather than sending an email
- getting up and collecting your printing rather than waiting for someone to bring it to you
- breaking up your sitting time at least every half-hour; just standing up regularly uses your muscles and expends excess energy; the less you sit around the healthier you can become.

Rather than being time-consuming or restrictive, taking every opportunity to put a little more physical activity into your day can be quite creative and invigorating. It requires little or no planning. The most exciting thing is that there are an endless number of options to try. The only thing that is limiting is taking the time to get up and get going.

However, the most familiar form of physical activity is exercise, which is any activity that is structured, planned and repetitive.

Doing exercise is probably the easiest way to ensure you engage in enough physical activities to build your health and resilience against diabetes and its complications.

Some form of exercise is generally required to become really fit. A good strategy is to plan exercise as a part of your regular daily commitments, rather than have it as an optional 'add on' to do 'when you have time'. Exercise sessions can be structured into a weekly work and recreation schedule to ensure they become a regular habit.

There are many different kinds of exercise, from walking and swimming, yoga and Pilates, to sports and more formal programs in a gym. Exercise broadly falls into two main categories: aerobic and anaerobic. Each has its own benefits and limitations, and the greatest benefits are probably gained when you do some of both over the course of your week.

GETTING AEROBIC EXERCISE

Aerobic exercise simply means doing some sort of physical activity that burns fuel in your muscles, using oxygen as the catalyst, to provide the energy required for movement. Aerobic exercise involves activities performed at moderate levels of intensity for extended periods of time.

Most continuous activities of more than 3 minutes are aerobic exercises, such as brisk walking, jogging, cycling, swimming, rowing, dancing, aerobics, as well as sports such as football, soccer, squash and tennis. They're all good. The best one for you depends on your interests and enjoyment, but mostly whether you can stick with it.

A number of studies have demonstrated the health benefits of just brisk walking on a regular basis. For example, a regular brisk walking program can improve your fitness, lower your blood pressure, improve your blood lipid profile and lower your blood glucose levels. This is often the easiest way to take up exercise. It is simple, cheap and right there at the end of your legs. For example, when compared to doing nothing at all, some health benefits can be observed with as little as 1 to 2 hours of walking at a moderate pace every week. This is a good place to start and may be all you can do or fit in. It might include walking for pleasure, walking the dog, walking to work or the shops or walking as a break from work. After a while it will get easier and you'll find yourself walking further, faster and more often. This soon adds up to better fitness and to better health outcomes.

Pedometers that count each step (by registering impacts as your feet hit the ground) can provide a simple method to assess your current activity, as well as a motivational tool to become more active. Sedentary people will generally accumulate fewer than 5000 steps a day. Although everyone should have their own target based on their age and level of fitness, a general goal should be to try to walk at least 10,000 steps every day.

It is recommended that all adults with type 2 diabetes should undertake some kind of regular, **moderate-intensity aerobic exercise** on 3 to 5 days of each week — not just on the weekend. Physical activity is best spread out across the week so that there is no longer than 2 or 3 days between each session. Ideally you should get some activity on most days. In total, you should aim to get at least 2 to 3 hours of aerobic exercise across every week, divided into sessions of about 30 to 45 minutes each.

Each session can be further divided into smaller blocks of 10 to 15 minutes each, with a rest period of 5 minutes between each segment or spread at intervals through the day to fit your exercise into your daily routine. As your fitness improves, the duration of each segment can gradually become longer or the rest period between each segment can become shorter. However, you have to ease into it. If you've been inactive for a while you can't go hard at it immediately. Some tips on getting started are listed later in this chapter.

Although the first target is 2 to 3 hours per week, better health outcomes are seen with longer and more frequent workouts; again, you have to build up to this. But while more is better, even a small increase in your level of activity provides some protection and benefit when compared to doing nothing at all.

The exercise you choose doesn't need to be very hard. But it needs to be enough to tax you and your muscles. This is why it is called moderate-intensity and is the key goal of your aerobic exercise. But how intense this really is will be very different in different people.

There are a number of different ways to judge this. For example, you can use a simple scale:

- level 0 is sitting down
- level 10 is the highest level of effort possible
- to exercise at moderate intensity you need to aim for 5 or 6. If your exercise program is under the care of professional trainers, they will often determine the best program for you based on formal measures of your fitness. This can also be used to track your progress and provide quantitative motivational goals.

One of the most common tests of fitness is the **VO2 max** (also known as aerobic capacity, endurance exercise potential). This test is done by putting you through a graded exercise on a treadmill, bike or rowing machine (often referred to as an ergometer). The test starts easy and gets harder and harder until you reach your limits. While you are working away, the volume and composition of air breathed is directly measured, and how much oxygen you have used is calculated. Moderate-intensity activity should see you exercising at about 60 per cent of your VO2 max.

Another common way to judge the required intensity of an activity is to check your heart rate. When you start any physical activity, your heart rate will increase; the greater the intensity of the activity, the greater the increase in your heart rate. A rough guide to establishing an appropriate training intensity is to work at around 60 to 70 per cent of your age-adjusted maximal heart rate.

Your maximal heart rate can be estimated using the following formula:

Maximum heart rate = 220 minus your age (in years).

So if you are 60 years old, your maximal heart rate should be around 160 beats per minute. Then when you are exercising at moderate intensity, your heart should be racing at around 60 to 70 per cent of this figure, or between 100 and 112 beats per minute. This is also known as getting into 'the zone'. Many people find checking their heart rate while exercising the most convenient way to ensure they are getting a good aerobic workout.

It is important to note that these formulae apply only to healthy people and cannot be applied to those with heart disease and on certain medications that slow the heart. When prescribing appropriate exercise intensity, a number of other factors must also be taken into consideration, including age, health status, and current fitness and activity levels. Consequently, all those with diabetes should seek advice from their physician or diabetes care team, an accredited exercise physiologist or a suitably qualified allied health professional, to set a target that is just right for them (see 'Starting an exercise program' detailed below).

Although aerobic exercise is associated with improved health and wellbeing in people with type 2 diabetes, it does have some limitations when performed on its own. While aerobic training increases the capacity of the heart and lungs it may not have much effect on muscle strength or bone mass, both of which buffer the impacts of diabetes. Aerobic exercise also may not use up as much extra fat and glucose when compared to the same amount of strength training, although it can be undertaken for longer periods and more frequently to make up any difference. On the whole, aerobic exercise is best used as one component of a balanced exercise program that also involves some anaerobic exercises.

ANAEROBIC EXERCISE

The phrase 'anaerobic exercise' describes undertaking short bursts of intense exertion at nearly 100 per cent effort, like sprinting or weight lifting. Because the energy required for this kind of activity is at or above the maximal ability to supply oxygen to the muscles, anaerobic exercise must rely on fuel stores already present within the muscles themselves. These stores are limited and maximal exertion cannot be sustained for more than 2 to 3 minutes before exhaustion sets in. But by specifically burning these muscle stores, anaerobic exercises set in motion adaptations that build strength, endurance and size of muscles. However, its success does not require you to become bulky or muscle-bound.

By exhausting your muscles' fuel stores, they respond by filling up again on glucose and fat which is drawn out of the bloodstream. And this means less work for insulin and often less medication.

The workload on the body during this kind of exercise is much higher when compared with that during aerobic exercise, like jogging or swimming. This means anaerobic exercise will be able to burn more energy and can have a greater impact on your metabolism and fat stores. However, it also means that special precautions must be taken by those with diabetes when undertaking this kind of exercise program (see below).

Strength training

Strength or resistance training is the best known form of anaerobic exercise. This is where your muscles move against an opposing force that resists their movement (known as resistance). The force resisting you may be the force of gravity (e.g. weights, push-ups and squats), elastic resistance (e.g. rubber tubing) or hydraulic resistance as used in many exercise machines.

For your resistance training to be effective you must do enough in a session to fatigue your muscles.

Generally, muscles are repeatedly worked at 65 to 75 per cent of their maximal capacity (**known as one repetition maximum or 1RM**) until the point of fatigue. This usually means 8 to 12 repetitions of a specific activity, which is called a set. To maximize the benefits, the last few repetitions of each set are supposed to be hard. If you can do more than 12 repetitions of the exercise then you are not using enough resistance.

When starting out, one set of each exercise is all that is required. This is gradually built up to three sets of each exercise, with a recovery period of 1 to 2 minutes between each set, to provide the best stimulus to increase muscle strength.

The beauty of such programs is that they are self-adjusting. Even if you have little strength, activities can be planned to be in keeping with your 1RM. As the body strengthens and adapts it will become easier to lift the same weight, so the applied resistance must be progressively increased to ensure you are continually strengthening your muscles and maximising the benefits of the exercise. This is usually done by gradually increasing the training intensity, duration, frequency, time or a combination of some of these parameters. For example, if you do not want to increase a weight, slowing the exercise down will increase the amount of work you are doing.

There are a number of different strength programs available. A typical program would generally consist of 8 to 10 different exercises that are specifically chosen to increase the strength of a range of muscle groups, but in particular the large muscles of the legs, buttocks, trunk and upper back.

Strength training is best conducted at least 2 or 3 times each week, on alternate days so the muscles have a chance to regenerate and become stronger as a result of repeated sessions. If you want to do your strength training every day, it is advisable to split the program into two segments (e.g. upper body on Monday, Wednesday and Friday and lower body on the Tuesday, Thursday and Saturday) so each muscle group has two days to recover between each session.

When undertaking a strength program it is also important that each exercise is performed with the correct technique and that this is maintained throughout the set. This is known as **form**. This ensures that any activity achieves its desired outcomes and is performed safely. Loss of form, especially at the end of a set when muscles are tiring, not only reduces the effectiveness of an exercise but may also be dangerous.

Interval training

While aerobic fitness relies on continuous activity, additional fitness gains can also be achieved in already active people by alternating short bursts of vigorous exertion with intervals of lower activity. This is known as **interval training**. Interval training is not overly difficult and can be built up gradually according to your individual requirements. It may, for example, involve incorporating short periods of jogging as part of a basic walking program and progress to including multiple sprints of 100 to 200 metres with alternate periods of walking or jogging. Swimmers may include a couple of faster laps followed by slower laps. The high-intensity phase should be long enough and strenuous enough that you are out of breath by the end. Recovery periods (the slower, less intense periods of exercise) should be only long enough to result in a partial recovery before the next faster interval is begun. You should start with 10 to 15 minutes of warming up, followed initially by burst–recovery repeats totalling some 15 to 20 minutes, then end with a 10- to 15-minute period of cooling down. This is performed as part of training 2 or 3 times a week.

Interval training is more effective in burning fat than sustained moderate-intensity activity for the same or longer period. However, interval training is certainly more strenuous than continuous aerobic training, and generally requires increased levels of motivation. It should only be attempted by already active people and, in the context of diabetes, under the supervision of a doctor or appropriately trained exercise instructor.

Flexibility training

Although flexibility training (stretching exercises, yoga) has no direct effect on glucose control, it does help to improve and maintain the range of motion of your joints. This allows you to participate more easily, and with less pain, in other activities that can improve your health. As a result, most programs also incorporate an element of flexibility training, in addition to aerobic and anaerobic components.

STARTING AN EXERCISE PROGRAM

Whenever you plan to start a new exercise program, it is important to take it slowly and stick within your limits. If you are getting started after a period of inactivity, exercising on alternate days is a good place to begin, with a day of recovery between each exercise day. The recovery days may also be used to incorporate another exercise type, such as strength or flexibility training.

The pre-assessment

While regular physical activity has an enormous number of benefits for those with diabetes, it also has risks. This is not a reason to remain a couch potato, but the demands of exercise may be different in different people. To ensure that any risks are minimised and to allow for appropriate exercise prescription, it is recommended that all those with type 2 diabetes undertake a careful screening assessment of their health and fitness before commencing any new exercise program. This may be conducted by a doctor, diabetes educator or exercise specialist. However, everyone in your diabetes care team should be updated on your plans, as exercise potentially impacts all aspects of diabetes care, from your feet to your mind and everything in between.

People with well-controlled diabetes or stable heart conditions do not need formal medical clearance before beginning a low to moderate physical activity program. However, it is essential for all those with complications, those with difficult diabetes management, and in those who are unsure as to their risks. The kind of things a pre-assessment will look out for include risks for 'hypos', heart disease, high or low blood pressure, and foot damage.

Risks for hypos

During and after exercise, blood glucose levels can fall as muscles draw in glucose from the bloodstream. This is why exercise is so effective in controlling glucose levels in diabetes.

The majority of people with type 2 diabetes have glucose levels that are high enough to buffer the effects of exercise. However, some of the medicines that lower glucose levels in people with type 2 diabetes have the potential to cause **hypoglycaemia** when combined with exercise. The solution is not to avoid exercise, but to plan it better with the help of your physician or diabetes care team. For the minority who do experience these 'hypos' with exercise, they can be mostly prevented by better coordinating their physical activity with their medication. For example, not exercising straight after taking your medication can be useful. Some people also find it useful to carry some carbohydrate-rich snacks which they can eat in case they get caught up in physical activity that is more vigorous or more prolonged than originally planned. Another strategy is to eat your snack if glucose levels are already less than 5.6mmol/L (100.8mg/dL) before starting your activity. Alternatively, simply delay exercise until blood glucose levels are high enough to start.

Risks for heart disease

Any physical exertion places demands on the heart. While such demands can result in beneficial adaptations, in some people with type 2 diabetes the blood supply to the heart is a limiting factor. In particular, those with heart disease may be limited in their ability to undertake physical exertion. How this occurs is discussed in detail in Chapter 10. Because heart disease is very common in those with type 2 diabetes, before starting any new exercise program all people with diabetes should undergo some assessment of their heart. This may simply mean seeing your doctor, or you might need to undergo an exercise stress test (see earlier in this chapter) to see how the heart copes with physical stress and how safely exercise might be conducted on your own.

Risks for high or low blood pressure

As exercise increases the output of blood from the heart, this can cause an increase in blood pressure levels in some people, especially in those who already have high blood pressure. Rapid rises in blood pressure may lead to heart attacks and strokes and should be avoided where possible in people with type 2 diabetes (see Chapter 10). Such rises can usually be prevented by changing the dose or timing of blood pressure medications. People with uncontrolled hypertension should not begin an exercise program until their blood pressure has been effectively managed.

Some people with type 2 diabetes may also experience a profound fall in blood pressure with exertion. In particular, when diabetes damages the nerves that regulate blood pressure levels, blood pressure levels may be quite brittle and fall significantly with prolonged standing or moderate physical exercise. This may also be seen in some people taking blood pressure-lowering treatments which block the pathways required to keep the blood pressure up. Some doctors will ask you to monitor your blood pressure at home, or carry a continuous monitor for 24 hours (known as **ambulatory blood pressure monitoring**) to look out for falling blood pressure (see Chapter 8).

Risks for foot damage

Diabetes affects circulation to the feet and their ability to sense pain or pressure. This can lead to progressive damage to the feet and is discussed in detail in Chapter 12. Physical exertion can place significant demands on your feet, especially when undertaking activities like walking, running, dancing and other step exercises. Every time your foot strikes the ground it feels the force of nearly twice your body weight.

Everyone with diabetes should undergo regular assessment of their feet anyway. Many integrated diabetes care centres now offer these services under one roof.

Before starting any new exercise program particular attention should also be given to ensuring your feet are appropriately protected. For most people this will involve wearing supportive shoes and socks that fit well and do not rub or restrict the circulation. Appropriate shoes should have plenty of room around the forefoot and toes, but be snug enough around the heel to prevent rubbing and blisters. The wrong type of shoe or one that fails to control excessive foot movement can cause pain, blisters or injury.

Good foot hygiene before, during and after exercise is also important. Regularly inspect your feet for damage and change (rather than stop) your physical activity if necessary. It is also useful to consult with a podiatrist regularly, to ensure you haven't missed any early signs of problems and also to keep the nails trimmed, as foot problems with exertion can begin with pressure around sharp nail edges and/or ingrown toenails. A podiatrist can also recommend a specific shoe type or a pair of orthotics to take unwanted pressure off your feet. For people at high risk for foot problems, such as those with insensitive feet or those with previous foot ulcers, more care should be taken in choosing activities that minimize the risk of foot damage — swimming, aquarobics, cycling, rowing, resistance training, etc. are all good choices.

SUPPORT IS OUT THERE — GET HELP

Exercise is rewarding but it is not easy. In fact, it is supposed to be demanding. This means it can be hard to accomplish and sustain on your own. People generally have greater success with exercise when they have supervision and encouragement from someone else, be that an exercise physiologist, trainer or a local club. Even friends and family can make a real difference in keeping you going strong. There are lots of great programs and resources out there to support you and help you reach your goals. Most of these can be accessed through your diabetes care team and may be subsidised as part of your diabetes care.

Exercise is about doing the right activity in the right doses and at the right pace to achieve your individual goals and needs. No matter what the ads say, there is no generic solution. Different people have different needs, likes and dislikes. Don't be bullied into a gym membership or doing something outside your comfort zone. The exercise program you select needs to become part of your new lifestyle so it must be convenient and enjoyable. When starting out make your exercise program practical, realistic and achievable so that it complements your existing lifestyle without requiring too many changes. When beginning an exercise program after a period of inactivity or unaccustomed exercise, start slowly and stay well within your current capabilities. Set yourself modest but realistic goals, and keep updating them as you get fitter.

It is also important to follow the results of exercise and stay on the right track. Chart the average distances and times of a walking/jogging program and see how you have improved. Keep a record in a diary. Document how weights increase as you undertake your strength program. Watch how your waistline shrinks with a tape measure or changes in your belt size.

Observe the health improvements, like lower blood pressure or cholesterol levels. Enjoy and monitor your progress over time. This can serve as a motivational tool. But, most importantly, it keeps you connected with your exercise and helps you to stay alive.

6

PILLS AND INJECTIONS

Understand

- Most people with type 2 diabetes eventually reach a point where some medicines are needed to prevent their glucose levels from rising dangerously.

- Medicines are not an alternative to a good diet and regular exercise, and work better when all are combined.

- There are a number of different medications used to lower glucose levels in people with type 2 diabetes. Each has their benefits as well as the potential for unwanted side effects. Different treatments may be suited to different people and different circumstances.

- The longer you have diabetes, the more likely it will be that insulin may be required. This does not mean you have failed in any way. Type 2 diabetes is a progressive condition in which your ability to make and use insulin declines and ultimately becomes exhausted.

Manage

- Learn how your medications work to get the best out of each.
- Make it easier to remember to take your medications by establishing regular routines and using pill packs.
- Coordinate your medications with your diet and lifestyle to ensure the maximum effectiveness of each.
- Discuss with your doctor some of the new options for managing type 2 diabetes and how they might work for you.

A number of different medications are now available to help your body regulate its blood glucose levels. They are not a substitute for a good diet and a regular amount of physical activity. Equally, having to take pills or injections does not mean you're doing something wrong. Most people with type 2 diabetes eventually reach a point where some medicines are needed to prevent their glucose levels from rising dangerously. This is simply the nature of the disease. Over time your pancreas becomes less able to make the insulin it needs to keep glucose levels under control, so it needs more help. The longer you have diabetes, the more likely it will be that you will need one or several different types of medication to keep glucose levels under control. Your doctor will advise which medications may be right for your particular needs. It is important to remember that different treatments may be suited to different people and different circumstances.

This chapter refers to the major classes of medications used to control glucose levels in people with type 2 diabetes and gives the chemical (generic) names of pills and injections rather than their brand names. These chemical names are usually displayed on the packet, under the brand name in smaller writing. There are many different brands and formulations of various products, and these often vary in different countries. If you can't make out or find the chemical name of your medication and how it fits into this chapter, please consult your doctor, pharmacist or diabetes care team.

It is important for everyone with type 2 diabetes to know what medications they are taking and how they work to get the most out of them.

METFORMIN

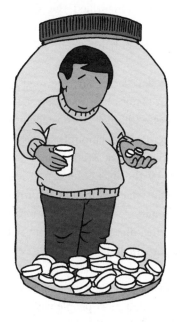

Most people with type 2 diabetes eventually reach a point where some medicines are needed to prevent their glucose levels from rising dangerously. This is simply the nature of the disease.

Metformin is the most widely used pill to treat diabetes. Between half and two-thirds of all people with type 2 diabetes take metformin, either alone or in combination with other pills or insulin. It is widely considered to be the first choice of medical treatment to improve glucose control in people with type 2 diabetes. Metformin is thought to have particular advantages for those who are overweight. Recent data have suggested that metformin can also modestly reduce the risk of heart disease, strokes and possibly some cancers, beyond its effects on glucose levels.

Metformin was originally developed from natural compounds found in French lilac (also known as goat's rue or Galega officinalis). Extracts from this plant have been used as a traditional treatment of diabetes and other ailments since the Middle Ages. Subsequent studies identified the specific chemicals (known as **biguanides**) that gave it the ability to lower glucose levels. Metformin is the only biguanide used for the treatment of diabetes.

One of the reasons glucose levels remain elevated in people with type 2 diabetes is that insulin fails to suppress the production of glucose by the liver (see Chapter 1). Consequently, the liver continues to make and secrete large amounts of glucose even when glucose levels are already high. Metformin works by reducing glucose production by the liver. Metformin also increases the body's sensitivity to the effects of insulin, improves the uptake of glucose by muscle and slows the absorption of glucose from a meal. When taken as directed, metformin will reduce your HbA1c by between approximately 0.5 and 1 per cent.

To work effectively most people will need to take 2 to 3 grams of metformin every day. Consequently, metformin tablets will usually be the biggest tablets in size that most people with type 2 diabetes will take. Some people find them difficult to swallow. A metformin syrup formulation taken as drops can be helpful if swallowing the big metformin tablets is a problem for you.

The other commonly reported side effects from metformin include gastrointestinal disturbances (e.g. nausea, diarrhoea, cramping and flatulence). These side effects will affect around one in five people using metformin to some degree but they are usually mild, only seen when using high doses or transiently when first starting metformin. The likelihood of developing side effects can usually be reduced or avoided by taking the following steps:

- Your doctor will start you at a low dose, often only one pill at night to begin with.

- Your doctor will increase your dose of metformin very gradually (e.g. increase by one pill every fortnight until reaching your target dose).
- Take your metformin with or after meals rather than before meals.
- The dose of metformin can be divided through the day to reduce side effects, or extended release (XR) formulations of metformin can be used. These have become preferred for the initial treatment of type 2 diabetes. This is mostly because of the convenience of a once-daily treatment that doesn't need to be coordinated with meals and achieves roughly the same level of glucose control as standard metformin, which you have to take twice or three times a day.
- Do not use too much metformin. Because metformin is removed from the body by the kidneys, people with type 2 diabetes with impaired kidney function will require lower doses to maintain safe levels and prevent side effects (e.g. 1 gram per day instead of 2–3).

Despite these simple manoeuvres, about 10 per cent of people with type 2 diabetes are still not able to take metformin because of its side effects.

More seriously, metformin has been associated with an extremely rare but life-threatening condition known as **lactic acidosis**. It is still controversial whether metformin is the instigating cause or whether it exacerbates this condition when it is caused by other things such as heart failure, liver or kidney failure. For this reason, those with a heart condition, a heavy alcohol intake or impaired kidney or liver function should only use metformin with caution and close supervision by their doctor. Metformin should also be temporarily stopped during any major illness (e.g. acute gastroenteritis, heart attack, bone fracture) and prior to major surgery or procedures that might precipitate a sudden fall in kidney function, such as imaging of the arteries using injections of dye (known as contrast angiography). Assuming no problems, metformin can be started again once you have recovered from your procedure.

Unlike with other anti-diabetic medications, low blood glucose levels (hypos) are seldom observed when metformin is used on its own. This is because it does not increase insulin levels or interfere with the body's responses to hypoglycaemia. Metformin also has the advantage over other agents in that it does not cause weight gain and in some people with diabetes it may reduce their weight slightly. Metformin may also be preferred for women with both diabetes and polycystic ovary syndrome (PCOS) as it modestly improves their PCOS symptoms as well as fertility.

SULPHONYLUREAS

Sulphonylureas are currently used by about one-third of all people with type 2 diabetes, mostly in combination with metformin. They are by far the most common 'second-line' agent for treating diabetes after metformin, because of their low cost, their effectiveness in rapidly lowering glucose levels and their long history of use in the treatment of type 2 diabetes.

The anti-diabetic effect of sulphonylureas was discovered quite by accident during World War II, when it was found that some sulphur-containing antibiotics (known as sulphonamides) caused low blood glucose levels in animals. These were then tested in people with type 2 diabetes with outstanding results.

Within 10 years sulphonylureas became the first widely used oral medications for the treatment of type 2 diabetes, providing the first real alternative to insulin injections.

A number of different sulphonylureas are currently available. There are many different formulations, brand names and manufacturers. However, in common, the chemical name of sulphonylureas usually begins in the prefix 'gli-' including:

- glipizide
- gliclazide
- glibenclamide (also known as glyburide)
- glibornuride
- gliquidone
- glisoxepide
- glyclopyramide
- glimepiride.

By and large, all of these sulphonylureas have comparable actions upon glucose levels. However, certain sulphonylureas may be suited to certain people because of their differing mode of clearance from the body, duration of action and risk of hypoglycaemia.

Sulphonylureas all work by triggering the release of insulin from the pancreas, which then works to lower glucose levels as detailed in Chapter 1. Sulphonylureas have the advantage of producing a rapid improvement in glucose control once treatment is initiated. When taken as directed, sulphonylureas will reduce the HbA1c by between 0.5 and 1 per cent in most people with type 2 diabetes.

Although effective, sulphonylureas have a number of disadvantages, including:

- Hypoglycaemia. Sulphonylureas can cause low blood glucose levels in some people with type 2 diabetes by stimulating insulin production and release in excess of their requirements, especially if they are missing meals or undertaking unplanned or excessive physical activity. (This is discussed in more detail in Chapter 7.)

• Weight gain. Sulphonylureas can cause modest weight gain (2–3 kg/4½–6½ lb) in some people. This is mostly seen in the first few months after sulphonylureas are started, and it usually doesn't get worse when treatment is continued. Weight gain is caused by increasing your insulin levels, whose job it is to get glucose and fat out of the bloodstream, at the expense of increasing your fat deposits.

• Exhaustion. Some doctors think that by stimulating the pancreas to make more insulin all the time, without a break, sulphonylureas can progressively burn out the capacity for insulin production over time (known as beta-cell exhaustion). This may be one reason why there can sometimes be a gradual loss of glucose control achieved with sulphonylureas with their long-term use over time.

In a small number of people (less than 10 per cent) sulphonylureas are completely ineffective in controlling glucose levels when used on their own. This may be because the ability to make insulin is completely exhausted already.

Other uncommon side effects of sulphonylureas include headache, abdominal upset and allergic reactions. Sulphonylureas can sometimes interact with alcohol to produce unpleasant hangover-like symptoms in some people about 10 minutes after drinking and sometimes lasting several hours.

SGLT-2 INHIBITION

Another way to reduce an excess amount of glucose in the bloodstream is to allow it to pass harmlessly into your urine. This is exactly what normally happens when glucose levels are too high — it spills over into the urine. This is the reason why people with diabetes may pass large amounts of slightly sweet urine (hence the term 'diabetes mellitus' which means 'siphon of honey').

It is possible to further enhance the loss of glucose into the urine by blocking the pathways that would normally retrieve it from the urine. It has been known for over a century that the bark of pear, apple, cherry and other fruit trees contains a chemical that causes glucose to be lost into the urine. This compound also inhibits the absorption of glucose from the intestine. More recently, companies have developed more selective chemicals that only block the kidney pathways. These drugs (known as **SGLT-2 inhibitors**) have just recently become available for the management of type 2 diabetes.

There are currently three different SGLT-2 inhibitors available for the treatment of diabetes, which have in common a chemical (generic) suffix '-gliflozin':

- dapagliflozin
- canagliflozin
- empagliflozin.

When used as directed, these agents lower HbA1c levels by between 0.5 and 1 per cent. Because they have no effect on insulin release they do not cause hypoglycaemia, and glucose will not spill into the urine if blood glucose levels are low anyway. By losing the excess calories contained in glucose, this treatment may also be associated with some weight loss (1–2 kg/2¼–4½ lb) and a reduction in body fat (as the body burns fat to make up for sugars lost into the urine). There are also modest reductions in blood pressure, similar to that achieved by taking a diuretic (see Chapter 8).

However, having glucose in your urine has its downside too. It means passing more urine more frequently, which can be an issue in those with a troublesome bladder. It can also increase the risk of genital fungal infections (known as thrush), although this is typically mild and easily managed when you are on the lookout for it (see chapter 18).

Recent long-term studies have confirmed not only the safety of this strategy in people with type 2 diabetes, but have also shown that it can reduce the risk of heart and kidney complications. Indeed, in one study the risk of dying from any cause was reduced by a third. Such positive data will likely see these agents become a central part of diabetes management over the next few years

INCRETIN AGONISTS

Incretins are natural hormones made by the intestine that act to amplify the amount of insulin released from the pancreas when eating. This is why they are called incretins (because they are made by the intestine and act to increase insulin production). Over half of the insulin made by the pancreas in response to a meal is directly related to the amplifying effects of your incretins.

In people with type 2 diabetes, the incretin effect is about half what it should be, further adding to the burden of making enough insulin to keep glucose under control. Unlike sulphonylureas, incretins do not stimulate the production of insulin directly. In fact, they only work to amplify insulin production when there is another signal to stimulate it, such as food or elevated glucose levels. They don't work when glucose levels are low because insulin production is naturally suppressed. There is no signal to amplify, so incretins do not cause hypoglycaemia unless combined with an excess of sulphonylureas or insulin.

While the human body has its own incretins (called GLP-1 and GIP), their effect is not very powerful or long lasting. This is possibly because the human body is evolutionarily adapted for grazing on carbohydrates (small amounts of food more often) rather than eating large amounts at once. But this is not true for other animals.

For example, in the Sonoran Desert in the United States lives a venomous lizard, the Gila monster. It eats only once every month or two. And when it does, it goes to town, eating up to one-third of its body weight. In the desert you never know when your next meal is coming so you have to make the most of it. But what is most remarkable about this lizard's adaptation to its 'binge eating' lifestyle is that it secretes a powerful incretin into its saliva that is able to remarkably boost insulin release from its pancreas several fold to allow it to better cope with eating large amounts in one sitting.

This lizard incretin is similar to the one found in humans, but subtly different in that it works much better and for longer. And not only for lizards. When injected into humans, a chemical made to look like just like this lizard incretin is also able to amplify insulin release and improve glucose control. It also suppresses appetite and slows the absorption of glucose following a meal, by reducing the rate at which the stomach empties. These two features of incretins also mean that using these injections can bring about weight loss (on average 2–3 kg/4½–6½ lb).

These agents are also known as GLP-receptor agonists because of their similar mode of action to the human incretin,

GLP. There are a number currently in clinical development for the treatment of diabetes, all of which have in common a chemical (generic) suffix '-tide':

- exenatide
- liraglutide
- lixisenatide
- albiglutide
- dulaglutide
- semaglutide.

For each, injections are required. Short acting ones are taken twice daily, one hour before both breakfast and dinner. Once daily and once weekly injections are also now available for longer-acting forms of these medicines. Even longer delivery using implantable pumps is also now possible, allowing for refills only every 3 to 6 months. Each of these formulations has comparable actions on glucose levels, reducing the HbA1c by an average of one per cent in most patients. However, the longer acting ones appear to achieve slightly better control than the shorter acting ones, although this may be due to compliance and tolerability more than any mechanism of action.

Although injections can be used in most settings, they are often added to the treatment of people with type 2 diabetes who are also injecting basal insulin, to reduce the risk of hypoglycaemia and weight gain that often accompanies adding more insulin (see below). In the near future, combination injections of insulin and an incretin will become available to further enhance their ease of use.

Apart from the need to inject, the key disadvantage of these injections is their action on digestion. While slowing the stomach down is a great idea for a venomous lizard that eats once a month, in humans this same effect can upset the stomach in many people. In most cases any discomfort settles gradually over the first month of treatment. When starting off using this kind of medication it is usual to begin with a small dose and then slowly increase the amount you take over a month to limit these side effects. The longer acting formulations (which are generally used in lower doses) cause fewer stomach side effects. Recent clinical studies with these agents have also demonstrated the potential for reducing the risks from heart and kidney complications in people with type 2 diabetes.

DPP-4 INHIBITORS

DPP-4 is an enzyme that breaks down your natural incretin hormones. One of the reasons that the injectable incretins detailed above have such powerful effects on human metabolism is that they are partly resistant to DPP-4, so they hang around long enough in high enough levels to get the job done.

However, you can achieve the same sort of effect by inhibiting the DPP-4 enzyme that breaks down your own incretins (using pills known as gliptins). In essence, by raising your own incretin levels, this tricks the insulin-producing cells of the pancreas that the last meal was much bigger than it really was, so it makes proportionally more insulin as a result.

There are currently only five different DPP-4 inhibitors available for the treatment of diabetes, which have in common a chemical (generic) suffix '-gliptin':

- sitagliptin
- saxagliptin
- linagliptin
- vildagliptin
- alogliptin.

Through inhibiting DPP-4, these pills will elevate your natural incretin levels three- to fivefold and thereby further amplify the amount of insulin released from your pancreas after eating or in response to elevated glucose levels. This has roughly the same effect as injecting a GLP-1 agonist, reducing the HbA1c by half to one per cent on average in most people with type 2 diabetes.

Gliptins are mostly used largely as 'second-line agents' in people already taking metformin, as an alternative to sulphonylureas or insulin, although they are effective on their own as a first-line therapy.

The key advantage of gliptins is that they have few side effects and are the best tolerated of all diabetes medications. Gliptins can be taken in tablet form once (or at the most, twice) daily. They can be taken any time of the day, with or without food and do not require coordination with meals or physical activity. Again, this is because they are amplifiers not stimulators of insulin release. They only work when there is a stimulus, such as a meal or having high glucose levels. But if glucose levels are low, there is no signal to make insulin so there is no incretin effect and no risk of hypoglycaemia when used on their own. Gliptins also do not cause weight gain and may bring about weight loss of 1 to 2 kilograms (2¼–4½lb) in some people.

While the gliptins have a number of advantages for glucose control, and large clinical trials have confirmed their safety, it remains to be established if these agents can reduce the complications of diabetes. This is in direct contrast to other strategies that, despite their higher rate of side effects, have demonstrated significant benefits over and above glucose control.

GLITAZONES

Thiazolidinediones (also known as 'glitazones' or TZDs) were introduced to diabetes care over a decade ago, with much fanfare and great expectations. Glitazones are able to increase the body's sensitivity to the glucose-lowering actions of insulin in muscle and the liver, in a manner different (and complementary) to metformin. When taken as directed, glitazones reduce the HbA1c by 0.5 to 1 per cent in most people with type 2 diabetes.

In some people, glitazones are an extremely effective way of controlling blood glucose levels when other drugs are not working. And like metformin, hypoglycaemia is not seen when glitazones are used on their own or with metformin.

There are currently only two different glitazones available, which have in common a chemical (generic) suffix '-glitazone':

- rosiglitazone
- pioglitazone.

Unfortunately, the risk of serious side effects has limited the use of this glucose-lowering medication. Glitazones can cause fluid retention which leads to weight gain, ankle swelling and even heart failure in susceptible people. Some studies have suggested rosiglitazone may also modestly increase the risk of heart attack. It is generally recommended that people with type 2 diabetes known to have heart disease should use some other kind of medication to control their blood glucose.

Some studies have also suggested glitazones may increase the risk of vision-threatening eye disease and some cancers when compared to other therapies. Glitazones can also thin your bones, which increases fracture risk in susceptible people, especially older women possibly by as much as double. Taken together, the side effect profile of glitazones (as opposed to the comparative safety of other classes of medication for treating diabetes) has seen a steady decline in their use in people with diabetes. However, for some people with type 2 diabetes the benefits of glitazones on their glucose control may outweigh the potential for harm.

MEGLITINIDES

Meglitinides (known as 'glitinides' or 'glinides') are quick-acting pills that are used to swiftly lower glucose levels after eating. They are taken with the first bite of each meal and rapidly stimulate the release of insulin from the pancreas, through some of the same pathways used by sulphonylureas with which they should not be combined. Glitinides work fast and only for a short time (less than 4 hours). This rapid increase and fall in insulin levels effectively reproduces what happens in healthy people who eat a meal, when insulin levels rapidly rise after each meal and fall as all the food is digested.

There are currently only two different 'glitinides' available, which have in common a chemical (generic) suffix '-glinide':

- repaglinide
- nateglinide.

When taken as directed, glitinides will reduce the HbA1c by 0.5 to 1 per cent in most people with type 2 diabetes. They are very effective in people who have a large rise in glucose levels after meals, but whose glucose control is fine at other times, including during the night.

However, their rapid action can also be a disadvantage as it can quickly cause a rapid drop in glucose levels and hypoglycaemia if not taken appropriately and coordinated with a meal (see Chapter 7). Because of the need to take these tablets three times a day and carefully coordinate them with your meals, glitinides are only sparingly used and generally reserved for selected and fastidious patients. Some people also experience gastrointestinal disturbances (e.g. nausea, abdominal pain, indigestion) with glitinides.

ACARBOSE

Acarbose is a natural product derived from cultured bacteria. Most of the glucose you get from your diet comes from the digestion of starch contained in carbohydrate-rich food. Acarbose temporarily blocks the enzymes that digest starch, meaning that instead of being broken down immediately and entering the body, it takes much longer for glucose to get into the body from each meal. This effect is much like converting a high GI meal into a low GI meal. This slower rate of absorption better matches the limited rate of insulin secretion typical in people with type 2 diabetes.

Since it only works briefly, acarbose is taken three times a day at the start of each meal. Although acarbose modestly lowers blood glucose levels after meals, it does not cause hypoglycaemia when taken on its own as it does not interfere with the body's ability to make glucose. However, if someone is having a hypo due to other anti-diabetic medications they are also taking, acarbose can prevent consumed starchy foods from raising glucose levels enough to treat the hypo. Consequently, if someone taking acarbose is having a hypo they must eat pre-digested sugars such as glucose tablets or fruit juice, rather than starchy foods, to reverse the fall in glucose levels.

But while preventing the digestion of carbohydrates, acarbose allows more starch to reach the lower parts of the intestine, where it is happily digested by bacteria. This releases gas, and sometimes lots of it. This will cause significant flatulence in most people and result in bloating, discomfort or diarrhoea in others. These side effects can usually be reduced by starting at a lower dose (25mg once a day) and gradually increasing over a month (to 100mg three times a day). Symptoms will generally settle after a month or two of regular use. However, some people will not be able to tolerate these effects at all. As a result, acarbose is not widely used in the management of type 2 diabetes outside of developing countries.

Some studies have suggested that acarbose reduces the risk of colon cancer, partly through nourishing your healthy gut bacteria. Acarbose may also have other useful effects on clotting, blood pressure and lipid levels. This has been suggested as one reason it appears to modestly reduce the risk of heart attack and stroke in those with diabetes, over and above its effect on lowering glucose levels.

INSULIN

Insulin is the most important regulator of blood glucose levels in the human body. If glucose levels are too high, then insulin is not doing its job. For nearly a century it has been recognized that injecting insulin can reduce glucose levels and maintain glucose control in people with type 2 diabetes.

All people with type 1 diabetes must take insulin due to irreversible damage to the insulin-producing cells of their pancreas.

In some people with type 2 diabetes, the different medications that assist in the release of insulin or its actions are not enough to maintain glucose control. If this happens your doctor may consider starting insulin.

This does not mean you have failed in any way. Type 2 diabetes is a progressive condition in which your ability to make and use insulin declines and ultimately becomes exhausted. The longer you have diabetes, the more likely it will be that insulin may be required.

Injecting insulin is the most effective way to lower your glucose levels. When taken as directed, insulin injections will reduce the HbA1c by 1 to 2 per cent in most people with type 2 diabetes. The insulin injection works in the same way as the insulin made naturally in your pancreas — it stimulates the removal of glucose from the bloodstream and its storage in the tissues of your body, as well as stopping the liver making more glucose.

Insulin is injected into the fat under the skin (known as a subcutaneous injection). The best place is usually the fatty areas on your abdomen or thighs. You might think injections are difficult, painful or embarrassing, but it is actually quite easy to become proficient. The needles used to inject the insulin are very small. Most people say the injections are less painful than pricking the finger to test blood glucose levels. Most insulin syringes are very discreet. Many are indistinguishable from large fountain pens with a cartridge of insulin inserted like an ink cartridge. These make insulin injections quite straightforward since drawing up the medicine into the syringe is unnecessary. You just need to dial up the dose you want to use, and inject.

There are many different insulin formulations that vary in how rapidly they deliver insulin and how long they continue to provide it. These will suit different people and situations. The most common varieties include:

- rapid-acting insulin which is injected immediately before meals, one to three times a day
- intermediate and long-acting insulin (also known as

basal insulin) which is injected once a day, usually at bedtime or breakfast

- a mix of short- and long-acting insulins (known as pre-mix insulin) which is usually injected twice a day.

It is common to start out insulin injections for someone with type 2 diabetes with a low dose (8–10 units) of intermediate or long-acting insulin at bedtime or once in the morning (for those who have high glucose levels during the day). This is then slowly adjusted in small increments (e.g. 2–4 units every 2–4 days) as required to get control of glucose levels. The final dose usually ends up being between 20 and 40 units a day but can vary considerably between different people. This period of adjustment is quite intensive and always requires frequent contact with your diabetes team. You will generally also need to keep taking some or all of your oral anti-diabetic medications, to help the injected insulin to work effectively.

Because insulin is able to lower your glucose levels, no matter what level they are, blood glucose levels can sometimes fall to very low levels in people using insulin injections and cause a hypo (see Chapter 7). Hypos may be more likely when you are starting out, when the right dose and timing are first being assessed. This is also why the slow supervised start to insulin detailed above is so important. The chance of having a hypo is also increased in people who don't take their medications regularly, and those whose diet or lifestyle are irregular (different levels of physical activity, different amounts and types of food, skipping meals, trying to catch up by taking insulin after a meal, etc.). But while hypos can sound scary, most can be prevented by good diabetes management.

Starting insulin is also often associated with increased

appetite and unwanted weight gain (often between 2–5 kg/4½–11 lb). This occurs because insulin's main job is to drive glucose out of the blood by making and storing fat. Some new specially modified forms of insulin seem to cause less weight gain while achieving the same or better glucose control.

COMPLEMENTARY THERAPIES

All of the medicines detailed in this chapter are backed by scientific evidence that demonstrates their effectiveness in people with diabetes. However, there are also many other products that are marketed for those with type 2 diabetes to improve your glucose control. You will see them every day in the pharmacy, in the supermarket or on the internet. It is appealing to think that they may help you to better manage your glucose levels. However, none of these should be considered 'alternative medicines' for the management of diabetes. In fact, there is evidence of significant health risks when such remedies replace standard-of-care treatment.

The most widely sold supplements for diabetes contain **trace elements**, including chromium, zinc, magnesium and/or vanadium. But while each of these minerals has been reported to have effects on glucose levels in some studies, this has not been borne out in other studies and larger trials. At best the effects are very modest, lowering the HbA1c by less than 0.3 per cent.

Plants and their extracts have been used in traditional (folk) medicine for the treatment of diabetes for thousands of years. In fact, the most widely used medicine for lowering glucose levels, metformin, was originally derived from a traditional diabetes remedy. While a number of different herbs have been shown to lower glucose levels in some people, their effects are small at best and quite variable. They will not work in the majority of patients (unlike known diabetes medications). The long-term effectiveness and the potential for serious side effects of many of these herbs remain to be clarified. At present there is no evidence to recommend their use in people with type 2 diabetes.

Some herbs reported to have glucose-lowering effects include:

- American ginseng (*Panax. quiquefolius*)
- aloe vera
- bitter melon or kerala (*Momordica charantia*)
- cinnamon (*Cinnamomum verum*)
- ivy gourd (*Coccinia indica*)
- fenugreek or methi (*Trigonella foenum-graecum*)
- garlic (*Allium sativum*)
- holy basil (*Ocimum sanctum*)
- gurmar or gymnema (*Gymnema sylvestre*)
- nopal or prickly pear cactus (*Opuntia streptacantha*)
- huang lian (*Rhizoma coptidis*)
- Russian tarragon (*Artemisia dracunculus*)
- vijaysar or petrocarpus (*Petrocarpus marsupium*)
- guduchi or amrit (*Tinospora cordifolia*)
- zarchik (*Berberis arista* root)
- skeels (*Syzygium cumini*).

7

SWINGING LOW

Understand

- The brain requires a constant supply of glucose to function. If glucose levels fall below 3mmol/L (54mg/dL), then the brain's functions can become impaired.
- Most people with type 2 diabetes have little or no risk of having a hypo.
- Some of the medicines that lower glucose levels in people with type 2 diabetes have the potential to cause hypoglycaemia under certain circumstances. The most common reason for a hypo is that there is too much insulin for your prevailing glucose level.

- In the minority of people with type 2 diabetes who experience a hypo, changes to their lifestyle and medications can significantly reduce the risk of further episodes.

Manage
- Talk to your doctor about your risks for having a hypo, based on the type of medication you are using and the targets for your treatment.
- If you are at risk, develop and execute an action plan of what you would do in the event of a hypo. Always be prepared.
- If you suspect a hypo, get on and treat it, since the risks of failing to treat a hypo outweigh those of unnecessary treatment.
- Take special precautions to make sure you don't 'swing low' when driving.
- Limit the amount of alcohol you drink and always combine alcohol with food.

Your brain needs a continuous supply of glucose to function. And not just a little. Over half of all glucose made by the body is subsequently used by the brain. For the brain, glucose in the blood is just as important as the oxygen in the air you breathe. The brain cannot last more than a few minutes without it. The brain can't make its own glucose. Instead, it requires a continuous supply of glucose in the bloodstream to keep it going.

It's easy to keep your glucose levels up while you are eating. But you can't eat all the time. And when you're not eating, the body must still maintain roughly the same glucose levels as always. To achieve this, a healthy pancreas directs a coordinated response to keep your glucose levels steady. This response includes:

- stimulating the synthesis and release of new glucose from the liver
- releasing fat from its stores, which is then used as an alternative fuel source by most organs (except the brain) — this effectively spares glucose for exclusive use by your brain
- suppressing the release of insulin, whose job it is to lower glucose levels and put fat back into storage — this is precisely the opposite of what is needed when glucose levels are already falling or low.

Because of these safety mechanisms, dangerously low glucose levels cannot occur in healthy people, even in those who undertake prolonged fasting or go on fad diets that are very low in energy. Your metabolism is programmed to look after your brain and its best interests.

Most people with type 2 diabetes have too little insulin and their body makes too much glucose (see Chapter 1). This is why their glucose levels are generally too high. Consequently, in people with type 2 diabetes who are not on any glucose-lowering medications there is little or no risk that glucose levels will fall too low (known as hypoglycaemia).

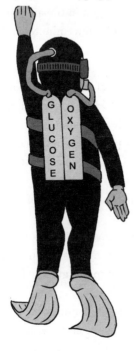

For the brain, glucose is just as important as the oxygen in the air you breathe. The brain cannot last for more than a few minutes without either.

Diabetes does not cause hypoglycaemia. Hypoglycaemia can only occur if one or all of these protective mechanisms fails to kick in when glucose levels are falling. The most likely trigger is that there is inadvertently too much insulin present when glucose levels are already low. This can sometimes occur in people with type 2 diabetes if they are also taking medications that increase their insulin levels (sulphonylureas and meglitinides) or are injecting insulin itself. The other medications used to treat diabetes do not increase insulin levels when glucose is low, so can't cause hypoglycaemia on their own.

Hypoglycaemia can also occur in people with type 2 diabetes if glucose production by the liver is suppressed when it should be turned on full to keep your glucose levels up when they are falling. For example, alcohol suppresses the production of glucose by the liver. So if levels are already swinging low with your medication, they are likely to swing lower and swing faster if you have also been drinking.

WHAT HAPPENS WHEN GLUCOSE LEVELS FALL TOO LOW?

To protect against low glucose levels, the human body triggers a number of 'early warning' symptoms including:

- hunger
- looking pale
- sweating
- palpitations (pounding heartbeat)
- increased pulse rate
- tingling sensation (known as parathesia), often around the lips
- shaking/trembling
- headache
- nausea.

These symptoms are collectively experienced as what is commonly termed a **hypo**. The severity of these symptoms partly depends on how low the glucose levels go and how rapidly they fall. Generally, the body's warning symptoms first kick in as glucose falls below 3.5 mmol/L (63 g/dL). However, some people can experience no warning signs until glucose levels fall to much lower levels. For example, older people with type 2 diabetes generally experience warning signals for a hypo at lower glucose levels than in younger people.

At least initially, these warning symptoms of hypoglycaemia may be mild and readily ignored, especially if your mind is focused on other matters. Many of these symptoms might also occur for reasons other than hypoglycaemia in people with type 2 diabetes. For example, low blood pressure has very similar effects on the body and the brain when compared to those caused by low glucose levels. However, if it is a hypo, all these symptoms will be rapidly improved by taking sweet food or drinks, making it usually possible to quickly distinguish low glucose levels from other causes of illness.

Not all people will experience the same warning signs with a hypo, which are often unique to any given person. For the minority of people with type 2 diabetes who experience hypos as a result of their treatment, it is important for them to become familiar with their own signals that tell them their glucose levels are low and the scenarios in which they occur, and use them to recognize that it is time to do something about them (see 'How do you treat hypoglycaemia?' later in this chapter).

If these early warning symptoms pass unheeded and glucose levels drop further, the brain becomes starved of the glucose (energy) it needs, and all of its functions begin to slow down. This can lead to:

- faintness
- drowsiness
- loss of attention/concentration/performance
- delayed reflexes
- confusion/impaired judgement
- anxiety/moodiness/shakiness

- blurred vision
- disturbed sleep/nightmares
- slurred speech
- unsteadiness.

Rarely is a hypo so incapacitating to the brain that you need the assistance of others to get right again. It is very unusual to completely lose consciousness. But it is hard to do the simple things you need to do to fix low glucose levels if your brain is starved of the glucose it needs to work properly. And this means you may need help. For the minority of people who suffer lots of hypos, carrying or wearing some form of identification that clearly states you have diabetes and you are on medication that can cause hypos may be appropriate.

These symptoms of brain 'slow down' are not generally seen unless glucose levels fall below 3 mmol/L (54 mg/dL). But some people with diabetes may experience this slow down at higher glucose levels, especially if glucose levels have been falling rapidly. This is why it is better to treat a suspected hypo than to wait and see what the glucose level is.

However, one of the biggest problems about hypos is the lengths some people feel they need to go to in order to avoid them. Hypos are scary. Anyone who has experienced one knows how upsetting they are, and how important it is that you do everything in your power to prevent them from occurring again. Consequently, the fear of hypoglycaemia is one of the most important barriers to good glucose control and is a key reason why current treatments cannot achieve the level of glucose control seen in people without diabetes. For example, hypos can be a major reason to compromise your glucose control and accept values where the risk of hypoglycaemia might be lower.

Sometimes the fear of hypoglycaemia can also restrict the

things you feel you can do, including exercise or social activities. But it does not have to be this way. As discussed in the previous chapter there are now many new medications for managing diabetes that don't increase the risk of hypoglycaemia. So rather than compromise, it is possible to tailor the right medications for the right patients.

WHAT TRIGGERS A HYPO?

As detailed above, hypos can occur in people with type 2 diabetes if they are also taking medications that increase their insulin levels (e.g. sulphonylureas) or are injecting insulin itself. However, even with these medications the risk of hypos is low, and the majority of people with type 2 diabetes have glucose levels that remain too high and even taking these medicines does not lead to hypos.

That said, hypos may sometimes occur, especially in the following circumstances:

- If you inadvertently take too much (dose) of these medications.
- If you inadvertently take these medications at the wrong time or wrong time interval.
- If you accumulate too much of these medicines in your system (as may occur in people with kidney disease).
- If the medicines you take are acting quicker than you expect, such as if you accidentally inject insulin into muscle (instead of fat) which can also sometimes lead to faster absorption of insulin and drop glucose levels faster than planned.
- Whenever your doctor adds new diabetes

medications to your management, a period of extra vigilance is warranted as their effects cannot always be anticipated. Sometimes they work too well, and some reduction in therapy may be required to reduce the risk of having a hypo.

- As your health improves with good diabetes management, it is common for your medications to get better at lowering your glucose levels. In fact, it is quite common to become more 'sensitive' to the actions of insulin. This is one of the key benefits of good diabetes control. However, when insulin works better, some people find that the high doses of the medications they needed before may become too high, and some dose reduction is required in order to prevent hypoglycaemia.

- Changing lifestyle. Even when taking the right medications, at the right time and in the right doses, it is also possible to drop glucose levels too much by failing to coordinate diabetes management with your lifestyle. Some common precipitants of a hypo involve irregular or changing lifestyle circumstances, such as missing or delaying a meal or meals, or radically changing your diet (e.g. eating meals that contain less carbohydrate than usual, or fasting — see below).

- The stress of being unwell, for whatever reason, changes the amount of insulin your body needs. It also often changes the amount and type of food you eat. Under these circumstances it is common for glucose control to get out of hand, with more highs but also sometimes a greater risk for hypos. If you become unwell it is important to alert your diabetes team early, so that your medications can be adjusted accordingly.

• As mentioned earlier in this chapter, drinking too much alcohol or drinking alcohol on an empty stomach can suppress the production of glucose by the liver. This is an essential buffer for low glucose levels, so alcohol increases the risk and severity of hypoglycaemia. If you are intoxicated it may also be hard for you (or anyone else) to recognize you are low and start treatment in a timely fashion. Having diabetes does not mean you have to give up drinking. However, moderation is important in people with diabetes, especially those who experience hypos. It is also often recommended in this setting to eat some carbohydrate-rich food if you are drinking as a safeguard against falling glucose levels later on.

Apart from careful adjustment of medication, it is often thought that the problem of hypoglycaemia can simply be avoided by eating more often, and in particular by regular snacking between meals. However, this is usually unnecessary and is an important source of unwanted calories and weight gain. Many so-called 'snacks' provide as many calories as a normal meal. Certainly, in those people prone to hypos, having healthy snacks available can be useful in the event of unforeseen activity or changes in the timing or amount of meals. But overeating to prevent hypoglycaemia is never a solution.

Another way some people try to avoid having hypos is to limit their physical activity. Certainly, excessive physical activity (commonly more prolonged or more vigorous than what you are used to) may sometimes also trigger a hypo in those who can't buffer falling glucose levels because of their treatment.

Blood glucose is normally used up by any physical activity, and at a greater rate during vigorous exercise. This is why it is so effective in controlling glucose levels in type 2 diabetes. But it is also why it can sometimes lead to hypos in some circumstances.

Exercise not only uses up glucose, it can also slow the emptying of food from the stomach so that sugars from food may be delivered more slowly than expected. Exercise also slows down the body's ability to make and release glucose, so low glucose levels may still occur many hours after physical activity.

The solution is not to avoid exercise. The majority of people with type 2 diabetes have glucose levels that are high enough to buffer the effects of exercise and never get close to significant lows. For the minority who do experience hypos with exercise, they can be prevented by better coordinating physical activity and medication.

For example, don't exercise straight after taking your medication. Another solution may be to eat a carbohydrate-rich snack if blood glucose levels are less than 5.5 mmol/L (100 mg/dL) before starting your exercise.

DIABETES AND FASTING

Many people wish to undertake periods of fasting as part of their religious observance, such as during Navratri or Ramzan. Fasting may be required for brief periods or longer durations. Many people observe fasts on certain days every week. Fasting is not only important for their spiritual wellbeing, but it also an important part of their identity, culture and relationship with friends, family and community.

Intermittent fasting has a number of benefits for health, including self-discipline, sympathy, purification and breaking bad habits, such as smoking. It can also contribute to waist loss and improve control of lipid and blood pressure levels. However, having type 2 diabetes can sometimes make fasting complicated. This is mostly because some medications used for the management of type 2 diabetes are predicated on eating food and the insulin required to deal with the sugar load. So if you are not eating, your insulin requirements will be reduced, so insulin injections or medications that increase insulin levels (e.g. sulphonylureas) may need to be carefully adjusted in consultation with your physician and diabetes care team.

It is never a good idea to simply stop medicines when fasting. Many medications used to treat type 2 diabetes have no risk of hypoglycaemia, so need little or no adjustment during a fast. Sometimes your physician can pre-emptively switch you to such agents if you wish to undertake regular or prolonged fasting. However, during Ramadan, any medications will need to be long acting to be taken before dawn and/or after dusk.

Most people with well controlled type 2 diabetes should be able to fast, and with good planning and coordination it is usually not necessary to need an exemption. Some simple actions to reduce your risks of problems during a fast include:

- Getting good control of your glucose levels well before you start a prolonged fast.
- Getting a comprehensive check-up a few months before the onset of Ramadan or other prolonged fasts to establish your health and give time to fix any problems before commencing the observance.
- Refreshing yourself and your family about the awareness of symptoms and signs of a hypo,

including when you must break the fast (e.g. glucose levels less than 3.5mmol/L or hypo symptoms), and what to do in an emergency (see below) and why it is legitimate to do so.

- If you have had hypos before, it is important to carry with you at all times information that you have diabetes, with an emergency contact number and some glucose just in case, to be able to take care of hypos.

- Some doctors recommend that you should monitor blood glucose levels more regularly than usual if you have had problems with hypos before, although it remains controversial if self-monitoring prevents hypos or improves individual tailoring of treatment. If your sugar levels are less than 4.0mmol/L on the morning of a fast you should seriously consider breaking the fast for the day.

- During Ramadan, when meals can be taken at pre-dawn (Suhur) and sunset (Iftar), high fibre, low GI foods have an advantage for prolonged glucose control (discussed in Chapter 3). High GI foods such as dates (which are traditionally used to break the fast) can cause both sharp rises in blood sugar and equally sharp falls subsequently.

- Some people with diabetes will require an exception from fasting, such as those with unstable control, complications or frailty. They may not feel comfortable in asking for it, but it is entirely appropriate with their faith and does not represent a moral failing on their part.

DIABETES AND DRIVING

There are some other circumstances where special preventive management for hypoglycaemia is also appropriate. One of the most important is when planning to drive a car, particularly on long journeys.

Most people with type 2 diabetes are healthy and are able to drive without restrictions. Some countries have specific restrictions on your fitness to drive that prevent you driving a car if you have a high risk of hypoglycaemia. Other countries allow you to drive only after a medical certificate has been received and this may need to be updated every few years depending on the medication you are using and the presence of other complications, including eye problems and heart disease.

If you have experienced a hypo, you'll know it's not something you'd want to happen while you are driving. So for those people with type 2 diabetes who are at risk for hypos there are some simple precautions you can take before and while driving to minimize your risks and keep you and others safe:

- Have a meal before setting out on a long journey.
- Check your glucose levels before driving and every 2 hours while driving.
- Never get behind the wheel if you have low blood glucose levels or are experiencing symptoms, even if it is not far to home.
- Be proactive about treating falling levels — don't wait until you feel symptoms.
- Although snacking all the time can be a problem, having a supply of snacks which you can safely and easily reach while driving is a good precaution for a long journey.
- Never drink and drive, as alcohol makes hypos more likely and more severe.

HOW DO YOU TREAT HYPOGLYCAEMIA?

You should always intervene if you experience symptoms suggestive of a hypo. Measuring your blood glucose level first can be informative. It will usually be less than 3.5mmol/L (63mg/dL). But if you suspect a hypo it is better to treat it immediately, since the risks of not treating a hypo outweigh the risks associated with unnecessary treatment.

If you are having a hypo, immediately take any one of the suggestions below:

- **20g of glucose (tablets, powder or five to seven jelly beans, depending on their size)**
- **1 tablespoon of jam/honey or table sugar**
- **half a glass of fruit juice or a regular soft drink (not 'diet' drinks).**

If symptoms persist, repeat the dose in 10 minutes.

When your symptoms have resolved, give the glucose another 10 minutes to be fully absorbed, then eat a carbohydrate-rich snack (e.g. a piece of fruit, glass of milk, a tub of yoghurt, six small dry biscuits or a sandwich), or if your next main meal is nearly due then just start early.

This should then be followed up with your diabetes care team so that changes can be made where necessary to your medication, diet or physical activity. In most cases repeat episodes can be prevented without having to rely on treatment to save the day all the time.

8

UNDER PRESSURE

Understand
- The level of blood pressure that represents hypertension has been broadly defined as a systolic blood pressure of 140mmHg or higher or a diastolic blood pressure 90mmHg or higher.
- Hypertension is at least twice as common in people who have type 2 diabetes as in those who do not have diabetes.
- High blood pressure is an important cause of complications in people with type 2 diabetes. For every 1mmHg

increase in the systolic blood pressure, the long-term risk of heart attack or stroke will increase by 2 to 3 per cent.

- Most people with type 2 diabetes need medications (known as anti-hypertensives) to control their blood pressure levels and reduce their risk of complications.

- Diet and lifestyle changes can not only lower blood pressure levels but also reduce the need for medication(s) and improve their effectiveness.

Manage

- Get your blood pressure checked every time you see your doctor, even if you don't have high blood pressure or are not receiving medication.

- Obtain an accurate assessment of what your blood pressure is really doing over the course of your day with ambulatory monitoring, and use it to target and achieve comprehensive blood pressure control.

- Lose that waist. For every 1 kg (2¼lb) of weight you lose, your systolic blood pressure will go down on average by approximately 1 mmHg.
- Recognize the stress you may be under, and get some assistance in managing it. Find time to relax and make constructive lifestyle changes that help prevent stress.
- Take your medication. A common reason for high blood pressure is non-compliance. Drugs don't work unless you take them.

High blood pressure (hypertension) is an important cause of complications in people with type 2 diabetes. Heart disease, stroke, poor circulation to the legs, eye and kidney damage are more common in people with high blood pressure than in people whose blood pressure is under control. This is partly because high blood pressure causes wear and tear on the walls of the major blood vessels that supply these parts of the body. Its mechanical effects can be likened to the effects of traffic on a road — the greater the pounding of the traffic, the more heavy trucks that roar along its surface, the more likely it is that potholes will occur and that accidents will happen. This is the same for blood pressure, except the accidents are called heart attacks and strokes.

High blood pressure has similar effects on the heart. Literally, the heart is put under pressure. This means it has to work harder to move all the blood around the body, just as it gets harder to put air into a balloon as the pressure inside it increases. In the short term, this extra work causes the heart to grow larger in an attempt to cope with this extra load. However, these extra demands come at some cost. Bigger hearts are also more vulnerable to the effects of poor circulation, such as occurs in type 2 diabetes.

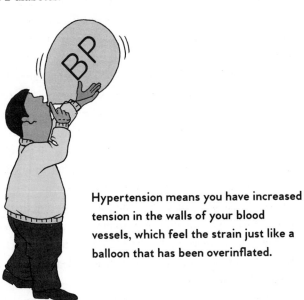

Hypertension means you have increased tension in the walls of your blood vessels, which feel the strain just like a balloon that has been overinflated.

Yet high blood pressure can be prevented and/or treated. Lowering blood pressure will lower the stress on the surface of your heart and blood vessels, just like preventing the passage of heavy trucks will protect a road. In fact, sustained control of blood pressure is one of the most important ways to protect your heart, brain and other organs.

WHAT IS BLOOD PRESSURE?

In order to move all your blood around your body once every 4 minutes, your blood must flow fast and never stop. The force of the flowing blood is known as the **blood pressure**. This pressure is not insubstantial (as anyone who has cut themselves accidentally or seen too many horror movies will easily appreciate). However, the pressure of blood is kept in check by the **tension** in the elastic walls of your blood vessels. A similar tension can actually be seen in the walls of a balloon that has been fully inflated, where its 'elastic recoil' resists the expanding pressure of the air so that the balloon stays roughly the same size.

The highest pressure in any blood vessel is generated by the force of contraction of your heartbeat (known as **systole**). This pressure peak is known as the **systolic blood pressure** and is what you feel as your pulse. Systolic blood pressure can be simply measured by using a pressurised cuff to block off the circulation in the arm. When the cuff pressure is higher than the systolic blood pressure, no blood will flow into your arm, which is why it tingles. But as the pressure in the cuff is lowered, there comes a point at which the blood begins to flow again, when the pressure in the cuff is overcome by the force of your heartbeat. This is the systolic blood pressure and is usually between 120 and 140 mmHg in most adults.

The lowest pressure in a blood vessel is known as the **diastolic blood pressure**, as it corresponds to the point (known as **diastole**) at which the heart is relaxed and busy filling in order to get ready for its next contraction. Diastolic pressure is usually around 70 to 80mmHg when measured using a blood pressure cuff.

When recording the blood pressure, it is common to report

the systolic over the diastolic blood pressure, so that '130 over 80' means a systolic blood pressure of 130mmHg and a diastolic pressure of 80mmHg. The difference between systolic and diastolic pressures is called the pulse pressure, as this is a measure of how forceful your pulse seems to be when it is felt at your wrist.

Blood pressure levels are generally higher in men than in women. However, following the menopause this difference is reversed as blood pressure levels rise more rapidly when the protective effects of sex hormones on the blood vessels decline.

The pressure inside your blood vessels is determined by a number of different factors including:

- The volume of blood. Just like air in a balloon, the more air the more pressure. In the same way if there is more fluid retained in the body, for the same space, the pressure in your arteries can increase. Similarly, when people lose large amounts of blood, such as after surgery or following an accident, their blood pressure is also often low.

- The strength of each heartbeat. During each contraction of the heart, a small volume of blood is squeezed out. The stronger the heart squeezes, the higher the pressure it is able to generate. Equally, if the heart is not pumping well, the blood pressure can be low, such as in some people with heart failure (see Chapter 10).

- The elastic recoil of the blood vessels. Blood vessels have strong elastic walls. These distend in response to the increase in pressure associated with each pulse of pressure generated by your heart. You can sometimes actually see this bulging as the pulse passes through blood vessels in your neck or arms. This stretching is very important as it provides the energy that will help maintain blood pressure after the pulse has passed. This is because after being stretched out by the pulse, the elastic rebound/recoil of the arteries then creates an inward pressure. This pressure serves to maintain the continuous flow of blood until the next contraction of the heart. One of the best known changes in the blood vessels of people with type 2 diabetes is known as **hardening of the arteries**. This literally means that blood vessels are less compliant or less able to distend. So when each pulse comes along in a hard artery, the systolic pressure will be higher, as instead of distending like a balloon the increased volume with each pulse has nowhere to go. However, diastolic pressure does not tend to rise in hardened arteries, as less distension also means less recoil. This means that hardening of the arteries usually causes an isolated elevation in systolic blood pressure, which is the most common change in the blood pressure of adults with type 2 diabetes.

- The resistance to flow. Pushing fluid down a large pipe is much easier than pushing the same amount of fluid down a series of small tubes. What makes it hard is known as resistance. The higher the resistance to flow, the higher the pressure needed to overcome it. Resistance in your blood vessels is determined in part by the changing diameter of small blood vessels in your circulation (known as resistance vessels). If these vessels constrict, the blood pressure goes up as there is more resistance to the flow of blood. To keep flow constant it takes more pressure to overcome more resistance. By contrast, when resistance vessels dilate, the pressure needed to make the blood flow is reduced. Many medications that lower blood pressure chiefly work by dilating resistance vessels (known as vasodilators).

Because high blood pressure is damaging to blood vessels, and low blood pressure is not good either (as it means less blood supply and the oxygen and nutrients it contains), the human body contains a number of mechanisms that keep the blood pressure levels within relatively narrow confines. These sense when the blood pressure is falling, and activate pathways to increase the output from the heart, retain fluid and constrict blood vessels supplying non-essential organs to prop up the blood pressure. Equally, if blood pressure rises, the pathways to dilate blood vessels, remove fluid and restrict the heart's functions become active.

Even so, blood pressure doesn't stay absolutely the same all the time but varies slightly depending on a number of factors:

- Position. Blood pressure is usually a little lower when standing up than when sitting or lying down. This is because blood pools in the legs when standing, so less blood gets back to the heart and the pump pressure falls. However, this drop is usually very small because it immediately triggers a reflex response to cause the constriction of resistance blood vessels, and an increase in the heart rate. In some people with type 2 diabetes, their systolic blood pressure can drop very significantly when they stand (more than 20mmHg). This is known as **postural** or **orthostatic hypotension** and in some cases is experienced as dizzy spells or fainting. This drop in blood pressure on standing may be because some medications and/or diabetes itself can interfere with the reflexes required to keep the blood pressure up. Dizziness on standing may also be experienced by people who are dehydrated, anaemic or hot, because such reflexes are already fully active and can't increase further.

- Sleep. Systolic blood pressure is generally 10 to 20 per cent lower during sleep when compared to daytime levels. This is known as **nocturnal dipping**. People who don't experience a nightly fall in blood pressure of at least 10 per cent (known as **non-dippers**) have higher rates of complications from their diabetes. Whether this is because blood pressure is not falling at night or because non-dippers have other problems with their blood pressure control is unclear. Nonetheless, some doctors advocate their patients take their blood pressure medication in the evening so that its greatest effect may be at night and first thing in the morning.

- Stress. In the short term, blood pressure levels are sometimes higher if you're excited, stressed or nervous. This is because blood pressure is controlled by the **sympathetic nervous system** (also known as the **fight or flight response**). When you are nervous or stressed, activation of the sympathetic nervous system makes your heart race and beat more strongly, while the resistance vessels constrict. This can sometimes lead to a surge in blood pressure. For example, the blood pressure when seeing your doctor is usually 5 to 10mmHg higher than it is when you are at home. This can sometimes make it appear to your doctor that you have increased blood pressure, even if you don't usually have it at other times (known as white-coat hypertension). However, there is good evidence that any surges in blood pressure may be very important for your health and wellbeing.

- Mornings. First thing in the morning, there is normally a surge in blood pressure of between 20 and 30mmHg associated with waking up, rising and becoming physically active after a night's sleep. This increase may be exaggerated in some people and may be one reason the risk of heart attacks and strokes is greatest in the two hours after getting up in the morning.

- Exercise. Although regular exercise can lower blood pressure levels over weeks or months of application, any sudden or excessive physical activity can cause a rapid rise in blood pressure in some people. This is why your doctor will usually take your blood pressure after at least 5 minutes of rest. This is also why, before starting an exercise program, a careful assessment of risk should be performed (see Chapter 5). Sometimes doctors counsel some people with diabetes to limit activity because of these concerns, especially those with poorly controlled blood pressure.

- Food. Different food or drink in your diet can impact the development and progression of high blood pressure over the long term. This is discussed in detail below. However, sometimes a meal can also affect blood pressure levels. This is because, when you eat, extra blood is diverted to your intestines to help absorb its nutrients. This can result in a small but significant drop in blood pressure after meals in some people with diabetes.

HOW IS BLOOD PRESSURE MEASURED?

People with type 2 diabetes should have their blood pressure checked every time they see their doctor, even if they don't have high blood pressure or are not receiving blood pressure medication.

Blood pressure measurements are usually taken when sitting, but measurements taken while standing are also worthwhile to check for the development of postural hypotension. This should be done at least annually or more often if you are experiencing symptoms such as dizziness when standing abruptly, or if you have other signs to suggest diabetes has damaged your nerves (numbness, feet problems, etc.). Blood pressure will sometimes also be measured in both arms to look for differences between the arms that could indicate narrowing of the arteries.

Measuring your blood pressure is usually performed by wrapping an inflatable cuff with a pressure gauge around your arm or wrist. This should fit snugly. If a cuff is too small, it will underestimate your blood pressure. Equally, if the cuff is too large it will produce a higher blood pressure reading than your true blood pressure. Different cuff sizes are available to accommodate for larger or smaller arms and ensure accurate readings.

The pressure in the cuff is then slowly increased until blood flow in the arm is temporarily prevented. In most people this is completely painless. However, some people experience unpleasant numbness or tingling when the cuff is maximally inflated. But it is only for a moment and subsides when the cuff is deflated. It will not cause damage to the arm. Air is then slowly released from the cuff. The point at which blood flow returns to the arm (the systolic blood pressure) can be gauged either by feeling or listening for the pulse. Normally, smooth flow through blood vessels makes no sound. But when the blood first returns to the arm after the cuff is slowly released, with each turbulent spurt of blood that comes down the artery a tapping noise can be heard with a stethoscope, in time with the pulse. When the pressure in the cuff falls below the diastolic pressure, the continuous flow to the arm is fully restored and the sounds of intermittent turbulent flow in blood vessels can no longer be heard; so diastolic pressure is gauged by the sound of silence. For this reason it is harder to measure accurately, especially in noisy environments such as medical practices or shopping malls.

Automated machines that inflate and deflate by themselves are also widely used. In these machines, a sensor (known as an **oscillometer**) is used to detect the return of blood flow to the arm. This can make it easier to detect changes in blood flow without needing to hear it. When standardised and used regularly, such machines are very valuable and are widely used in hospitals and medical clinics. Home oscillometers are also available. Results can vary significantly from machine to machine, but they are generally pretty reliable once standardised and calibrated. So if you have one, take it with you for your next check-up and compare its reading with that taken by your nurse or doctor to make sure they are close to one another. Using the same machine all the time is the best way to ensure that any changes measured in your blood pressure are real.

Ambulatory blood pressure monitoring is emerging as the best way to establish a diagnosis of high blood pressure and to determine the response to treatment in people with type 2 diabetes. Although the word 'ambulatory' makes you think that it means monitoring while you are walking (ambling), in fact this kind of monitoring means taking an automated blood pressure reading every 20 to 30 minutes while you are awake and every 30 to 60 minutes while you are sleeping. This gives a much more accurate picture of what blood pressure levels are over the course of a single day. It can detect any surges in blood pressure or any dipping at night or other times. Your blood pressure readings can also be matched with a diary noting what you were doing at the time, or how you felt. The average value of measurements taken during waking hours is often used to confirm a diagnosis of high blood pressure.

Although it might seem cumbersome to carry around a blood pressure device for a day and a night, the machines are surprisingly small and quiet. But the cuff still has to blow up; the most common complaint is that this disturbs your sleep, or that of your bed partner. But it is only for one night.

Home blood pressure monitoring is another way to confirm a diagnosis of high blood pressure. Home monitoring simply means taking your blood pressure twice a day for a week. The average value of all the measurements (ignoring the first day, which is usually higher as you are getting used to the plan) can be used to confirm a diagnosis of high blood pressure. The home monitoring method takes some application, but many people find it better as it does not mean blood pressure measurements through the night. However, this is also its downside, as it does not give information about what is happening at night. Nonetheless, it is still better than basing treatment decisions on just the blood pressure measurements taken when you go to the doctor.

HOW HIGH IS HIGH — WHAT IS HYPERTENSION?

All pressure applied to blood vessels causes some tension in their walls. This tension progressively leads to changes, or damage, in the way they function. The greater the blood pressure, the greater that damage. The point at which the risk of blood vessel damage is significantly increased is known as **hypertension**. This literally means you have increased tension in the walls of your blood vessels that feel the strain, just like the wall of a balloon that has been overinflated.

The level of blood pressure that represents hypertension is broadly defined as:

- **a systolic blood pressure of 140mmHg and/or higher or**
- **a diastolic blood pressure of 90mmHg or higher when measured on more than two occasions by a health professional using standard blood pressure-monitoring devices.**

These arbitrary thresholds used to define hypertension do not mean that if your systolic pressure is 139mmHg when you see your doctor, your blood vessels are not under stress. In fact, there is a continuous relationship between the level of tension in your arteries and the likelihood of heart attack, stroke and kidney disease. Any reduction in blood pressure will lower the risk of complications, even if you don't have high blood pressure levels.

Because blood pressures are generally higher when you go to see your doctor, lower blood pressure thresholds are used to define hypertension using at-home monitoring or using ambulatory monitoring:

- a systolic blood pressure of 135mmHg or higher and/or
- a diastolic blood pressure of 85mmHg or higher.

Using these criteria, three out of four adults with type 2 diabetes will have hypertension or need medication to prevent it.

Why is hypertension so common in people with type 2 diabetes?

Regardless of how it is defined, hypertension is at least twice as common in people who have diabetes as in those who do not. Diabetes has direct effects on blood vessels to increase the tension within their walls, including:

- increased volume of blood
- increased activity of the pathways that cause constriction of arteries
- increased responsiveness to these 'constrictor' signals
- reduced responsiveness to signals that cause dilation of arteries.

A number of other factors also contribute to high rates of hypertension in people with diabetes, including:

- Ageing. As you get older, systolic blood pressure levels gradually rise by about 1mmHg every two to three years of your adult life. By the time you retire, on average the systolic blood pressure is at least 20mmHg higher than when you were in your twenties. This is thought to be caused by progressive hardening of the arteries as the systolic blood pressure is more affected than diastolic pressure. This process is enhanced in people with diabetes and pre-diabetes. In effect this means that people with diabetes have arteries that are older than their numerical age.

- Ethnicity. Many of the populations at greatest risk of type 2 diabetes also have increased rates of high blood pressure. For example, people of African, Hispanic, Polynesian and other indigenous origins are at least twice as likely to develop hypertension if they also get diabetes.

- Genes. Blood pressure levels are influenced by your genetic make-up. High blood pressure tends to run in some families. The same families may also be prone to develop diabetes. Indeed, a family history of high blood pressure, especially at an early age, is a risk factor for type 2 diabetes and vice versa.

- Obesity. As discussed in Chapter 4, an enlarging waistline has a number of effects to raise the blood pressure and make it difficult to bring down. The dramatic effect of bariatric surgery on blood pressure levels stands as a testament to how important sustained weight loss is for the control of blood pressure in people with type 2 diabetes.

- Kidney disease. The kidneys are key regulators of blood pressure in the body because they control the amount of fluid in the system. If kidney function is impaired, as is often the case in people with type 2 diabetes (see Chapter 13) more fluid is retained and, just like too much air inside a balloon, the tension on the walls is also increased.

REDUCING YOUR BLOOD PRESSURE — DIET AND LIFESTYLE

There are many simple things that you can do to prevent the development of high blood pressure. These are equally applicable to the many people who already have high blood pressure, in whom diet and lifestyle changes can not only lower blood pressure levels but also reduce the need for medication(s) and improve their effectiveness. Many of these interventions are also beneficial to people with type 2 diabetes beyond their actions on blood pressure control, and are discussed in greater detail elsewhere in this book. Among the most important are:

- Weight control (see Chapter 4). Losing a few kilos can make a real difference for many aspects of your health, including your blood pressure. For every 1kg (2¼lb) of weight you lose, your systolic blood pressure will go down on average by approximately 1 to 2mmHg (e.g. losing 10kg/22lb in weight will usually lower your blood pressure by 10–20mmHg, which is as much as would be achieved by taking blood pressure-lowering medications). Some of this benefit to blood pressure may disappear with time, however, especially if the weight goes back on.

- Regular physical activity. If your blood pressure is normal, regular physical exercise can reduce the chance that it will rise as you age. In those with high blood pressure, getting regular exercise can lower your blood pressure and improve your response to blood pressure-lowering medications. There are many different forms of exercise that will work on blood pressure. The most effective programs include an element of aerobic exercise such as brisk walking, climbing stairs, jogging, bicycling and swimming. Where appropriate, it is recommended that everyone with diabetes tries to get at least 30 minutes of aerobic exercise on all or most days of the week. Like the effect of weight loss, the blood pressure benefit is not sustained if you don't keep it up.

- Smoking cessation. Smoking is a catastrophe for people with type 2 diabetes. If the risk of heart disease, stroke and other complications was not already increased, smoking significantly kicks it along. One of the many reasons for this is that smoking raises blood pressure levels. The nicotine contained in tobacco acts to constrict blood vessels. During each cigarette, blood pressure levels rise between 20 and 30mmHg. Even though they may fall again when you are not smoking, these surges in blood pressure are extremely damaging to blood vessels and the heart.

- A diet rich in fruit and vegetables can also help control blood pressure. Use them to replace high fat or high calorie foods that are associated with higher blood pressure levels.

- A diet rich in oily fish and omega-3 oils can reduce your blood pressure. Including oily fish in your weight-loss diet can also help reduce blood pressure more effectively than weight loss or fish intake alone. Fish oil supplements can also reduce blood pressure but they need to be regularly taken in very large amounts (e.g. greater than 5g a day) to have a substantial effect. These doses are not easy to stomach because of the fishy aftertaste, and it can be hard to sustain taking this large a number of pills over a long period of time.

- A diet rich in fibre. Current recommendations say you should aim for at least 30g of total fibre each day. On average most people with diabetes consume less than half this amount, mostly as breakfast cereal and bread. Just by replacing refined products with wholegrain equivalents you can more than double your intake of total and soluble fibre. For those who find dietary change difficult, there are now a number of simple and highly palatable fibre supplements. Regular use of fibre supplements has been shown to have a number of useful effects in people with diabetes, including lowering blood pressure levels (see Chapter 3).

- Stopping alcohol excesses. Excessive alcohol intake (more than five standard drinks per day) is linked to the development of high blood pressure. For this and many other reasons, it is really worth moderating your alcohol intake.

- Not too much caffeine. Caffeine is the most widely consumed stimulant in the world. Caffeine is found in coffee, tea and many 'energy' drinks, and acts by blocking receptors in the brain whose job it is to dull your brain's activity. So by preventing dulling, it stimulates the brain. This stimulation also modestly increases systolic blood pressure levels. The effect on blood pressure is most pronounced in non-coffee drinkers and immediately after having a cup. A moderate daily intake of coffee (two to three cups a day) is not associated with an increased risk of high blood pressure, mostly as you quickly become tolerant of its effects. However, a higher intake (more than five to eight cups a day or more than three espressos every day) seems to be more of an issue, especially in those who already have problems with high blood pressure.

- Not too much salt. It remains controversial whether all people with diabetes should reduce the amount of salt they eat. However, people who habitually eat large amounts of salt have an increased risk of high blood pressure and its consequences.

- Deal with daily stress. Stress is an unavoidable part of modern life, be it physical, environmental, mental or spiritual stress. But chronic activation of stress response pathways leads to higher blood pressure, especially in those whose blood pressure is already difficult to control. Indeed, the increases in blood pressure seen in most people as they get older are not seen in those who live stress-free lives (such as cloistered nuns). This suggests that accumulated stress may be at the core of many blood pressure problems. Interventions to reduce or manage stress, such as relaxation, meditation, avoidance, disclosure and support networks, and can all be very effective in some people (see Chapter 16).

MEDICATIONS TO LOWER BLOOD PRESSURE

Medications (also known as anti-hypertensive agents) are needed by over two-thirds of people with type 2 diabetes to control their blood pressure levels. There are many different types of anti-hypertensive drugs. All can be effective in lowering blood pressure. The choice of which one(s) to prescribe depends on your individual requirements.

Angiotensin-converting enzyme (ACE) inhibitors

ACE inhibitors are the most commonly used agents for blood pressure control in people with type 2 diabetes. There are many different types, brand names and manufacturers. However, what they do have in common is that the technical or generic name of ACE inhibitors usually ends in the suffix '-pril'.

ACE inhibitors came about by chance. The first ACE inhibitor was generated on the basis of chemicals found in the venom of the Amazonian pit viper, *Bothrops jararaca*, which lowered the blood pressure of its prey before devouring it.

ACE inhibitors all act to inhibit the angiotensin-converting enzyme (ACE), whose job it is to generate 'constrictor' signals in blood vessels and break down molecules that might signal blood vessels to relax. Consequently, by inhibiting ACE, blood vessels are able to dilate more easily and tension/pressure within them falls. ACE inhibitors also appear to have beneficial effects in diabetes beyond lowering blood pressure, especially in the heart, eyes and kidneys. This may be because the same signals that ACE inhibitors modify in blood vessels are also important for the development and progression of diabetic complications.

ACE inhibitors are generally well tolerated with only a few side effects experienced in some people, most notably headaches, cough or tickling sensation in the throat. Some people can put up with these without needing to stop taking this medication, but for others it can be a significant problem, meaning they have to look to other kinds of medication to lower their blood pressure. Rarely, ACE inhibitors can cause allergic reactions, including rash or more serious swelling of the face, lips, tongue or throat (known as angioedema). This side effect is more common in African or Caribbean patients, although it is still very uncommon.

Angiotensin-receptor blockers (ARBs)

These medications also block the effects of the angiotensin, a key constrictor signal in blood vessels. But rather than inhibiting the enzyme that generates angiotensin (which is what ACE inhibitors do), these agents impede its ability to trigger constriction of blood vessels by blocking its major receptor. Like putting a protector into a power socket to prevent a child accessing it, these agents sit in the socket to stop angiotensin plugging in. These ARBs are able to sit there for a long time, usually over a day, meaning that they have prolonged blood pressure-lowering activity and once-a-day treatment is usually all that is required.

Again, there are many different formulations, brand names and manufacturers. However, what they have in common is that the generic name of angiotensin-receptor blockers usually ends in the suffix '-sartan'.

Although they have different mechanisms of actions, recent studies suggest that ACE inhibitors and ARBs are not significantly different in terms of their actions on blood pressure and protecting the heart and other organs in diabetes. However, ARBs appear to be slightly better tolerated than ACE inhibitors and do not cause cough or angioedema.

Calcium-channel blockers

These are very effective anti-hypertensive medications that reduce blood pressure by dilating blood vessels and thereby reducing resistance to blood flow. They are second only to the ACE inhibitors in their popularity for treating high blood pressure in people with type 2 diabetes, and are often used in combination with ACE inhibitors or ARBs for the management of high blood pressure. The most common class are the dihydropyridine calcium-channel blockers, which are denoted by a generic name that ends in the suffix '-dipine'.

Calcium-channel blockers are especially effective in people with hardening of their arteries, where stiffness in the blood vessels drives up the systolic blood pressure.

Calcium-channel blockers are also long acting, meaning that many can provide good blood pressure control with a single daily dose. Calcium-channel blockers are generally well tolerated by people with diabetes. However, some people find swelling of the ankles, headaches, flushing and constipation troubling, especially at higher doses.

Diuretics

Diuretics are safe, effective and inexpensive medications that have been used for many years and have been proven to reduce blood pressure and improve health outcomes. They are more effective in combination with other anti-hypertensive agents, and are generally used this way in people with type 2 diabetes.

Diuretics make you lose more salt (and water) in your urine, thus lowering your blood pressure in the same way as releasing air from a balloon lowers its pressure. For this reason they are widely known as **water pills** or **water tablets**. Many also have modest vasodilator effects similar to the calcium-channel blockers detailed above, which may be their major mechanism of actions when given in low doses.

The low doses used by most people with diabetes mean that they seldom make you go to the toilet too frequently and/or dry you out excessively. However, higher doses of diuretics can have these drawbacks. But in most people with diabetes, especially those who also have heart failure or swollen ankles, this drying out action can also be quite beneficial and help to relieve symptoms as well as improve blood pressure control. Excessive urination can also lead to the loss of important chemicals in the urine, such as potassium and magnesium, and increase levels of uric acid which may cause gout. In some individuals, diuretics can also interfere with their glucose control.

Beta-blockers

Beta-blockers lower the blood pressure by blocking stimulation signals from the sympathetic nervous system. Again, there are many different formulations and manufacturers. However, in common, the generic name of beta-blockers usually ends in the suffix '-olol'. As detailed above, when you are nervous or stressed, activation of the sympathetic nervous system makes your heart race and beat more strongly, while the resistance vessels constrict. Being overweight or having kidney or heart disease can also activate the sympathetic nervous system and cause high blood pressure through over-activity of the same pathways. Beta-blockers prevent these signals so are able to slow the pulse, making your heart beat less forcefully. These actions are also useful not only to lower the blood pressure, but to reduce stress on the heart. Consequently beta-blockers are generally used in someone with diabetes who has angina, heart failure and some disturbances in their heart's rhythm. Beta-blockers can also be used to treat glaucoma and resting tremors (e.g. troublesome shaking hands). In addition, some studies suggest that those people who are prone to sympathetic induced surges, such as after smoking, may be better protected by beta-blockers.

However, such individuals would be best protected by stopping smoking.

Overall, the side effect profile of beta-blockers is generally not as favourable as other blood pressure medications. For example, some people experience tiredness, low mood, sleep disturbance, weight gain or impotence with beta-blockers. Breathing problems can also be exacerbated in some people. Beta-blockers can also interfere with glucose control and the body's response to hypoglycaemia.

Other treatments to lower the blood pressure

SGLT-2 inhibitors that are used for lowering glucose levels in the blood can also modestly lower blood pressure levels in people with diabetes, especially those on other blood pressure lowering agents.

For people with high blood pressure that is resistant to medication, a number of surgical options are becoming available, including radiofrequency renal denervation that stops the kidneys from driving up blood pressure levels.

ALL TOGETHER NOW

Most people with type 2 diabetes will need some medication to keep their blood pressure under control. A small number will get away with just one tablet, but for the majority two or three different classes of medication will be required in combination with diet and lifestyle interventions. This is certainly worth the effort. For every 1mmHg decrease in your systolic blood pressure, the long-term risk of heart attack or stroke will fall by 2 to 3 per cent. This means that if you have high blood pressure and you can safely reduce your systolic blood pressure by 10mmHg, your risk of a heart attack or stroke will fall by between 20 and 30 per cent. In fact, that sustained control of blood pressure is the most important way to protect the heart, brain and other organs in people with type 2 diabetes.

9

ESCHEW THE FAT

Understand

- One of the most efficient ways to
  reduce your risk of complications is
  to aim to improve the levels of fats
  and cholesterol in your blood (known
  collectively as 'lipids').
- The most widely used class of
  medication in the treatment of type 2
  diabetes is the statins, which inhibit the
  manufacture of cholesterol by the liver,
  so LDL cholesterol levels fall in the
  blood by between 20 to 50 per cent.
- LDL cholesterol levels in your blood
  are only partly determined by the

fats in your diet. The majority of the cholesterol in your bloodstream is made inside your body.

- HDL cholesterol works to remove cholesterol from your blood vessels and so protects them from atherosclerosis.
- Although diabetes can affect the level of LDL and HDL cholesterol in the blood, by far the greatest change is the overproduction of triglyceride-rich particles.

Manage

- Get the best out of your statin by taking it in the evening.
- Reduce the amount of saturated fat and increase the amount of soluble fibre in your diet to improve your lipid levels beyond what can be achieved by medicines alone.
- Avoid any food that contains trans fat. For people with type 2 diabetes there is no safe intake of trans fats.
- Get up and get active. This will improve

many aspects of your health, including your lipid levels.

Fats are one of the most important building blocks of life. However, they can also be the foundation of poor health, especially in people with type 2 diabetes. Fat has a number of characteristics that make it unhealthy in excess. It has twice the calories of sugar or protein, so that for the same weight of fat, more goes to your waistline. Likewise, cholesterol can be a means to a sticky end by clogging the walls of blood vessels, contributing to their narrowing and stiffening, and ultimately increasing the risk of heart attacks and strokes (see chapters 10 and 15). High levels of fats and cholesterol in the blood are also associated with kidney, foot and eye disease in people with type 2 diabetes.

One of the most efficient ways to reduce your risk of complications from diabetes is to aim to improve the levels of fats and cholesterol in your blood (known collectively as your **lipids**). All people with type 2 diabetes should have a blood test to look at their complete lipid profile when they are diagnosed and at regular intervals thereafter (at least annually). This blood test is sometimes taken after a period of fasting (no food or drink, except water, for 12 hours), which in practical terms means the test is done first thing in the morning before any breakfast. This is so that your lipid levels aren't confused with those of your last meal. The results of this important test will be used to determine the best strategy to get your lipids under control and reduce your risk of future problems.

Lipids are mostly transported around the body in special waterproof containers known as **lipoprotein particles** (because they are particles made up of lipids and proteins). Lipids must travel in containers because oil does not dissolve in water. If you tried it, it would just congeal on the surface, where it would be unusable. The same goes for lipids. These particles come in different sizes and densities and have different functions in the body. For the purpose of your blood test, these lipid particles can be broadly classified into three basic types:

1. low density lipoproteins (LDL) = bad

2. high density lipoproteins (HDL) = good

3. triglyceride-rich lipoproteins = ugly

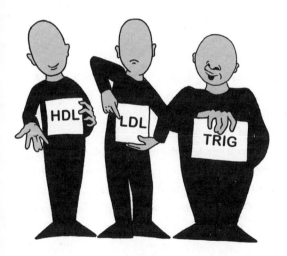

Cholesterol is moved via the bloodstream using three different types of particles: good, bad and ugly.

WHY IS LDL CHOLESTEROL BAD?

Most of the cholesterol that circulates in your bloodstream is contained in low density lipoproteins (LDL) and is therefore known as LDL cholesterol. The cholesterol contained in these LDL particles in generally considered to be 'bad cholesterol'.

This is because high levels of LDL cholesterol are associated with an increased risk of heart attack, stroke and other diseases of the blood vessels.

At the same time, there is good evidence that lowering LDL cholesterol can reduce this risk. For every 1 mmol/L (39 mg/dL) you lower your LDL cholesterol, the risk of a heart attack lowers by between 20 and 25 per cent. This is readily achievable through diet, exercise and other lifestyle changes and, for those who are at high risk, regularly taking LDL-lowering medications.

All people with type 2 diabetes should make lowering their LDL level an important priority, even if their levels are relatively normal. This is because any lowering of the LDL cholesterol in the blood also means a lowering in the amount of cholesterol in your blood vessels, and this in turn means a lower risk of heart attack and stroke (see chapters 10 and 15).

LDL levels aren't usually any higher in people with type 2 diabetes when compared with those who don't have diabetes. However, there is often an excess of small, dense LDL particles. These are the 'baddest of the bad (cholesterol)' because of their increased ability to deposit cholesterol into your blood vessels and not respond to signals to return any excess cholesterol to the liver. Consequently, all people with type 2 diabetes will benefit from lowering their LDL cholesterol level even if it is not too high, because it will also help eliminate these 'very bad' LDL particles.

The main job of LDL cholesterol is to transport cholesterol out of the liver and deliver it to any areas of the body that need it to build new membranes. Areas that are damaged or inflamed need more cholesterol to rebuild, so they capture LDL particles and utilize their store of cholesterol. For example, when blood vessels are stressed, damaged or inflamed they also accumulate cholesterol which they take from LDL particles. The accumulation of cholesterol in the walls of blood vessels progressively leads to narrowing and instability of blood vessels and leads to heart attacks and strokes.

Too much bad (or very bad) cholesterol in your blood means that cholesterol can be easily taken up into your blood vessels and in greater amounts. But if you can successfully lower your LDL cholesterol, it means that the important triggers to accumulate cholesterol in the blood vessels, such as diabetes, high smoking or blood pressure, have much less to work with. And this means less heart disease.

HOW CAN YOU LOWER LDL CHOLESTEROL?

The great majority of the cholesterol in your bloodstream is made inside your own body. Cholesterol is an important component of healthy function, so the human body has enzymes to make the cholesterol it thinks it needs. Each day, you usually make about 1000mg of cholesterol, and take in only another 250mg from your diet. The body even recycles cholesterol from the bile in your intestines so there is no unnecessary wastage.

This means that LDL cholesterol levels in your blood are only weakly determined by what you eat. But it also means that blood levels can rise to dangerous levels if your liver makes too much LDL cholesterol, even if cholesterol-rich foods never touch your lips. Consequently, reducing your LDL cholesterol is all about reducing the amount of cholesterol made by the liver, while at the same time improving your diet.

There are many different **lipid-lowering medications** that act to reduce the amount of cholesterol made by the body and thereby reduce LDL cholesterol levels in the blood.

Most people with type 2 diabetes will need lipid-lowering medications to keep their LDL cholesterol levels as low as possible.

The most widely used type of medication to treat lipids is the **statins**. Statins work by partly inhibiting the manufacture of cholesterol by the liver. So LDL cholesterol levels fall in the blood by between 20 and 50 per cent. To make up for the shortfall, the liver then actively takes back any harmful cholesterol from where it is deposited. This is known as vascular remodelling and is a key benefit of statin therapy.

There are many different brands and formulations of statins, and these are often different in different countries. Each has a chemical (generic) name that ends with the suffix '-statin'. A number of different statins are currently available, including:

- atorvastatin
- fluvastatin
- lovastatin
- pitavastatin
- pravastatin
- rosuvastatin
- simvastatin.

These chemical names are usually displayed on the packet under the brand name in smaller writing. Each of these statins will reduce LDL levels, although they vary slightly in how much it will be reduced and their potential for side effects (see below).

Statins were first identified by Japanese biochemists looking at chemicals made by fungi to defend themselves against other organisms. They discovered that some of these chemicals also blocked the ability to make cholesterol, and these became the first statins. Other fungi, including oyster mushrooms and red yeast koji (a traditional Chinese dish in which rice is fermented in the presence of a specific red mould), also naturally contain a statin, and consequently have the ability to modestly lower cholesterol levels in the blood. However, today all statins are synthetic relatives of the original natural compound.

Although effective at lowering LDL cholesterol levels in the blood, statins are not without their problems. Some people cannot take statins because of troublesome side effects. The most common problems are muscle aches and pains, which are experienced by over one-third of people taking statins, especially those people on high doses. The risk of suffering these muscle pains with statins is partly genetically determined because some people do not have the ability to break down statins efficiently. There is no easy means to prevent muscle aches and pains with a statin. The response is not the same for all statins, meaning that if you have muscle pains with one statin it does not mean you will have the same problems with another statin. So your doctor will often ask you to try another statin if the side effects from one are troublesome. However, many people either have to use smaller doses of a statin, where symptoms are better tolerated, or discontinue it altogether. Recent studies suggest statins may modestly increase the risk of diabetes. However, statins themselves have no major effects on the glucose control of people who already have diabetes.

There are a number of ways to get the best effect out of your statin and maximize your reduction of LDL cholesterol.

Good timing

Statins are usually taken once a day. However, most cholesterol production by the liver occurs at night. So the most efficient way to reduce cholesterol production is to take your statin in the evening. This can add a further 10 per cent reduction to LDL cholesterol levels. The other advantage of taking your statin at night is that the peak chemical concentration coincides with the time you are least likely to experience side effects, when you are asleep.

Ezetimibe

While statins tell the liver to make less cholesterol, the body tries to make up the shortfall by extracting more cholesterol from your intestines (both that contained in your food and the bile released to digest it). So LDL cholesterol levels don't fall by as much as they could. Taking ezetimibe tablets effectively halves the reabsorption of cholesterol. It doesn't do much on its own, but in those already taking a statin, taking ezetimibe as well can reduce LDL cholesterol levels by a further 20 to 25 per cent. Some statins now come mixed with ezetimibe in the same capsule, so that using ezetimibe may not mean taking any extra pills. When taken together, the combination of a statin and ezetimibe is able to reduce the risk of heart attack and stroke in people with diabetes significantly more than a statin alone.

Sterols

Some foods contain natural chemicals with a structure very similar to cholesterol (known as **plant sterols/stanols** or **phytosterols/stanols**). This means they are able to compete with cholesterol for absorption from the intestine, so that less cholesterol is taken up from your diet. Sterols are naturally high in many vegetable oils, nuts and legumes, which can be effectively used as a meat substitute in an everyday diet. But sufficient naturally occurring sterols are hard to get while at the same time trying to limit your overall food intake. So a number of companies have deliberately enriched their foods with sterols to increase their potential health benefits, including margarines, yoghurts, salad dressings, cheeses, breads and even orange juice. These can be hard to find in the shops and tend to be more expensive than standard products, but will further lower your LDL cholesterol levels if you are on a statin. Plant sterol supplements are also available from health food stores. Both supplements and fortified foods only have a modest effect and work best when taken regularly in combination with statins and in high doses (more than 2g per day).

Dietary fibre

A diet high in fibre, and in particular soluble fibre, can also have beneficial effects on LDL cholesterol levels, as well as a number of other health issues. It is thought that soluble fibre causes the liver to make more bile acids from cholesterol, thereby diverting it away from making LDL cholesterol. Dietary fibre can be obtained from a variety of sources, especially wholegrain cereals, fruit and vegetables as well as from nutritional supplements (see Chapter 3).

A low cholesterol diet

Most people will only lower their LDL cholesterol by 5 to 10 per cent at best when going 'cholesterol-free' in their diet. However, in people who are already taking statins, the machinery to capture cholesterol from the intestine is significantly ramped up. This means a low cholesterol diet is also much more effective in those people taking statins.

It is recommended that all those on a statin should also limit their intake of cholesterol-rich foods, including:

- Meat and dairy. Any meat that contains high levels of animal fat will also contain cholesterol, especially those parts that are visibly fatty, such as the skin and the liver. Substituting lean cuts or vegetable protein (like legumes) is one useful way to lower your LDL cholesterol levels.

- Some low fat foods are paradoxically high in cholesterol, including egg yolks, coconut, palm oils and prawns/shrimp. Reducing your intake of these can also lower your LDL cholesterol levels.
- Most foods will now have a label stating how much cholesterol the food contains. Read the label and where possible pick the product that contains the lowest amount of cholesterol.

A low fat diet

LDL cholesterol levels are also partly determined by the mix of other fats in your diet. Fats come in many forms. Most have three chains of fatty acids lined up like cricket stumps and linked at the top by glycerol, like the bails. You could also say it looks like the letter 'E'. This complex is called a **triglyceride** (because of its three — tri — chains). Over 90 per cent of the fats you eat, and almost all that you store in the body, are in the form of triglycerides.

The length of the stumps (fatty acid chains) and the type of bonds between elements in the chain determine its physical properties and its role in the body. If a fat chain contains no double bonds, it has the maximum possible number of hydrogen atoms that can be attached to it. So it is said to be (fully) **saturated**. This chemical arrangement results in a straightening of its molecular structure, allowing it to pack in tightly. This means saturated fat can be solid on the knife, but easily melts with a small amount of heat on your toast. It also means saturated fats have a greater energy density than unsaturated fat. For this reason, most of the fat you store in the body is in the form of saturated fat, which is slowly broken down between meals to ensure a constant energy supply.

Unsaturated fats are those fats that have (one or many) double bonds, which effectively introduces a kink into their structure. This kink prevents them from stacking efficiently. This makes unsaturated fats more difficult to make solid, so they are generally liquid (an oil) at room temperature. But in your body, unsaturated fats are more flexible in their use, so some of them are essential for good health.

Most foods contain a mixture of saturated and unsaturated fats. Foods that are rich in saturated fat are also often high in cholesterol. But in addition, eating lots of saturated fat also triggers an increase in LDL cholesterol levels in the blood.

So any foods that are high in saturated fat will be able to increase your cholesterol levels even if they claim to be 'cholesterol-free'.

Equally, LDL cholesterol can be lowered by reducing your intake of foods that are high in saturated fats, including:

- Limit full-fat dairy products (especially whole milk, yoghurt, cheese and ice-cream) and/or substitute low fat varieties instead.
- Choose lean cuts of meat and remove all visible fat before cooking. The meat of grass-fed animals and free-range birds also contains lower levels of saturated fat than the conventional bulk (grain) fed stocks.
- Eat skinless chicken.
- Where practical, substitute animal protein with vegetable protein, e.g. substitute legumes for ground mince so you use half as much mince in your spaghetti Bolognese.

- Substitute animal meats with seafood and fish.
- Limit your intake of eggs, especially egg yolks. Up to five eggs a week may be acceptable for people with diabetes as part of a healthy diet. But for those with high LDL levels, further moderation should be considered.
- Limit your intake of processed foods, which often contain a significant amount of hidden fat with the addition of butter, oils and lower quality non-lean meat (e.g. pies, pasties, fish and chips, commercial cakes and biscuits/cookies).
- Limit your use of butter in cooking and/or use margarine rich in polyunsaturated or monounsaturated fat.
- Where possible, cook without oil. Where oils are necessary, use products rich in **monounsaturated fats** (MUFAs) such as those found in Mediterranean countries. These are also associated with lower LDL cholesterol levels. Whether this is a direct effect or just because MUFAs replace saturated fat in the diet is still unclear. The most common MUFA in the Mediterranean diet is **oleic acid**, which is found in vegetable and seed oils, nuts, avocado and some meats. Tea oil and olive oil contain more MUFAs than normal canola oils, which are in turn greater than sunflower, peanut, corn and soybean oils. However, on the market now are many oil products which are naturally high in oleic acid (greater than 70g per 100g, or 70 per cent) and comparable in content to olive oils.

Avoid trans fats

Trans fats are an unnatural form of unsaturated fat that has been realigned with a straight backbone. This means that even though it is really unsaturated, it looks and behaves more like the straight chain of a saturated fat. Most trans fats are deliberately created during the processing of vegetable oils (by hydrogenation) to make them solid at room temperature, melt on baking (or eating) and more resistant to going off (rancid) when compared to animal fats such as butter. Prolonged deep-frying can also generate trans fats, which are then transferred to the foods you are eating.

Trans fats increase heart disease partly by raising bad (LDL) cholesterol levels and lowering good (HDL) cholesterol levels and increasing levels of inflammation. Saturated fat does the same thing, but trans fats are much more potent at it. In fact, for the same amount, trans fats increase the risk of heart disease more than any other component of your diet. This is not just the case for those who eat a lot of them — even a small intake may be sufficient to begin increasing your risk of heart disease. There appears to be no safe limit for trans fats.

The only real way to avoid trans fats is to avoid foods containing them, or choose foods in which the processing has specifically prevented their formation. One source of trans fats is deep-fried fast foods, especially those re-using cooking oils. Steer clear of any processed foods that have any trans fats listed on their nutritional contents. Many commercial bakery products, packaged snack foods, and products made in vegetable ghee contain trans fats. There are much safer choices if you have diabetes, including many trans-fat free oils. If a product doesn't know about its trans fat content, then it doesn't care about you, and should be avoided.

WHAT IS GOOD CHOLESTEROL?

Not all cholesterol is bad. About 20 to 30 per cent of cholesterol in your blood is contained in small, dense packages known as high-density lipoproteins (HDL). HDL particles perform a number of jobs that are important for the health of blood vessels, including:

- soaking up excess cholesterol from the walls of blood vessels and transporting it back to the liver for excretion, storage or recycling (known as reverse cholesterol transport)
- transferring their signalling proteins to other particles, which allows them to dump their fatty cargo safely back into the liver, rather than getting stuck in your blood vessels
- HDL also contains antioxidant molecules and may also have beneficial effects on clotting and inflammation.

These helpful actions partly explain why HDL cholesterol is considered to be 'good cholesterol'. Certainly, people with high levels of HDL cholesterol have a lower risk of heart disease and stroke, and those with low HDL levels have more problems with cholesterol deposits in their blood vessels.

HDL cholesterol levels are often low in people with type 2 diabetes. This is partly because HDL particles get used up faster when trying to deal with all the other changes in fat metabolism.

Many of the things you are already doing as part of your routine diabetes management will be improving your HDL cholesterol levels, as well of other aspects of your health. These include:

- Losing excess waist. Being overweight or obese is associated with reduced HDL cholesterol levels. Every 1kg (2¼lb) in weight you can lose means a better waistline and better cholesterol (see Chapter 4).

- Increasing your level of physical activity will increase HDL levels, especially in those with low levels. Regular aerobic exercise seems to have the best effect. This action seems to correlate with the ability of exercise to help you lose weight. However, it is not instantaneous and it may take many months to see any significant change in HDL. But then, good things take time.

- Stopping smoking is important for many reasons, one of which is its impact on HDL cholesterol. Smokers have lower HDL levels, while stopping smoking will increase HDL levels by 10 to 20 per cent on average.

- Drinking alcohol, in moderation. It is well known that those who regularly drink alcohol have higher HDL cholesterol levels when compared to those who don't drink at all or drink only occasionally. This does not explain why the risk of heart attack and stroke is also a little lower in people who drink small amounts of alcohol on a regular basis when compared to teetotallers. Moreover, this association does not mean that non-drinkers should now start drinking alcohol to raise their HDL or lower their risk of heart disease, now that they have diabetes. A little tipple can easily become more if the bottle is there within reach. It is far healthier to never drink at all than go down this slippery slope. Irregular heavy drinking bouts, even if accompanied by usual moderation, can undo any benefits and contribute to high blood pressure and hypoglycaemia in some people on glucose-lowering medications. Alcohol is also a good source of excess calories (just think 'beer belly').

- Substituting unsaturated fats into your diet (instead of eating saturated and trans fats) will also help raise your HDL cholesterol levels.

- Fasting. Prolonged periods of fasting can result in a modest but significant rise in HDL cholesterol. This is often lost after returning to normal habits, but may represent one of the many health benefits of regular fasting observed in certain cultures. Remember, fasting in someone with diabetes should always be undertaken with caution and in consultation with your physician and diabetes care team. These issues are discussed in detail in Chapter 7.

- Medications to raise HDL cholesterol. Because of the importance of HDL, a number of different medicines have been developed to try to raise HDL cholesterol, especially in those with type 2 diabetes. At the present time, though, there is no evidence that their specific actions on HDL cholesterol confer any benefits in people with diabetes. Moreover, niacin (vitamin B3) can raise glucose levels in some people with diabetes.

WHAT ARE TRIGLYCERIDES DOING IN YOUR BLOOD?

The most important store of energy in the human body is fat. As discussed in Chapter 2, this energy store is mostly in the form of triglycerides, which you bank in your fatty tissues under your skin and around your waistline. When you are eating, these energy stores are built up. But when you are not eating these stores are slowly broken down and used to provide the energy for life.

Because triglycerides don't dissolve in water, to reach our fat stores they must be transported in lipoprotein particles alongside cholesterol. Most triglycerides are made by the liver, which converts any excess energy in the diet into triglycerides, packages it into particles and ships it off into the bloodstream so it can be dumped into our fat stores, for later use when we are not eating. These particles are made up of mostly triglycerides, with some cholesterol and very little protein, so they have a very low density (and are therefore also called very low density particles or **VLDL cholesterol**).

Excess fat in your diet also needs to be packaged and sent off. After digestion, the intestine packages fat for the body in a different kind of very, very low density particle (known as a **chylomicron**).

Although type 2 diabetes can affect the level of LDL and HDL cholesterol in your blood, by far the greatest change in your lipid levels is the over-abundance of these ugly triglyceride-rich particles. This is because insulin does much more than just look after your glucose levels.

After a meal, when there is lots of glucose, this is the time to build up your fuel stores. So insulin also signals the body to take up triglycerides as well as glucose, and store them until their energy is needed later. Insulin also signals the liver to stop making new triglyceride-rich particles. After all, you have just eaten. In the same way, and for the same reasons, it also tells it to stop making glucose.

When insulin levels are low, such as between meals, triglycerides are broken down and released into the bloodstream. This is important for two main reasons. First, triglycerides can be used by the liver to make new glucose and thus sustain blood glucose levels for the sake of your brain. Second, this fat provides an alternate fuel source for the working of your muscles, liver, heart and many other organs. Many others that is, except for your brain, which cannot use fat so gets preferential treatment. And when other organs use fat for their metabolism, this frees up glucose for your brain, allowing it to keep running (on glucose) even if you've missed a meal or two.

However, in those with diabetes there is not enough insulin (function) to keep metabolism under control. So not only do glucose levels rise, but there is also not enough insulin to support the healthy uptake of fat or to stop the liver, which keeps cranking out triglyceride-rich particles. This means that triglyceride levels are elevated in the blood of people with type 2 diabetes as well as glucose, especially after meals. People with diabetes are two to three times more likely to have elevated blood triglycerides than people without diabetes. These triglyceride-rich particles are bad for you in a number of ways:

- HDL particles get used up trying to deal with them, so as triglyceride levels rise, levels of good (HDL) cholesterol fall.
- Because of their large size, these triglyceride-rich particles are prone to get stuck in the walls of blood vessels, which contributes to atherosclerosis and

ultimately heart attack and stroke (see chapters 10 and 15).

- In extreme cases, these lipid particles are deposited under the skin as itchy, whitish lumps, known as xanthomas.

How can you lower your triglyceride levels?

Again, many of the things you are already doing as part of your routine diabetes management will be improving your triglyceride levels, as well as other aspects of your health. These include:

- losing excess weight
- undertaking regular physical activity
- achieving and maintaining good glucose control
- reducing the saturated fat in your diet
- avoiding trans fats in your diet (see above).

In addition, there may be other things you can do to keep your triglycerides down that you might not immediately think of doing, including the following.

Avoiding sweetened beverages

Fructose is a sugar that is naturally present in ripe fruit. It is also present in large amounts in many carbonated beverages and fruit juice mixes. It is also added to many prepared foods as a preservative and sweetener. Any fructose we eat is rapidly converted into triglycerides by our liver, allowing us to make the most of fruit when in season. This means that immediately following the intake of high-fructose drinks, triglyceride levels can rise quite dramatically. In those with already elevated levels and/or difficulty clearing away triglycerides, the excess fructose in sweet drinks can still be a cause of rising lipid levels, even when they contain no fat.

Increased intake of omega-3 fatty acids

Fats are more than just the means to a sticky end. Some fats are also essential for good health, and must be found in the diet. The best known of these are the omega-3 polyunsaturated fatty acids, of which the most important nutritionally are alpha-linolenic acid (ALA) from plants, and eicosapentaenoic acid (EPA) and docosahexaenoic acid (DHA), which are found in high levels in oily fish. Their potential health benefits explain why it is often recommended that people with diabetes consume a meal of oily fish (such as salmon, herring, mackerel, anchovies, sardines and to a lesser extent tuna) two or three times every week, to keep up their omega-3s. Although enjoyable for some, many find that this is difficult to achieve. These doses of omega-3s contained in fish generally will not be enough to lower triglycerides, although they can have other beneficial effects. If you can't get enough from fish, eating fortified foods with added amounts of omega-3 fat can prove useful, including bread, mayonnaise, yoghurt, orange juice, pasta, milk, eggs, infant formula and even ice-cream.

Many people also take supplements that contain the required amounts of omega-3, such as **fish oils** and **flaxseed (linseed) oil**. Clinical trials have demonstrated that fish oil supplements can lower blood triglyceride levels in people with diabetes by about one-third. However, the dose required to achieve any significant change in your triglyceride levels is high (more than 2g per day) and can leave a 'fishy' aftertaste. But while triglycerides are strongly associated with all the complications of diabetes, it also remains to be established whether omega-3 supplements actually reduce your chances of developing these complications.

Moderation of alcohol

Those people who regularly drink heavily often have elevated triglyceride levels. This partly reflects the extra calories that come with drinking as well as the direct effects of alcohol. Some of this rise in triglycerides will improve once any excessive alcohol intake is stopped.

Medications to lower triglycerides

Because of the potentially toxic effects of triglyceride-rich particles, the potential value of medications to specifically target this kind of lipid have been widely studied in people with type 2 diabetes. The best studied are the **fibrates**. Again, there are many different brands and formulations of different products, and these often vary in different countries. Each has a chemical (generic) name that contains the letters 'fibr'. Only three fibrates are currently available, including:

- fenofibrate
- gemfibrozil
- bezafibrate.

These medicines are able to lower triglyceride levels by between 20 and 40 per cent in people with type 2 diabetes, when used on top of standard treatment with a statin and other dietary modifications detailed above. In people with high triglyceride levels, treatment with a fibrate has been shown to prevent heart attacks. It also may reduce the risk of eye, nerve and foot complications. Fenofibrate can be used in people who are taking a statin, so is the preferred fibrate for people with type 2 diabetes. By contrast, gemfibrozil and bezafibrate may interact with your statin in a way to increase the risk of side effects including muscle pain and damage, so is only used on its own, in people who can't use a statin.

10

DIABETES IN MY HEART

Understand

- Heart attacks are a common complication of type 2 diabetes, and are sadly the major cause of death.
- Good management of your diabetes is able to reduce your chance of having a heart attack by over half.
- Heart attacks are caused by the erosion of an unstable surface of a blood vessel supplying the heart, which causes it to become completely blocked by a clot.
- Many heart attacks in people with type 2 diabetes are silent. The first sign may be shortness of breath, ankle swelling

or other signs of heart failure.

- The changes in your blood vessels that lead to a heart attack are reversible when the risk factors for atherosclerosis are addressed.

Manage

- Get your levels of bad (LDL) cholesterol as low as possible. Even if your levels are not high, less cholesterol means less chance of heart disease.
- Treat high blood pressure levels and maintain smooth control over them.
- Stop smoking as a matter of priority and encourage others in your environment to do the same as it may also affect your health.
- Undertake a comprehensive risk factor assessment with the help of your diabetes care team to calculate your individual risk of a heart attack, and the benefits that can be achieved from each treatment.
- Become familiar with the warning

signs of a heart attack. Have an action plan for what to do in the event of a heart attack and when to call for an ambulance.

All parts of the body depend on the flow of blood for their survival. If this flow is blocked, even for a brief period, any parts downstream from the blockage suffer and may die. When this blockage occurs in the blood vessels that supply the heart (known as the **coronary arteries**) it is called a **heart attack** (also known as **myocardial infarction** or **MI**). When a blockage occurs in blood flow to the brain it is called a stroke (also known as a **cerebrovascular accident**; see Chapter 15). Together, heart attacks and strokes may be the most important complications of having type 2 diabetes, accounting for over half of all deaths in people with diabetes.

The burden of heart disease among patients with type 2 diabetes is substantial. Many years of life are lost, while quality of life for survivors is greatly reduced. Between one-third to half of all adults with type 2 diabetes will currently have heart disease. Approximately 1 to 3 per cent of people with type 2 diabetes experience heart attacks and strokes every year. Overall, this risk is at least twice that observed in people who do not have diabetes.

Finding ways to prevent or reverse this process is therefore an integral part of diabetes care.

And it does work! If you have diabetes today, the risk of having a heart attack or stroke is less than half what it was for those with type 2 diabetes twenty years ago. With modern diabetes care, it is anticipated that heart attack rates will continue to fall.

This chapter will look at the key opportunities you have to look after your heart and, with it, your life.

WHAT CAUSES HEART ATTACKS?

Think of your blood vessels as roads that allow for the steady flow of traffic along major arterials to smaller streets and then back again in a round trip. Like any carriageway, the health of these roads is important for maintaining this flow. If the surface stays flat, traffic flows smoothly and easily gets to where it needs to go. Over long periods of time, changes occur under the surface of our roads, causing them to thicken and soften. This is known as **atherosclerosis** and is the start of the process that eventually leads to heart attacks and strokes.

These changes do not occur equally in all parts of the road. Streets that get damaged fastest are the ones that have the extra pressure of heavy trucks or turning vehicles. The same occurs in our arteries, where the large blood vessels under the greatest pressure are most vulnerable, especially where vessels divide and blood flow turns a corner into the heart or the brain. When atherosclerosis affects the coronary blood vessels that supply the heart, it is known as **coronary heart disease** or **CHD**.

Years may go by as the structures underneath the surface become progressively unstable in spots. The surface may even start to bulge a little bit (known as **plaque**). But still the surface remains intact and the traffic keeps flowing. Then one fateful day, usually after a particularly large truck passes (or another stressful event), the surface breaks and a pothole occurs. The next car falls into the pothole. The car behind it hits the first car and a major pile-up ensues, completely blocking the road. This is precisely what happens if you have a heart attack. A coronary artery becomes clotted because of an erosion or rupture of its protective surface.

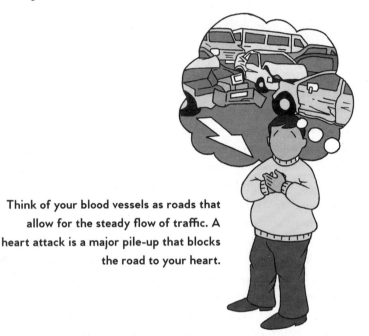

Think of your blood vessels as roads that allow for the steady flow of traffic. A heart attack is a major pile-up that blocks the road to your heart.

In most people with diabetes, a heart attack or stroke is the first sign that there is anything wrong with their arteries.

If this blockage can't be quickly cleared, then everything further down the road relying on the traffic getting through will suffer. Unlike damage to your skin, heart muscle and brain cells cannot grow back, so any significant loss of blood flow always means some permanent loss of heart function. But if the clot is dissolved and traffic flow can be quickly restored, any permanent damage can be prevented or kept to a minimum.

Sometimes surface erosions and ruptures are limited and

the resulting clot is so small that any obstruction is partial. Such events do not cause a heart attack, as sufficient blood flow is still maintained along the artery for the heart to survive. But as each clot is incorporated into the wall, the road is progressively narrowed and further compromised in its ability to handle more than a trickle of traffic.

As with a road, if you lose a lane or two things only really come to a head at 'rush hour', when more traffic wants to use the road. The same occurs when the heart needs more blood flow, such as with physical exertion or other stresses that get the heart racing. In such circumstances any narrowing in the coronary artery can suddenly become limiting. This is experienced as chest pain (known as **angina**) and is often a forerunner of more complete and more serious blockages in the future.

WHAT IS YOUR RISK OF A HEART ATTACK?

Although having diabetes increases your risk of heart attack, the personal risk for a heart attack varies considerably between people with diabetes. In younger people with diabetes, their risk is quite small, so even with the doubling in risk associated with having diabetes this doesn't add up to much. However, for older individuals with type 2 diabetes, or those with other risk factors such as high blood pressure, high total cholesterol or smokers, any doubling in their (already elevated) risk caused by diabetes has a much more substantial effect in absolute terms.

It is recommended that all people with type 2 diabetes should undergo a comprehensive risk factor assessment with the help of their diabetes care team to identify whether more intensive management can result in the greatest absolute benefits. A range of different 'risk calculators' is available. Each combines a number of key factors to estimate your personal risk of having a heart attack. Your doctor will be able to plug into these various factors about your history, your symptoms and signs, as well as results of your blood tests to calculate your personal risk.

While these calculators can be used to inform you about your risks, more importantly they can be used to estimate the benefits that could be achieved from interventions designed to lower your risk (see below). For example, if prescribing lipid-lowering medication to reduce your cholesterol levels is able to reduce your risk of having a heart attack by between 20 and 25 per cent, then the risk in someone who has a 5 per cent risk of a heart attack in the next five years is reduced by this medication to around 4 per cent. In absolute terms the 1 per cent reduction is quite small and may not be worth the side effects or the cost of the medication. By comparison, for someone who has a 50 per cent risk of a heart attack, lipid-lowering medication has over ten times the benefit (by reducing their risk by over 10 per cent in absolute terms, to less than 40 per cent). In this situation, more aggressive treatment and targets have greater gains — more bang for your buck. In this way it is possible to put real numbers on what you are achieving with management of your diabetes.

HOW TO PREVENT HEART ATTACKS?

The scenario of progressive change under the surface of your blood vessels, eventually leading to their loss of integrity, is preventable. In fact, it may even be partly reversible. There are now a number of different opportunities to look after your blood vessels and keep their traffic flowing for many years to come. Some of these opportunities include the following.

Reducing the LDL cholesterol levels in the blood

Large deposits of cholesterol under the surface of our blood vessels are the most important reason arteries become weak and eventually break down. A number of different factors cause cholesterol to accumulate in the walls of the coronary arteries. However, each requires LDL cholesterol to be present in the blood in the first place (see Chapter 9). LDL cholesterol is also known as 'bad cholesterol' because of its strong association with heart disease. Even though most people with type 2 diabetes do not have very elevated LDL cholesterol levels, by reducing your circulating levels of LDL cholesterol you also reduce the risk of a heart attack or stroke. For every 1mmol/L (40mg/dL) you lower your LDL cholesterol, your risk will fall by betwen 20 and 25 per cent. This can be readily achieved with a combination of diet, physical activity and appropriate use of lipid-lowering medications, such as statins.

Raising the HDL cholesterol in the blood

The body has a way to safely transport cholesterol out of blood vessels and back into the liver. This function is performed by HDL cholesterol particles (also known as 'good cholesterol'), which is discussed in detail in Chapter 9. Diabetes reduces HDL levels, meaning that this beneficial action is also reduced in people with diabetes. The higher your HDL cholesterol the greater your capacity to offset the effects of bad cholesterol, particularly with regards to the development and progression of heart disease, so that individuals with the highest levels of HDL cholesterol have a lower risk of heart disease and strokes. There are a number of different ways to increase HDL levels, again mainly through a combination of a healthy diet, physical activity and appropriate use of lipid-lowering medication.

Reducing elevated triglycerides in the blood

The greatest change in lipid levels in the blood associated with diabetes is the increase in triglycerides. In those with elevated triglyceride levels, treatment with the triglyceride-lowering drug fenofibrate is able to reduce the risk of heart attacks. It does not appear to have the same benefits in people who do not have high triglycerides or in those who already have heart disease. However, it may have other beneficial effects for your eyes and your feet, regardless of your lipid levels.

Reducing systolic blood pressure

The tension on the walls of our arteries is just like the pressure of traffic on the surface of a road: the greater and heavier the traffic, the more likely that the road will become progressively damaged and potholes will eventually occur. One simple way to keep your blood vessels in better shape for longer is to reduce this stress placed on blood vessels by lowering the blood pressure. Just as when the number of heavy vehicles on main freeways is reduced, the road will last longer. In those with hypertension, for every 1mmHg decrease in systolic blood pressure, the long-term risk of a heart attack is reduced by between 2 and 3 per cent.

Systolic blood pressure levels to less than 140mmHg can be achieved in most people with diabetes with regular exercise, healthy diet and medication. The benefit of targeting even lower blood pressure levels remains controversial. While it does not seem to further reduce the risk of heart attack, the risk of stroke can be substantially reduced by lowering blood pressure below 140mmHg. This may be particularly important in women, people of an Asian background and those with atherosclerosis in the arteries that lead to the brain.

Good glucose control

In people with diabetes there is a continuous relationship between blood glucose and the risk of a heart attack. This begins around an HbA1c of 7 per cent (53mmol/mol). The higher your glucose levels above this target and the longer that this exposure occurs, the higher your risk of having a heart attack. Keeping your glucose levels under control reduces your chance of having a heart attack by at least 10 to 15 per cent.

The benefit of good glucose control appears to be greatest in those recently diagnosed with diabetes, in people with poor diabetes control, and before they develop heart disease. In fact, the effect of glucose control achieved in the early years after being diagnosed with diabetes has a significant influence on the subsequent risk of complications in the years following. A period of good glucose control at the start of your diabetes can result in a reduced risk of heart disease and other complications that persists for over a decade later, even if this good control is no longer maintained. Equally, a period of lax control at the beginning can cast a pall over your future. This is known as the **legacy effect** or **metabolic karma**.

In those who already have heart disease, the benefits of aggressively targeting lower glucose targets in terms of reducing the risk of further heart attacks or death appears to be much smaller, or potentially not significant 'after the horse has already bolted'. However, this does not mean that glucose control has no part to play in the prevention of other complications (such as kidney and eye disease).

New medications for lowering glucose levels, including SGLT-2 inhibitors and GLP-1 agonists, appear to have additional benefits in reducing the risk of dying from heart disease over and above their actions on glucose levels. How this works remains to be established. But in those at high risk of dying from heart disease (e.g. those who have had a prior heart attack or have other complications of diabetes) these additional advantages are one important reason these medicines may be preferred over other ones used for controlling your glucose levels.

Stop smoking

Smoking significantly increases your risk of a heart attack as well as other complications from your diabetes. Toxins contained in cigarette smoke stress the surface of blood vessels, as well as increase your blood pressure and cholesterol levels. Even passive smoking puts your heart at risk. So encourage your partner and your workmates to stop as well!

Stopping smoking may be one of the most important things you can do to reduce your chances of complications from type 2 diabetes.

But it's hard to do on your own. Smoking is a powerful addiction that is understandably hard to break. Like managing diabetes, the best chances of quitting for good come if you can get some help. There are lots of people and effective therapies that can help you stop smoking. Individually, they won't work the same for everyone, or in all cases. But it is usually possible to find one that will work for you. Talk to your doctor or call your local 'quit smoking line' to find out the options that best suit your needs.

One of the big concerns about stopping smoking is weight gain. Weight gain after quitting is real but fortunately it's usually small and temporary, and the health benefits of quitting more than make up for this. As you begin to feel healthier, and are able to become more active, weight levels will often return to previous levels, or lower.

The good news is that if you can quit for good, you can reverse some of the damage caused by smoking. If you can keep off the cigarettes for more than a decade your risk of heart attack and stroke are almost as low as those of a non-smoker. And there will be many other benefits along the way, so start looking at the options now.

Waist management

Waist management is a key component of diabetes management and is discussed in detail in Chapter 4. In people with type 2 diabetes, getting rid of excess fat is helpful for many reasons. One of the most important is that it can reduce the incidence and improve your outcomes from heart disease. This is achieved partly by improving risk factors for heart disease such as control of glucose, blood pressure and cholesterol levels. But over and above these gains, moderate and sustained weight loss (i.e. 7 to 10 per cent of your body weight for at least a year) will also reduce your risk of having a heart attack.

Increased physical activity

Regular physical activity has positive effects to decrease the risk of heart attack. These include helping to maintain weight loss, improving glucose, lipid and blood pressure control, elevating mood, optimizing blood flow and reducing blood clotting. These benefits are discussed in detail in Chapter 5. There are a number of different ways to stay active, from an increase in daily lifestyle activities (such as walking or climbing stairs) to more structured forms of exercise in a gym. One isn't really better than another. For your heart, what seems to matter is that you are regularly doing something physical, and sticking at it. Gym membership is useless if you never go. Even if you are 80 years old, carefully starting a regular exercise routine for the first time reduces your risk of heart disease. Even if you already have diabetes, physical activity will improve your health compared to remaining on the couch. It is better late than never.

Stress management

There is no doubt that stress can be a killer. In particular, it is well known that a high level of stress is a major risk factor for heart attacks. Overall it has been estimated that up to one-third of all heart attacks may be attributable to chronic stress. For some people, stress is as detrimental to their health as being overweight or having high blood pressure. Those individuals feeling the tension of stress are at greater risk of suffering a heart attack. For example, those with persisting negative emotions (depression, anxiety or anger) have two or three times the risk of a heart attack than those without the added stress.

The stress that sets your heart pounding could come from many different sources; whether this is a major life event, job or family stress, mental, spiritual or physical stress is of less importance than its effects on you and your heart.

All stress increases the work of the heart, increases the blood pressure, raises cholesterol and glucose levels, and increases blood clotting. It is also hard to focus your mind on diabetes control when your attention is stuck somewhere else.

There are many effective ways to limit unwanted stresses, by augmenting resources and your ability to cope, or modulating the stress response itself. These include relaxation, hypnosis, disclosure, conditioning, avoidance and other behavioural interventions. There are also medications that can be useful in some individuals suffering from chronic stress. The most important step is identifying that stress is a problem, and getting help finding your way around it (see Chapter 16).

Thinning the blood

When a heart attack occurs, a thick clot is responsible for blocking an artery supplying the heart. Another way to reduce the chance of a major pile-up is to thin the blood, much like increasing the distance between cars on a freeway. If there is an accident it is less likely to block the whole road, and will perhaps only affect a single lane. For those at very high risk of heart disease, such as those who have previously experienced a heart attack, regularly taking drugs that slow the clotting process (such as aspirin, dipyridamole or clopidogrel) can reduce the risk of a heart attack by between 20 and 25 per cent.

The use of aspirin in people who have never had a heart attack or stroke is controversial. Combined data from clinical trials suggests that aspirin has only a small or no net effect when used in all people with diabetes who don't currently have heart disease. But even in the absence of active heart disease, aspirin therapy is warranted in people with diabetes who have a sufficiently high risk of having a heart attack, such as those who also have high blood pressure, high cholesterol levels, kidney disease, advanced age, who continue to smoke, and those with a strong family history of heart disease. In such cases your doctor may recommend taking low-dose aspirin (75–150mg per day). Blood thinners should not be used in people with an increased risk for bleeding, such as those who have peptic ulcers or other problems associated with intestinal bleeding and those who need to take other medications that increase the risk of bleeding, such as warfarin or anti-inflammatory drugs.

A diet rich in omega-3 fats found in fish oils (see previous chapter) is also associated with a reduced risk of having a heart attack, possibly because of its effects on clotting. Menaquinone (vitamin K2), which is found in green leafy vegetables, yoghurt and some supplements, may also have beneficial effects on clotting and may lower the risk of having a heart attack.

DON'T IGNORE THE SYMPTOMS

There are now many different ways to rapidly restore blood flow along blocked arteries following a heart attack. These are most effective when delivered as close to the first moment of blockage as possible. The longer arterial blockage is left, the greater the damage to the heart and the more limited any recovery. Time is (heart) muscle.

If you or your doctor calculate that you are at risk of having a heart attack, it is imperative you are familiar with the warning signs of a heart attack, and have an action plan for what to do in an emergency and when to call for an ambulance.

It is always better to be proactive and report any sudden new symptoms rather than hope they will go away. This may be more lifesaving than any other intervention in diabetes. The symptoms of a heart attack may include:

- sudden tightness, pressure or (crushing) pain in the chest that spreads to the shoulder, arm or jaw and doesn't go away
- suddenly feeling short of breath, nauseous, sweaty or faint for no reason (even in the absence of any pain).

It is not unusual for people with diabetes to suffer a heart attack without experiencing any symptoms (known as a **silent myocardial infarction**). This is because the nerves that supply the heart may be damaged by diabetes and are therefore unable to transmit the signals of pain through to your brain. This is why any unusual symptoms should be investigated in anyone with diabetes at risk of heart disease.

Screening for damage

If you are experiencing chest pain or shortness of breath on exertion or other symptoms suggestive of heart problems, your doctor will often arrange additional tests to determine how well your coronary arteries are functioning, to identify the earliest signs of problems, and to direct the type and intensity of future treatments. Some of these tests may include:

- Exercise stress testing. You will be asked to pedal an exercise bike or walk on a treadmill to get your heart working hard. At the same time the health of your heart will be monitored by electrodes placed on the skin over your heart and on your arms. If the heart shows signs of stress with this workload, this is taken as a sign that the blood supply to the heart is not what it should be and further investigations are necessary.

- Dobutamine stress test. Instead of pedalling to get your heart working, in this test a chemical (dobutamine) is infused into your body to get the heart working hard. At the same time the health of your heart will be monitored by an ultrasound machine (known as an **echocardiogram**) or nuclear perfusion imaging (known as single photon emission computed tomography or SPECT scanning for short). Again, if the heart shows signs of stress with a workload, then this is taken as a sign that the blood supply to the heart is not what it should be and further investigations are necessary.

While symptoms can be an indicator of heart disease, typical symptoms are often masked in people with diabetes (known as **silent ischaemia**), especially those with advanced age or who are very overweight, and those with other complications affecting the eyes/kidneys or sensation in the feet. In such circumstances your doctor may also sometimes order these same tests of your coronary arteries (even if you feel fine) to be sure that nothing important is missed. Such testing may also be important before embarking on a program of vigorous exercise.

Road works are sometimes necessary

If the damage to the road becomes dangerous to vehicles, sometimes road works may be necessary. If you have severe damage to your blood vessels, each of these procedures can be lifesaving and life-prolonging. Such work may include scraping out any narrowing (known as **endarterectomy**) or making the road wider (known as **angioplasty**) and holding it open with a metal stent, or even building a bypass around the damaged area (known as **coronary artery bypass grafting** or **coronary surgery**). There is some data to suggest that early coronary surgery may be the preferred therapy in patients with diabetes when road works are required. However, such surgical interventions are also associated with significant health risks that are also greater in those with diabetes. So a balance between risks and benefits must always be struck between you and your cardiologist regarding what is the best approach for your specific problems.

HEART FAILURE AND DIABETES

Any damage to the heart has the potential to reduce its ability to pump blood around the body. This is known as **heart failure**. It commonly follows a heart attack, but other factors may also damage the heart and reduce its functions.

To try to maintain the same output from your heart even if it is damaged, the pressure of fluid returning to the heart also increases to make the heart fill better. This is the equivalent of a 'head of steam' in an engine. However, this back-up of fluid from a failing heart results in a number of signs and symptoms of heart failure, including the following.

- You may experience **shortness of breath**, particularly on exertion, as the ability of the heart to step up a gear is limited.

- You may also feel **short of breath when lying down**. This is because when you lie down more blood is able to return to the heart instead of pooling in your legs due to gravity. This means more work for it to do. And if the functions of the heart are impaired, there will be a greater back-up of fluid into your lungs, which affects your breathing.

- You might get swollen feet and lower legs (known as **oedema**) as more fluid backs up from the heart.

- Heart failure also results in the chambers of the heart becoming stretched and dilated. This can trigger irregular heartbeats or change the rhythmical beating of the heart (known as **arrhythmias**). These may be experienced as palpitations or dizzy spells.

- Eventually these compensations can no longer keep the heart pumping strongly, and as the output of blood from the heart falls, so does the blood pressure.

Low blood pressure levels (known as **hypotension**) are common in those with severe heart failure, and this may manifest as feeling dizzy, lightheaded or faint when standing up too quickly or when standing for too long.

People with type 2 diabetes are unusually prone to heart failure. Heart failure is four- to fivefold more likely in someone with diabetes than in someone without it. This is partly because heart attacks are more common, and are often recognized late in those with diabetes because of fewer symptoms. However, beyond coronary artery disease, diabetes can also have direct effects to reduce the function of the heart muscle to contract and relax properly (known as **diabetic cardiomyopathy**). For example, with long-standing diabetes and high blood pressure the heart can become stiffer. A stiffer, or non-compliant, heart can't fill with blood very easily (known as **diastolic dysfunction**). So to make sure it keeps filling and pumping, the pressure inside the heart must rise; in essence, force-filling the stiff heart with blood. This also leads to shortness of breath, particularly on exertion, as the time available to fill the heart is shorter the faster the heart is beating, so that heart stiffening becomes the limiting factor.

To examine the functions of your heart, your doctor might order an echocardiogram. This is just like an ultrasound scan that is used to look at a developing baby in the womb. Both techniques use sound waves and their rebound to determine structures beneath your skin. It this way it is possible to determine how much blood is squeezed out of the heart during each beat (known as the **ejection fraction**) and how easily it fills up afterwards.

Another feature of the heart in diabetes is that there is often damage to the nerves that are required to carefully regulate its functions. Approximately one-third of people with type 2 diabetes will have damage to the nerves that supply the heart. This damage can sometimes lead to unresponsive and/or unbalanced electrical activity. For example, when you exercise, your heart beats faster to cope with the extra demands of pushing blood to and from the exercising muscles. But if the nerves that relay these signals are damaged, the heart doesn't respond, so you stay stuck in first gear. This can also sometimes mean you don't have the energy to exercise, or that your heart stays fast all the time.

YOUR HEART WILL GO ON

It is hard to think about type 2 diabetes without also thinking about heart disease. It is very easy to become frightened. It is also easy to want to give up. But the heart is a surprisingly resilient organ. It has the capacity to compensate against all manner of calamities to keep the blood pumping. To some extent it even has the capacity for regeneration. There really are second chances in life.

For many people with type 2 diabetes this comes after their first heart attack, when things really hit home. But even after this kind of damage, your heart has the capacity to adapt and even improve its function. With time, the damaged area of the heart contracts to become a scar while the remainder of the heart expands to take over the work of the piece that has been lost. This is the time when other changes can also be made in your diet and lifestyle, and the targets for your treatment revised. For example, rather than stopping you in your tracks, there is good evidence to show that appropriate exercise training after a heart attack can help the heart recover and keep it safe for the future. This is best conducted as part of a total program known as **cardiac rehabilitation**.

Although rehabilitation is still possible after a heart attack, taking steps to get your risk factors under control will work even better without having had the heart attack in the first place. The changes of atherosclerosis that lead to heart attacks are reversible. The instability that ultimately leads to erosions in the surface of blood vessels is reversible. And the plan of diabetes management is to do all that is possible to reverse them.

11

DIABETES IN MY SIGHT

Understand

- The tissues of the eye are uniquely vulnerable to the effects of diabetes. It is normal for most people with type 2 diabetes to have some changes in their eyes.
- Of all the complications of diabetes, those that affect the eyes appear to be the most preventable through good diabetes management. A combination of good metabolic control, regular screening and vigilant management may reduce the risk of serious eye problems by more than two-thirds.

- Cataracts are two to five times more common in people with diabetes.
- Diabetic macular oedema is the major cause of vision loss in people with type 2 diabetes.
- It's often very hard to recognize that your own vision is declining.

Manage
- Maintain good control of your glucose, lipid and blood pressure levels.
- Get your eyes tested regularly by an eye expert (optometrist or ophthalmologist) so that interventions to protect the retina can be instituted in a timely manner when they are likely to be most effective.
- Report any sudden changes in your vision to your doctor or eye specialist as soon as possible.
- Don't just suffer dry or itchy eyes. Talk to your doctor about treatment options including drops or changes to your medication.

Clear and comfortable vision is easy to take for granted. Whether reading or working, driving or just watching television, good eyesight is very important to allow you to do the things you want to do.

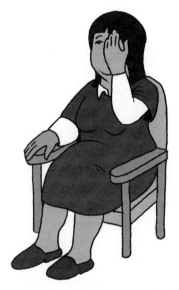

One of the things that most people know about type 2 diabetes is that it can affect your eyesight.

Diabetes is certainly a major cause of blindness in adults. However, diabetes seldom means going completely blind. Although this can rarely happen, the effects of diabetes on vision are usually more subtle. Rather than blocking an image entirely, diabetes more commonly reduces its qualities — its colour, its detail (contrast) and/or its sharpness (focus).

While the tissues of the eye are vulnerable to the effects of diabetes, at the same time, of all the complications of diabetes those that affect the eye appear to be the most preventable by good diabetes management.

A combination of good metabolic control, regular screening and vigilant management may reduce the risk of serious eye problems by more than two-thirds. Today, most people with type 2 diabetes retain excellent vision.

HOW DOES DIABETES AFFECT YOUR EYES?

To understand what diabetes can do to your eyes, it is first important to understand how the many different components of the eye contribute to your vision.

At its most basic, the eye works just like a digital camera. To get a clear image into your computer's memory (your brain), requires a number of steps. To take a clear photo with a camera, light must pass through the glass at the front that protects the inner workings of the camera. Light is then focused by the lens onto digital sensors at the back of the camera. This information is then packaged and relayed via cables back to the computer.

Roughly the same thing happens in the eye. For clear vision, light must pass through the cornea, the glassy dome on the front surface of the eye. It must be focused by the lens, and then activate the sensor (photoreceptor) cells of the retina. This information is then packaged and relayed via nerves back into the brain (computer).

Diabetes has the potential to disrupt any or all of these components and, with it, spoil the picture received by your brain.

Diabetes and the cornea

At the very front of the eye is a clear, glassy layer known as the cornea. This is just like the protective glass that covers the lens and workings of a camera. For the eye to work, this layer must be kept clean. Any smudges on the surface have the potential to distort images that reach the back of the eye.

Because your soft eye sticks out into the world, the front of the eye is normally very good at protecting itself from damage. A healthy eye is exquisitely sensitive to even the smallest speck of dust or a misplaced eyelash, causing you to tear up and blink rapidly until the irritation is cleared away.

Diabetes can sometimes affect the functions of the cornea (known as **keratopathy**). For example, diabetes often damages the nerves whose job it is to sense things that might be damaging. The same changes that lead to numbness in the feet (see Chapter 12) can also reduce the sensitivity of the eye to things that might damage it. And just like the feet, the cornea of people with diabetes is more prone to scratches, ulcers and infection. The cornea can also become thicker in people with type 2 diabetes, just like calluses on your feet that result from excessive pressure and repeated injury. At the same time, healing of the cornea may be slow in people with type 2 diabetes. This can represent a major problem after cataract surgery (see below).

Another common complication of diabetes is **dry eye syndrome**. As the name suggests, this results in your eyes becoming dry and easily irritated, making them feel itchy and burning, and more prone to becoming bloodshot. It can also make it hard to concentrate when reading, working or driving. Dry eyes are a common problem in all adults as they age, especially women, but they are far more common in people with type 2 diabetes. Tears normally form a thin film over the surface of the eye to protect the cornea from damage. Tear production lessens with age, and diabetes leads to a further reduction in the production and quality of tears, which makes dry eyes more likely. Certain medications used by people with diabetes (such as antidepressants, diuretics and some painkillers) also make dry eye more likely. But you don't have to put up with it. Dry eyes can be easily treated using eye drops (lubricants).

Diabetes and the aqueous humour

Between the cornea and the lens sits a thin layer of clear fluid, known as the **aqueous humour** (which is more like jelly than aqueous water). It is not merely a space-filler but plays an important role in maintaining the health of the eye. Its fluids provide nutrients and other useful things (such as antibodies and antioxidants) to the clear parts of the eye, where no blood vessels can go (otherwise they would get in the way of light and obstruct your vision).

This part of the eye also maintains the (low) pressure of the eyeball (of around 10–20mmHg), which ensures nutrients can flow freely into the eye. If pressure in the eye rises above this level, like pumping air into a balloon, it becomes harder and harder to fill and supply the eye with the factors it needs to remain healthy. Most vulnerable to any increase in pressure are the delicate nerves that relay signals from the retina to the brain. If pressure should rise in the eye, these nerves are the first to be damaged. This is known as **glaucoma**.

The most important risk factor for glaucoma is age. It is much more common in older people than younger ones. Glaucoma is also more commonly seen in women and in people with high blood pressure, migraine, short-sightedness or a family history of glaucoma. Diabetes may also increase the risk of glaucoma by damaging the blood vessels in the coloured portion of the eye (known as the iris) that control the drainage of aqueous humour from the eye and ultimately the pressure within the eyeball.

Glaucoma is usually painless. Nerve damage usually starts very gradually in the far corners of your eyesight (eventually producing what is known as **tunnel vision**). However, vision loss gradually works its way inward so that, like a silent thief, eventually all vision is ultimately lost if glaucoma goes untreated. Rarely, glaucoma can appear suddenly and painfully, if the outflow of the fluid from the eye is suddenly obstructed and pressure in the eyeball rapidly rises (known as **closed angle glaucoma**).

There are no simple ways to prevent glaucoma. However, it is possible for your eye specialist to detect raised pressure (greater than 20mmHg) in the eyeball using tonometry (see below). Sometimes characteristic changes of glaucoma can be seen in the back of the eye during a routine examination. If glaucoma is detected early enough, it is possible to slow its progression using eye drops (to reduce the production of aqueous humour and the pressure inside the eyeball) and pills. Laser treatments or surgery are sometimes also required to create a new passage for fluid to drain from the eye (known as trabeculoplasty).

Diabetes and the lens

Diabetes can also affect the lens in the eye. The lens sits in the middle of the eye and is about 1 cm in diameter. The job of the lens is to focus light coming into the eye by changing its shape/curvature (known as **accommodation**) so that any image that reaches the back of the eye is sharply defined with clear edges and contrast. When looking into the distance, the lens becomes long and flat. But when looking at objects close up, such as when reading or sewing, the lens must retract to become smaller and rounder to accurately focus the incoming light onto the retina.

Many people with type 2 diabetes experience blurring of their vision and/or difficulty in reading when their glucose control gets either better or worse. Often blurred vision is the first symptom of diabetes. This is not due to eye damage. In fact, these symptoms usually last only a month or two and settle once glucose levels are stable again. It is caused by changes in the focusing power of the lens, as the amount of stored sugars in the lens becomes mismatched with the amount of glucose in your blood. Although you might think you need a new pair of glasses, and these could help you to see for a short while, after a month or two you'll need a new prescription as your lens returns to balance. This is why it is recommended that you should only get glasses fitted when your glucose control is stable. Otherwise further changes in your glasses prescription may be needed.

A healthy lens is normally very elastic, allowing it to quickly and efficiently change shape. But with age the lens becomes progressively stiffer. And stiff lenses simply cannot easily change shape. This means the ability of the eye to focus on nearby objects also becomes progressively reduced (known as **short-sightedness** or **presbyopia**). Everyone will eventually have this problem to some extent as they get older.

Diabetes also makes the lens less flexible. So when ageing and diabetes combine, the result can be a more rapid decline in vision with age and/or problems beginning at a younger age. This progressive stiffening of the lens is a very slow process, so it may be hard to notice it yourself — sometimes it's only when people realize they are holding reading materials further and further away from them in order to focus. This is colloquially known as the 'short arm syndrome'. This is because, although holding books a little further away helps for a while, as the lens becomes stiffer you'll always need to hold things just a little bit further away. Eventually, your arms become 'too short' and some extra help is needed to focus on things close-up.

Lens stiffening does not always result in poor close-up vision. In some people, eyesight is maintained or may even improve as they get older (known as **second sight**). However, this does not mean that lens stiffening has not occurred. There's usually another factor at work, like being short-sighted to begin with, which means that instead of putting glasses on to read you now have to take your (distance) glasses off to see.

The most common treatment options for short-sightedness are to wear reading glasses, bifocals or contact lenses. Each of these treatments has its advantages and disadvantages, and is really a matter of individual preference. A number of new techniques have also been developed which can improve eyesight and help you avoid glasses or contacts. These are collectively known as **refractive surgery** and include surgically replacing the damaged lens, as well as newer techniques like inlays and laser therapy. The most common form of refractive surgery is known as **monovision**, where one eye is corrected for reading and other close-up work and the other eye is left to see things clearly in the distance. This can work quite well, but it does not work for everyone. Some people can feel uncomfortable with the changes in their vision as a result of this procedure.

The same changes that make the lens stiffer can also make the lens less transparent. This is known as a **cataract**. Cataracts are very common in everyone as they get older. At least half of all people will experience a degree of vision loss due to cataracts at some time in their life. But again, diabetes acts to speed up this process and increase its severity, so that cataracts are at least twice as common in people with type 2 diabetes.

Most cataracts are small and cause no or few symptoms like short-sightedness. They are often incidentally detected during routine eye examinations. Other early symptoms of a cataract may include things appearing less vivid with less contrast, especially in low light, as the cataract scatters the light entering your eye. Some people with cataracts also have difficulty telling colours apart, like blue and green, or may experience glare with bright lights, such as when driving at night. Eventually, cataracts can obstruct the passage of light into the eye and block your vision. Typically both eyes are affected, but usually one side is worse than the other.

Apart from age and diabetes, other factors also make cataracts more likely including cigarette smoking, excessive alcohol use, the use of steroids (as tablets but not as an inhaler for asthma) and excessive exposure to ultraviolet light (from sunshine or tanning lamps). Consequently, wearing sunglasses, wearing a brimmed hat and avoiding direct sunlight during the peak hours of ultraviolet radiation are important ways to reduce your risk of future cataracts, as well as other problems, such as skin cancer and wrinkles.

There are no medications or supplements that are able to prevent cataracts. Good diabetes control is able to modestly reduce your likelihood of developing cataracts but will not completely prevent them.

Surgery is currently the only cure for cataracts. The good news is that cataract surgery can restore working vision in most cases if it should ever get that bad. The procedure is relatively simple and is done one eye at a time. The most common form of surgery removes the damaged part of the lens (known as **lens extraction**) and replaces it with a synthetic substitute. However, synthetic lenses are not as flexible as a healthy human lens, so they tend to provide good vision only for either distance or close up, but not both. It is usually still necessary to use reading glasses for close work (or distance glasses to focus in the distance). Cataract surgery in people with diabetes can also increase the risk of macular oedema (a serious eye problem detailed later in this chapter). This means that your eyes must be very closely monitored if you have just had cataract surgery and treated pre-emptively with lasers at the first sign of trouble.

Diabetes and the retina

At the back of the eye there is a complex layer of sensor cells whose job it is to detect minute changes in the intensity and/or colour of light. This layer is called the **retina** and is the equivalent of film in a camera. This information is then transmitted to other cells in the retina, encoded (packaged) and then relayed back to the brain via nerve fibres which, in effect, connect the camera to the computer.

There are two main types of sensor cells, known as **rod cells** and **cone cells** because of their unique shapes. Each eye contains over 100 million rod cells, whose job it is to work in low light, to tell the difference between light and dark. They are very sensitive to light, so don't provide much help to your vision during the day. But at night or in dim light, these rod cells are the most important in determining whether or not you can see.

There are also about 7 million cone cells in each eye. The cones respond to bright daylight and take care of high-resolution colour vision. But unlike the rods, they are not sensitive enough to work in the dark. This is why things look almost black and white at night. However, the amount of light in most homes means that both rods and cones contribute to what you are able to see at night-time. There are blue, green and red cones which are each sensitive to light at different wavelengths. If you are born missing one of these types of cells, you are **colour blind**.

Different parts of the retina have different functions because of the make-up of rod and cone cells and their density of packing. In the middle of the retina where light is most focused (known as the **fovea**), cone cells that specialize in sharp detail and colour are densely packed in a hexagonal mosaic pattern, very much like a honeycomb. If diabetes damages these cone-rich parts of the eye or scatters the light reaching the centre, then one of the earliest signs is a reduction in colour vision or discrimination between colours.

The further out you go from the centre of the eye, the less dense the sensor cells are packed and the more the rod cells, which specialize in detecting small amounts of light under low light conditions, become the dominant type of cell. Damage to these areas will therefore preferentially affect your night vision.

The health of the retina is partly determined by the capacity of the small blood vessels in the eye to supply enough nutrients and oxygen for cells to survive. Type 2 diabetes is able to progressively damage these tiny blood vessels. These changes can be observed when looking into the eye. For example:

- Weakened walls of blood vessels can balloon out (to form **microaneurysms**).
- Weakened blood vessels can leak fat and fluid. These can look like tiny white flecks in the back of the eye (known as **hard exudates**).
- Damaged vessels are also very fragile and prone to bleed spontaneously (known as a **blot haemorrhage**).
- Damaged blood vessels also mean a reduced supply of oxygen and nutrients to parts of the retina (known as **ischaemia**). This can also disrupt the flow of nutrients along the nerves, which instead can build up and look like tiny wads of cotton wool in the retina (and are appropriately known as **cotton wool spots**).

Even with the best glucose control, it is normal for most people with type 2 diabetes to develop a small number of haemorrhages, exudates, spots and/or aneurysms in their retina (cumulatively known as **background retinopathy**).

The longer you have had diabetes, the more likely that some changes will be seen in the retina.

In general, these 'background' changes do not interfere with vision unless they become concentrated around the macula, where sensory cells are most densely packed. This may lead to swelling of the retina (known as **diabetic macular oedema** or **DME**), which can have serious consequences for eyesight. In fact, macular oedema is the most frequent cause of vision loss in people with diabetes. Without treatment approximately half of those who develop macular oedema will go on to lose at least two lines of reading on a chart over the next two years.

Since the macula is densely packed with cone cells, which provide fine detail and colour sensitivity, people with macular oedema may experience blurring of both distant and close-up vision, as well as difficulties in telling the difference between some colours. Although vision loss may appear to be rapid in those experiencing macular oedema, the processes that lead to macular oedema and vision loss are relatively slow and are often not perceptible until the very centre of the vision is itself affected at the fovea. Consequently, regular comprehensive eye examinations are important for the prevention of vision loss, so that interventions to protect the retina can be instituted in a timely manner when they are likely to be most effective. Some of these treatments may include the following.

- Focal laser treatment, where a laser beam is fired to help get rid of excess fluid or destroy unhealthy areas that promote the growth of new blood vessels. While this can slow vision loss, it rarely provides significant improvement to eyesight.
- Surgery, where part of the gel of the eye is removed and replaced with clear fluid. This is generally

reserved for those with severe haemorrhages or detachment that threatens the macula.

- Injections with selective antibodies that block the growth of new blood vessels which leak fluid into the retina.
- Injections of steroids into the eye that reduce leakage from damaged vessels. Although effective, this treatment may be associated with an increased risk of cataracts and raised pressure in the eyeball (see above).

When damaged blood vessels become blocked, this sometimes also triggers the growth of new blood vessels in the eye (known as **neovascularisation**) in an attempt to bypass the blockage and restore the flow of oxygen and nutrients. But far from being helpful, these new vessels promote scarring and even more damage to the retina (known as **proliferative retinopathy**).

The appearance of new blood vessels in the eye is also commonly managed by laser treatment, in which the unhealthy areas that promote their growth are cauterised using a high intensity beam of light. Typically, over a thousand tiny burns are made across the retina. This is generally not painful, although some people may experience discomfort which can be lessened with an injection of anaesthetic behind the eye.

The new vessels themselves are not targeted by the laser. Rather, the energy hungry rods and cones are destroyed, meaning there is more oxygen to go round and the signals to make new blood vessels are reduced. Without these signals, any new blood vessels stop growing and often partly or completely disappear. However, because the laser destroys some of the rod and cone cells, which detect incoming light in the eye, some loss of vision can occur with widespread treatment. For example, some people who have had laser therapy to their eyes complain of reduced peripheral vision, impaired night vision and/or lower contrast in their eyesight.

Rarely, the growth of new vessels continues despite laser therapy. In order to prevent more severe damage, in such cases surgery may be necessary to preserve or restore vision (known as **vitrectomy**). This involves removing part of the gel of the eye and replacing it with clear fluid.

As scar tissue associated with the growth of new vessels shrinks, it can sometimes pull and distort the retina, cause swelling (oedema) or, rarely, pull it right off the eyeball (known as **detachment**). These new vessels are also very fragile and prone to bleed spontaneously (or haemorrhage). This can sometimes lead to the appearance of dark spots in your vision, as clots in the retina block the light coming into the retina. Bleeding into the eye itself (known as a **vitreal haemorrhage**) can give the appearance of floating lines or webs. Very rarely, bleeding is so significant as to obstruct most of the light entering the eye, like a shade in front of your vision, so that only the difference between light and dark may be seen by the affected eye. For anyone with diabetes, these kinds of sudden changes in vision constitute a real medical emergency. Seeing your doctor or eye specialist cannot be put off until tomorrow.

Macular degeneration

Diabetes is not the only thing that can affect the retina as you get older. One of the most common causes of declining vision is **age-related macular degeneration** (AMD). AMD is caused by the accumulation of focal deposits (known as **drusen**) in the macula part of the retina. An in-growth of fragile blood vessels (that are also opaque) in response to the drusen further accelerates damage to the macula and ultimately leads to some loss of vision.

Again, because the macula is affected, AMD usually leads to problems in your central vision, detail, contrast and colour sensitivity. It does not lead to total blindness, as the macula only comprises a small part of the retina and the remaining (peripheral) retina remains unaffected. Usually, enough peripheral vision remains for you to see, so people often just dismiss AMD as a 'touch of old age'. But the loss of central vision can have a major effect on your functioning. For example, it may not be possible to read or recognize faces without central vision, although you will see they are there.

There are several risk factors for the development and progression of AMD. The most important is age. Around one-third of octogenarians have AMD. However, obesity, smoking, high blood pressure and high cholesterol levels also make AMD more likely as you age.

Although diabetes does not cause AMD directly, AMD is more common in people with type 2 diabetes because they are often overweight and have increased levels of blood pressure and cholesterol.

There is also some evidence that vision declines earlier and faster in people with AMD and type 2 diabetes than in those without diabetes.

The current treatment for macular degeneration involves laser therapy, although new options are being increasingly explored, including injections with selective antibodies or drugs that block the growth of new blood vessels. While these treatments may prevent further vision loss, at present no treatment is able to restore damaged nerves to the eye or improve eyesight once lost.

PREVENTING EYE DAMAGE IN DIABETES

Many of the things you are already doing as part of your routine diabetes management will be improving the health of your eyes, as well of other aspects of your health. There is good evidence that the techniques to control blood glucose levels and optimize lipid and blood pressure levels will reduce the risk of developing eye problems associated with diabetes. Some blood pressure-lowering drugs such as ACE inhibitors and angiotensin-receptor blockers may have additional advantages for preventing eye damage over other drugs (see Chapter 6). But even when you are on the right medications, and your glucose, lipids and other risk factors for eye problems are under control, it is still possible for diabetes to affect your eyes. This is why everyone with type 2 diabetes should get their eyes checked on a regular basis.

Regular eye examinations

It's often hard to recognize that your own vision is declining. This is why regular testing of your vision is an extremely important part of routine diabetes management.

Getting your eyes examined regularly by an eye expert (an optometrist or ophthalmologist) is the most important thing you can do to protect your eyesight. Don't wait until you notice problems with your vision. In diabetes, the damage to your eyes is insidious. There is no pain and few symptoms.

An eye examination should be done at least every year in people with type 2 diabetes, even if their vision is normal. Eye examinations will need to be performed more frequently if you have an increased risk of eye complications (e.g. if you already have early signs of damage, high blood pressure or kidney disease). An eye examination is a simple, painless procedure that is performed by your eye care specialist. A complete eye check-up may include the following.

- Examining the back of your eye (the retina). To do this, your pupils may need to be dilated with eye drops so that the entire retina can be examined in detail and sometimes photographed, to allow easy comparison with previous results. These drops can sometimes make your vision blurry for a short time, so don't drive from your appointment. Dilated pupils also make you more sensitive to bright light. This can be prevented by briefly wearing your sunglasses.
- Testing your visual acuity (e.g. letter charts).
- Testing the coordinated movement of your eyes in all directions (e.g. following a light).
- Cataract evaluation (e.g. shining a light into your eye and observing the 'red eye' reflection light bouncing off your retina).
- Testing the pressure in your eyeball (known as **tonometry**) to check for early signs of glaucoma).
- Checking your colour and night vision with special charts.
- Checking the health of the macula using an Amsler grid test. This involves staring at a black dot which sits inside a grid of intersecting lines. In healthy vision, all the lines around the dot will look straight and evenly spaced. If the lines appear bent, distorted or missing, then the macula is not doing its job.

Although most emerging problems can be picked up in a routine eye examination, sometimes things can change rapidly in your eyes. If this should ever happen, it is very important to report any sudden changes in your vision to your doctor or eye specialist as soon as possible. The early detection of sight-threatening changes in your eyes is very important, because it usually allows something to be done about it. There are a number of effective treatments for eye damage that are able to help preserve your eyesight. These treatments are most effective when damage is caught in its early stages. Don't ever shut your eyes to problems with your diabetes.

12

DIABETES ON MY FEET

Understand

- Changes in your feet are a common complication of longstanding type 2 diabetes, reflecting a reduced ability to heal combined with an increased propensity to become damaged.
- Foot ulcers precede at least eight out of every ten lower limb amputations in people with type 2 diabetes, so are worth preventing.
- Diabetes slowly causes damage to the nerves supplying the feet and lower legs, making them numb to injury, damaging pressure or rubbing from footwear.

- Damage to the nerves may also make the muscles in the foot weak or uncoordinated which can lead to deformities such as bunions, hammer toes or claw toes.
- Serious foot problems don't occur in everyone with diabetes, but extra special care should be taken in those people at high risk of developing a foot ulcer.

Manage
- Control glucose, lipids and blood pressure, and stop smoking to reduce your risk of complications from diabetes in your feet and everywhere else.
- Understand your personal risk for foot problems from diabetes, and the intensity with which you need to protect your feet.
- Don't go barefoot if you can avoid it. Without sensation you can't always rely on your feet to tell you when they are

in harm's way.

- Report any changes in your feet to your doctor or foot specialist as soon as they are identified. Don't ignore them and hope they will go away by themselves. Certainly don't try to treat them yourself.
- Take care of your toenails or get someone to do this for you.

Diabetes is important everywhere in the human body and nowhere more so than in your feet. While much is made of the amorous heart and the more glamorous brain, what gets you where you need to go is your connection with your feet. Looking after this part of your health can keep you mobile, independent and on your toes. In many cultures, the foot is regarded as an object of veneration. So should it be in diabetes.

Foot care is a key component of all diabetes management.

Changes in your feet are a common complication of type 2 diabetes. They reflect a reduced ability to heal, combined with an increased tendency to get damaged. The most dangerous changes result from a breakdown in the barrier formed by the skin, letting the dirty outside world under your skin and into your body. These may include cracks, fissures and foot ulcers (where the skin is completely lost over one particular area). One in seven adults with type 2 diabetes will develop a foot ulcer during their lifetime. Preventing foot ulcers is a top priority. This is because at least eight out of every ten lower limb amputations in people with type 2 diabetes start off with a foot ulcer. However, most foot ulcers are preventable by meticulous care of your feet.

When identified and treated early, most foot complications are also manageable.

WHY DOES DIABETES DAMAGE YOUR FEET?

Diabetes can make it more likely that you get foot ulcers and other foot complications in a number of different ways (usually in disastrous combination).

Diabetes slowly causes damage to the nerves supplying the feet and lower legs (known as **neuropathy**). This can make them numb to injury, damaging pressure or rubbing from footwear (known as loss of **'protective' sensation**). Nerve damage usually goes undetected, as it's hard to be aware of what you can't feel. However, some people experience numbness in their feet, as if wearing 'socks' or 'stockings'. Nerve damage can also sometimes be painful, producing a 'pins and needles' or burning sensation in your feet, which is often worse at night.

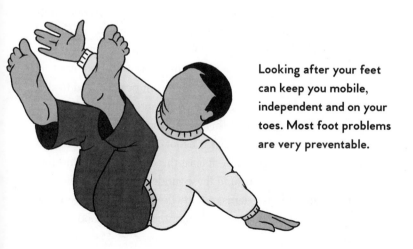

Looking after your feet can keep you mobile, independent and on your toes. Most foot problems are very preventable.

The presence of significant nerve damage may be identified by your doctor using simple clinical tools to examine if your feet can feel them or not:

- a small filament or wire may be used to test your sense of light touch
- a tuning fork may be used to test your sense of vibration
- a pin prick may be used to test your sense of sharpness
- warm and cold metal objects may be used to test your sense of cold.

A test of reflexes at the ankles is also sometimes performed. This is done by lightly striking the back of your ankle with a rubber hammer and seeing how the foot moves in response.

Some or all of these tests should be performed annually in people with type 2 diabetes to identify those who have lost their 'protective sensation', in whom a more meticulous program of foot care should be arranged (detailed later in this chapter).

Damage to the nerves may also make the muscles in the foot weak or uncoordinated. This can lead to bunions, hammer toes, claw toes or other changes in the shape of your feet (collectively known as **deformities**). These deformities create unnatural stresses and pressures on your feet, especially as your feet now don't fit into your shoes in quite the same way they used to. The extra pressure that arises from deformities can lead to skin thickening on the foot and cause corns and calluses, as well as blisters. Each is a sign that this area of the foot is being exposed to extra pressure. Overall, having a foot deformity increases your risk of getting a foot ulcer by at least threefold. In fact, most foot ulcers occur under or around these (under pressure) areas.

Diabetes can also damage both the small and large blood vessels that supply the feet, reducing the flow of blood, oxygen and sustaining nutrients to what is the furthest reach of your circulation. This is sometimes experienced as intermittent pain in the legs when walking (known as **claudication**) which is relieved by resting or elevating your feet. However, many people (possibly the majority) with poor circulation will not have any pain, especially if nerve damage is also present. The first sign may be a foot ulcer. Poor circulation can sometimes be detected by your doctor if they are unable to feel pulses in the feet or ankles, or hear blood flow in your feet using an ultrasound (Doppler) test.

Swelling of your feet (known as **oedema**) is sometimes seen in people with diabetes, especially those with kidney or heart problems, as well as those using some blood pressure-lowering medications. This makes your feet larger and tighter in your shoes (causing more rubbing and increasing the chances of getting a foot ulcer); in addition, swelling can sometimes become tight enough to reduce blood flow to the feet as well as interfere with healing.

Diabetes can also change the skin covering your feet, making it thicker, drier, less resilient and more prone to blisters or cracks (especially at the heel). Nerve damage can also reduce sweating in the feet. Areas of abnormally thick, dry skin (known as **calluses**) often form over areas of your feet that are subjected to extra pressure, such as alongside the big toe or under your heel. When these areas of thick, hard skin are compressed with walking or standing, they put even more pressure on the soft tissues underneath, causing further damage.

Visual impairment associated with diabetes (see Chapter 11) also makes minor trauma to the feet more likely to occur and less likely to be recognized early.

Finally, diabetes also increases susceptibility to **infection of**

the skin, by both reducing the ability to fight off bugs that get into the skin and deeper tissues through cracks or ulcers in the feet or into the toenails. Fungal infections usually start in the toenails or between the fourth and fifth toes, where the space is most compacted by pressure. These can set up local infections that, if left untreated, can spread. At its most severe, tissues in your feet can, rarely, be killed by infection (known as **gangrene**).

WHAT SHOULD YOU DO TO PROTECT YOUR FEET?

Many of the things you are already doing as part of your routine diabetes management will be improving the health of your feet, as well as other aspects of your health. These include optimal control of glucose, lipids and blood pressure, and smoking cessation. These are important for preventing complications of diabetes, everywhere. But it is especially the case for your feet.

Foot ulcers are not an inevitable part of diabetes. In fact, they only occur in a minority of people. This means that for most people with type 2 diabetes, nothing special is required to stay out of harm's way beyond common sense and regular assessment of the state of your feet with your diabetes care team. However, there are some people in whom foot ulcers are far more likely and for whom more can and should be done. This includes:

- people who have currently or have previously had foot problems (e.g. ulcers, calluses, deformities such as claw toes)
- people who have lost protective sensation in their feet
- people who have poor circulation to their feet
- people who have other complications from their diabetes.

In such people a formal program of foot care is appropriate, including some or all of the following.

Fastidious hygiene

People with type 2 diabetes who are at increased risk for foot problems should carefully wash their feet every day. However, they shouldn't soak them or put them in hot water.

Moist areas, such as between the toes, should then be dried carefully to reduce the risk of maceration or infection. Antifungal powders or talc may be useful in some people to keep moist areas dry and free of infection.

Moisturize dry areas

For dry areas of skin, like the heel and the outside of the foot, there is value in keeping the skin flexible and soft to prevent cracking. This can simply be achieved by regularly applying a non-alcohol-containing moisturiser to these areas.

Safety first

Check shoes for stones, sticks and other foreign objects that might hurt your feet, every time you put on your shoes. Without sensation you can't always rely on your feet to tell you when they are in harm's way. Many ulcers come from unnecessarily going barefoot. It may be just a short dash to the clothesline, but it's simply not worth the risk if you accidently tread on something sharp. You may feel uncomfortable or different when everyone else is barefoot. But it's important.

The right shoes

Many ulcers come simply from wearing poorly fitting or worn out shoes that rub the skin or cause pressure. Those at risk of ulcers should always wear shoes that are properly fitted to the shape of their own foot. Don't just go off the shoe size; it is invariably wrong. Only if the shoe fits should you wear it. A good fitting shoe is not when your foot fills the entire space. When buying a shoe, your longest toe should be no less than 1.5 cm (½ in) from the end of the shoe, to provide sufficient room for the toes to move when you walk. The ball of your foot should also correspond to the widest part of the shoe. Watch out for slip-ons — they are designed to be tight on the skin and toes (so they don't slip off!). Much better are laces or Velcro straps, which can be loosened according to the needs of your feet and tend to provide more room for the toes. They can also be loosened as the day goes on and the feet swell a bit. Shoes should be bought later in the day when feet have swelled, so the shoes will definitely accommodate and fit correctly.

Speciality shoe stores are usually better equipped than discount or department stores, which have often never heard about diabetes or think that shoes are just a fashion item. Many diabetes clinics now have foot specialists (podiatrists) who can help you to order the right shoes for your feet.

Therapeutic shoes look like any other shoe from the outside, but have a number of refinements that help to keep your feet healthy. These include:

- thick cushioning cork or pre-fabricated insoles that can be customised to your feet
- extra depth (or in-depth) to give more room for your toes
- rocker soles which decrease the pressure on the ball of the foot.

Extra cushioning (known as an **orthotic** or **orthotic insert**) can be useful if you have an increased risk of foot problems.

For example, if you have a callus on your foot this may be a sign of excessive pressure being placed at this point. To prevent it becoming an ulcer, orthotics can be made to specifically take the pressure off this area of skin.

The right socks

The right socks can also be important for keeping your skin dry and cool. Acrylic socks that are not tight/elastic and don't have rough seams can be useful for keeping the feet dry and cool. Some socks also have special padding. Always wear clean socks and throw out damaged, tight, frayed or thin, old ones.

Toenail care

Many foot problems begin in and around the toenails. This is partly because nails are hard and skin is soft. If the toes are placed under pressure, it is the skin that suffers the most. Thickened nails or sharp edges that dig in (without you feeling it) are often the opportunity infection needs to get started.

It is recommended that all people with type 2 diabetes should keep their toenails short by regularly having them trimmed, by themselves or others. This should always be straight across following the curve of your toes, but not too short to reduce the risk of in-grown nails. File any sharp edges with an emery board or nail file. Always have a podiatrist do this if you need help or are unsure, or can't see or reach the toes very well.

Keep a close eye on your feet

Inspect your feet every day for early signs of trouble or potential problem areas. Don't forget to check between your toes. Sometimes a mirror is helpful to see the entire bottom of your feet. Don't be afraid to show your doctor your feet. It's not unclean or rude. It may only take a few seconds to give you the all-clear but it could be life-saving.

It is also very important to report any changes in your feet to your doctor or foot specialist as soon as they are identified. Don't ignore them and hope they will go away. Certainly, don't ever wait for them to become painful. Some warning signs that there is something potentially problematic going on in your feet include:

- redness or skin discolouration, especially around corns or calluses
- swelling or change in the size or shape of your foot or ankle
- pain in the feet or legs at rest or while walking (but remember that you don't need to be feeling any pain for there to be a serious problem)
- blisters
- bleeding
- open sores (ulcers), no matter how small!
- hot or cold spots.

Avoid home remedies

Thinning areas of thick skin (a callus) on your feet can take the pressure off the skin that lies underneath. But this is not a task to be undertaken in your own 'bathroom surgery' or with over-the-counter 'corn cures'. Foot specialists (known as **podiatrists**) who have training in the management of the diabetic foot are widely available in most diabetes clinics and should be used in any situation where preventive management is appropriate.

HOW ARE FOOT ULCERS TREATED?

Each foot ulcer is different. Should one occur, it will need to be assessed and managed differently depending on the depth of the wound, the presence or absence of infection and healthy blood flow. This is a complex and delicate process and is best coordinated by wound specialists, often acting as part of a multidisciplinary team involving doctors, wound management nurses, podiatrists and other allied health professionals.

All ulcers will require regular cleaning and any dead skin and foreign material to be removed from the wound (a process known as **debridement**). Dressings are then used to create and maintain an optimal environment for healing, as well as to protect the wound from further damage. There are many different dressings available, all of which will be appropriate to different situations, including saline, disinfectants, gels and ointments.

If you have an ulcer, your doctor will often advise you to rest and limit your walking. This is not some idle request. Staying off your feet is sometimes vital for effective healing. Continued pressure to the bed of a wound can prolong healing or sometimes result in even more damage. It may seem excessive to be on crutches, using a walker or a wheelchair for just a little ulcer, but the complications of a non-healing ulcer may be far worse.

In many cases **off-loading devices** (such as padding, therapeutic shoes, orthotics, casts, walking aids, etc.) can relieve the pressure on ulcers and help with healing while you are maintaining your regular daily activities. Some can even be taken off at night or for a bath. Their only problem is that any walking without the cast, even for a short distance, can undo all the good of having rested your foot.

Antibiotics will sometimes be used to help an infection heal and prevent it from spreading. Antibiotic cream might be placed directly on the wound, tablets might be taken or an injection given. Antibiotic therapy on its own is always insufficient to heal an ulcer. And it's important to realize you can't just use any old antiseptic cream from the bathroom cabinet to fix such foot problems — some of these may be too strong for the feet of someone with diabetes and may do more harm than good. Antibiotic treatment is usually continued until there is evidence that the infection has resolved, but not necessarily until the ulcer has healed.

Surgery is sometimes necessary to help foot ulcers heal. This includes procedures to improve your circulation or to correct deformities. Very rarely, **amputation** of part or all of the foot may be necessary to save the rest of the foot or leg from gangrene. In most cases this outcome can be prevented.

13

DIABETES IN MY KIDNEYS

Understand

- The kidneys perform many important tasks in keeping you healthy that allow your heart, brain, bone and many other parts of your body to do the jobs they are supposed to do.

- At least every second person with type 2 diabetes has kidney damage, manifested by increased amounts of albumin in the urine and/or a reduced ability to filter the blood.

- Having kidney disease puts you at increased risk of other complications from type 2 diabetes, including heart, foot and eye disease and hypoglycaemia.

- Good glucose, lipid and blood pressure control in someone with type 2 diabetes can reduce the risk of kidney problems by over half.

- Although it is possible to have dialysis or sometimes receive a new kidney, the health of such people is sadly never as good as those who have their own kidneys functioning.

Manage

- Achieve and maintain good glucose control to keep your kidneys functioning for longer.

- Treat high blood pressure levels and maintain smooth control over them to protect your kidneys as much as your heart.

- Get even more serious about keeping your lipid levels under control. The most common serious complication of failing kidney function is heart disease, and

this can be partly prevented by good
lipid control.

- Get your kidney function checked at
  least annually.
- Encourage your friends and family to
  become organ donors. For those who
  develop kidney failure, this generous
  gift may be the gift of life.

The kidneys perform many important tasks to keep you healthy. You even have a spare one to make sure there is always enough capacity to deal with any extra demands and stand as insurance against any loss of function. In essence, good kidney function enables your heart, brain, bone and many other parts of your body to do the job they are supposed to do.

Impaired kidney function is a drag on everything else. The risks of heart, feet and eye problems, hypoglycaemia and many other complications are all increased in people with impaired kidney function.

The kidneys do their job partly by filtering the blood. Adults have about five litres (1 gal) of blood pumping around their body all the time. Every minute, about 1 litre (2pt) of this blood passes through the kidneys. Consequently, every five minutes all of the blood in the body has been filtered through the kidneys.

The filtered fluid then passes along a series of small tubes (or tubules) where any vital components (such as salt, water and glucose) are reabsorbed, leaving behind only waste (urine). This selective reabsorption system is so efficient that for every litre of blood that is filtered, less than a teaspoon of urine is made.

These tubules also actively secrete a number of toxins into the urine, to get rid of even more than could be filtered at any one time.

The kidneys' main priority is maintaining a strict balance of fluid inside the body. If only a small amount of fluid is drunk, the kidneys' priority is to keep hold of as much as possible, so urine production is reduced and the urine becomes more concentrated. Equally, if you drink a lot of fluid, the kidneys are able to release more water into the urine, which becomes lighter and more dilute. Either way, the amount of fluid in the body scarcely changes.

Often an early sign of diabetes may be passing urine more frequently, with more urgency, or having to get out of bed at night to go the toilet. This loss of bodily fluid makes you thirsty and as a result you also tend to drink more. In traditional Ayurvedic medicine, diabetes was known as *madhumeha*, from *madhu* (meaning sweet) and *meha* (meaning excessive urination).

When glucose levels in the blood are under control, any glucose that is filtered through the kidneys is very rapidly reabsorbed by the tubules so as not to waste this essential source of energy for your brain. However, the capacity for reabsorption in the kidneys is limited. After all, it should not be the kidneys' job to control glucose levels. And when glucose levels in the blood get any higher than 11 mmol/L (200 mg/dL), equivalent to an HbA1c >9 per cent (>75mmol/mol), too much glucose is filtered into the urine for the kidneys to pull it all back. So glucose spills over into the urine, dragging extra water with it. So even if you are dehydrated, the urine of someone with type 2 diabetes and poor glucose control can be surprisingly dilute, voluminous and frequent.

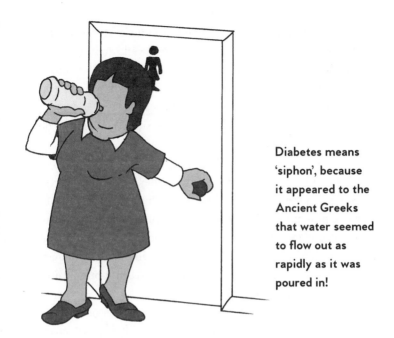

Diabetes means 'siphon', because it appeared to the Ancient Greeks that water seemed to flow out as rapidly as it was poured in!

Passing more urine is not a sign that your kidneys are damaged. In fact, it is a sign that your kidneys are doing their job. If you are able to get your glucose levels under control and maintain your HbA1c <8 per cent (<64 mmol/mol) for most of the time, then the twin problems of passing more urine and feeling thirsty will usually settle on their own.

HOW DOES KIDNEY DAMAGE AFFECT YOUR HEALTH?

Diabetes may result in damage to many parts of the kidney. The filter units of the kidney (known as glomeruli) are especially vulnerable. The kidneys usually have over a million of them.

They function in much the same way as a sieve: they hold onto the big things inside the blood (such as cells and big proteins) but allow the water (and any dissolved toxins) to filter down into the tubules and out into the urine. Like the damage to a sieve, damage to glomeruli can have two major effects:

- things can get through the sieve (and end up down the drain)
- the sieve gets clogged and it can't filter properly.

This is exactly what happens in the kidneys of people with type 2 diabetes. Firstly, instead of staying on the blood side of the filter, some proteins can leak into the urine (like pasta falling through a broken sieve and into the sink). The most common protein in your blood is **albumin**. So an early sign of kidney damage in diabetes is the presence of small amounts of albumin in your urine (known as **microalbuminuria**).

There is no pain or symptoms associated with microalbuminuria, so its detection relies on regular screening and urine testing (see below). About one-third of those with type 2 diabetes have elevated amounts of albumin in their urine. However, microalbuminuria is even more common in those who also have high glucose, high blood pressure and/or high cholesterol levels, as well those with established complications elsewhere (e.g. heart disease, eye, nerve or foot disease).

Secondly, just like a sieve, the filters of the kidney can progressively clog and become scarred over, reducing the ability of your body to filter fluid and clear toxins from the blood. This is a slow process and doesn't affect all filter units all at once. But any loss of filtering capacity means that the others have to take up the slack and work harder. This in turn causes them to burn out faster, causing more loss and more work for those remaining in a vicious circle. So by the time your kidney function becomes impaired it means that you have lost at least one kidney's worth of function. One in four people with type 2 diabetes will lose this much or more.

Although some decline in kidney function with age is inevitable, some people with type 2 diabetes are more likely to experience a more rapid fall in kidney function, including:

- people losing large amounts of albumin into their urine (as a marker of kidney disease and its severity)
- people whose blood pressure is very high and isn't easily controlled with standard medications
- people with heart disease
- people with eye problems from their diabetes
- people with foot problems from their diabetes
- people with anaemia (as a marker of kidney disease and its severity)
- people with an indigenous ethnic background
- people experiencing socioeconomic disadvantage.

As the function of the kidneys declines, to make up for any shortfall the kidneys send out signals to drive up the blood pressure. This is much like giving a car extra revs to get up a hill. The extra pressure means that more filtering can get done with fewer filters. However, this is at the expense of **hypertension**. This extra work also means they wear out faster.

One of the ways the kidneys increase **blood pressure** is by holding back more fluid from entering the urine. In addition to increasing blood pressure, this extra fluid can also lead to swelling of your legs or around your eyes (known as **oedema**). Fluid retention can also make some blood pressure-lowering medications less effective in people with impaired kidney function or increase the need for other medications that help you lose this excess fluid (known as **diuretics**).

Impaired kidney function also drives up lipid levels in the blood, which combines with high blood pressure and fluid retention to at least double the risk of heart attacks, strokes and other complications in people with type 2 diabetes who also have kidney disease.

The clearance of many medicines used to treat diabetes is also affected by impaired kidney function. Instead of being removed by the kidneys, these drugs hang around longer than they are really needed. This can sometimes mean more side effects from medications in those with impaired kidney function. For example, the kidneys filter and remove insulin from the body. But if kidney function is impaired, insulin stays around for longer, increasing the chances it will lower glucose levels too far and cause **hypoglycaemia**. So having kidney disease often means you need very careful assessment and use of the medications you are on in order to prevent any unwanted side effects.

The kidneys do much more than just pass water (and any dissolved toxins). The kidneys also regulate the levels of calcium in your bones. Damage to your kidneys can also result in bone thinning (known as **osteoporosis**), which when combined with normal thinning with age can increase your risk of fractures.

The kidneys also regulate the level of red cells in the blood, whose job it is to carry oxygen to all parts of your body for fuel. Damage to your kidneys will therefore sometimes reduce the concentration of red cells in the blood (known as anaemia), which is detected by a simple blood test.

HOW IS KIDNEY DISEASE DETECTED?

Regular examination of kidney function by your doctor can help identify early signs of trouble. This should be done annually in all people with type 2 diabetes, or more often if you have increased risk of kidney complications (e.g. if you already have early signs of kidney damage, high blood pressure or eye disease). This involves two separate tests, the glomerular filtration rate (GFR) and testing the level of albumin in the urine.

The glomerular filtration rate (GFR)

The GFR is estimated from the results of a standard blood test that measures the concentration of creatinine, an abundant natural chemical that is filtered and cleared by the kidneys. As kidney function declines, the level of creatinine rises in the blood. The amount by which it rises can be used to determine how far the filtration functions of the kidneys have fallen.

Albumin in the urine

The most practical test measures the amount of albumin in a urine sample from the first or second time you go to the toilet in the morning. Measurements of albumin in random urine samples (known as spot tests) are more variable and may be less accurate in determining your risks. Some doctors prefer to measure albumin in urine collected over 24 hours to document the total amount of albumin lost over the course of a day.

There is also normally substantial day-to-day variability in the amount of albumin in any one person's urine. For this reason an initial assessment of someone with type 2 diabetes will usually involve at least three urine tests taken over the first three to six months.

Once a level of albumin in the urine is established, further screening of kidney function can be undertaken annually. If normal amounts of albumin are detected at subsequent testing in someone with previously negative tests, they can simply be retested annually as part of routine assessment for complications, as it is unlikely that significant kidney problems have been missed. However, any new positive test is usually confirmed with additional tests performed during the subsequent three to six months.

HOW IS KIDNEY DISEASE PREVENTED AND TREATED?

Although kidney damage is very common in people with diabetes, in most cases it is possible to prevent serious decline in function or complete kidney failure. All of the different aspects of diabetes care will protect your kidneys from damage, and when performed together in someone with type 2 diabetes they can reduce your risk of kidney problems by over half.

Maintaining good control of your glucose

There is a strong association between how well you are able to control your glucose levels and your risk of kidney disease.

Achieving and maintaining glycaemic targets through a combination of healthy diet, regular exercise and medication significantly reduces the chances you will develop kidney disease.

Beyond their actions to lower glucose levels in the blood, some new medications such as SGLT-2 inhibitors, DPP-4 inhibitors and GLP receptor agonists also protect the kidney from damage. These kidney-protecting effects see such agents preferred in people at risk of kidney disease.

Maintaining good control of your lipids

High lipid levels are not just bad for the heart, but may be damaging to kidneys as well. Over and above their effects on heart disease, some studies have suggested that common medications used to lower lipid levels may also have beneficial effects on the development and progression of kidney disease.

Maintaining good control of your blood pressure

Getting your systolic blood pressure below 140mmHg is a key target for the prevention of diabetic kidney disease, as well as other complications. Although high blood pressure can be a result of kidney disease, in many cases high blood pressure may also precede the onset of kidney problems and contribute to its decline.

Some blood pressure-lowering drugs such as ACE inhibitors and angiotensin-receptor blockers may have additional advantages for preventing kidney damage over other anti-hypertensive drugs beyond their actions to lower the blood pressure. But the most important thing is to get rid of hypertension, in whatever way this can be achieved.

Early referral to a specialist

Sometimes, a kidney specialist can also assist in your medical care. This can be especially important for people with type 2 diabetes who have advanced kidney disease. Early planning for renal replacement, management of anaemia and other complications of failing kidney function is important. Waiting until you become unwell means that it is often harder to get your health back.

Kidney replacement

The accumulation of toxins that would otherwise be cleared by healthy kidneys can make people with severely impaired kidney function feel tired and weak, nauseous with a poor appetite, cold and itchy. Ultimately, toxins can accumulate to such an extent that a kidney transplant or some artificial means of clearing them (known as **dialysis**) is necessary in order to survive.

Diabetes is the single leading reason for needing to have dialysis and accounts for one-third to half of all people entering dialysis programs each year. A number of different dialysis options are now available, including **haemodialysis**, where a machine filters your blood through a direct connection to your bloodstream; and **peritoneal dialysis**, where fluid is rinsed through the abdomen allowing toxins to diffuse into the fluid and then be removed as fresh fluid is replaced.

Some people with type 2 diabetes may be candidates for a kidney transplant in the event their own kidneys fail. Transplantation involves major surgery in which a single kidney is removed from a live relative or a brain-dead organ donor who shares tissue features sufficiently similar to your own as to reduce the chances that your body will reject the new kidney (known as a match). This kidney is then connected to your blood and bladder, and will usually immediately function in filtering your blood and making urine.

Although kidney transplantation is a very effective way to save the life of people who develop kidney failure, it is not a perfect solution. There are never enough donors for everyone, and some people will wait many years on dialysis before a suitable match becomes available. By the time your kidneys fail, it is common to have many other problems with your health, including heart disease, which makes the stress of major surgery too dangerous for some people.

A number of medications are also required to prevent your body rejecting the new kidney and ensuring its survival. These can have serious side effects, including reducing your immunity, which opens the door to infection, cancer and other illnesses.

Although it is possible to have dialysis or sometimes receive a new kidney, the health of people receiving a kidney replacement is sadly never as good as those who have their own kidneys functioning. Consequently, it is much more important to protect your kidneys than to rely on modern medicine to get you out of trouble if your kidneys fail.

14

DIABETES IN MY BLADDER

Understand

- One sign of poor glucose control may be increased thirst along with passing urine more frequently, with more urgency, or having to get out of bed at night to go to the toilet.
- Some people with type 2 diabetes experience involuntary and inappropriate contractions of the bladder (known as an overactive bladder) that make you want to go to the toilet frequently and with great urgency.
- In other people, their bladder won't

contract enough to empty fully, causing urinary retention.

- Diabetes exacerbates the urinary symptoms of pelvic floor weakness (in women) and prostate problems (in men).

Manage

- Achieve and maintain good glucose control to slow the flow of urine, especially at night, and reduce irritability in the bladder.
- Don't suffer in silence with bladder problems. Ask your doctor for help.
- Strengthen up your pelvic floor by doing regular (Kegel) exercises.
- Establish a pattern of going to the toilet rather than being controlled by your bladder.

It is seldom appreciated by doctors that the bladder and its functions are pivotal for both productivity and quality of life. Yet it is well understood by people with type 2 diabetes, especially but not exclusively by women. Having to rush to find a toilet; having to get up many times at night; having to limit fluid intake in an attempt to stay dry — these are all common symptoms of people with type 2 diabetes if they are asked. Indeed, at least three-quarters of all people with type 2 diabetes will experience bladder problems to some degree. However, few complain without prompting, so these bothersome symptoms are seldom addressed as part of routine diabetes care. This needs to change.

ABOUT THE BLADDER

The bladder is a balloon-shaped organ that sits in the pelvis. It coordinates two opposing functions: stopping the flow of urine (storing it in the bladder) and starting the flow of urine (voiding it out).

All urine is made by the kidneys, from where it flows down into the bladder. Although it varies from person to person, the bladder's average capacity is between 300 and 400ml (10–13½ fl oz) before it begins to feel full. In other words, your bladder can contain about as much as a soft-drink or soda can. Near this point, the bladder signals to the brain that it is time to go to the toilet. These signals become more and more insistent as the volume of urine in the bladder gets closer to its capacity.

In infants, these signals trigger an automatic reflex to urinate. But in adults this reflex is held in check by sheer willpower. When you reach a toilet and are fully ready to go, you consciously release this hold, your pelvic floor relaxes and the bladder contracts, allowing the urine to flow. A healthy bladder will contract fully, leaving behind only a teaspoon of urine at most. This cycle will be repeated on average three to four times every 24 hours, without a drop ever being spilt.

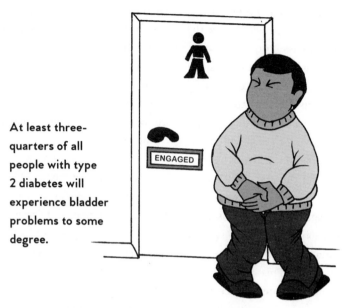

At least three-quarters of all people with type 2 diabetes will experience bladder problems to some degree.

WHAT DOES DIABETES DO TO THE BLADDER?

Diabetes has the potential to disrupt the coordinated functions of the bladder in a number of different ways. However, just as diabetes affects the heart, the eyes and the kidneys, the same process can also disrupt the coordinated functions of the bladder. This can cause a range of different symptoms in different people. Often people frequently overlook their bladder problems or put them down to just getting old.

Some people with diabetes experience involuntary and inappropriate contractions of their bladder before it is completely filled. This is known as an **overactive bladder** or **bladder instability**. These contractions suddenly make you feel the urge to urinate (known as **urgency**), meaning you have to go to the toilet many times during the day (known as **frequency**) or have to get up many times during the night (known as **nocturia**). Yet for each time you go, and despite all the urgency to get there, you don't pass more than a cup full. Sometimes you leak before you can stop it or get to a bathroom (known as **urge incontinence**).

The bladder can be jumpy like this for a number of reasons, such as if it is irritated with a bladder infection. However, diabetes itself can make the bladder more irritable, simply in response to having to deal with a greater urine output. It is thought that the bladder learns what's coming in diabetes and gets you to go sooner than would otherwise be necessary, in anticipation. This problem tends to be more common in those people who have recently been diagnosed with diabetes rather than those who have had it for many years. In other people with type 2 diabetes, their bladder may be underactive, which means it is less able to contract. This can lead to incomplete emptying of the bladder (known as **urinary retention**). The chance of still having over a cup of urine still left in your bladder after going to the toilet is at least ten times greater in those with type 2 diabetes when compared to those without diabetes. This problem tends to be more common in those who have had their diabetes for a long time rather than those who have only been recently diagnosed.

Urinary retention is often caused by nerve damage associated with diabetes that reduces the sensations the body uses to know it is time to go to the toilet. This nerve damage also disrupts the coordinated contractions that under normal circumstances empty the bladder completely each time you go.

A weak and underactive bladder may be experienced by its sufferer as a difficulty in starting to urinate or passing only a dribbling, weak stream of urine that falls off quickly. And if you can't empty your bladder fully it takes less time to be completely full again. This means you frequently have to go again and again to the toilet, through the day and night. So although your bladder may be inactive, you could be experiencing lots of bladder activity.

The longer urine is stored in the bladder, the greater the chance it will become infected, especially in women. So having urinary retention also leads to higher amounts of bacteria in the urine and a greater risk of **urinary tract infections** (known as **UTIs**).

A full bladder is also prone to unintentionally leaking small amounts of urine with coughing, exercising or other things that put stress on the bladder (this is known as **stress or overflow incontinence**). At least every second woman with type 2 diabetes will experience some urine leakage every month.

Women are more prone to this problem than men, due to the weakening of the pelvic floor during childbirth. The pelvic floor naturally forms a hammock across the pelvis that holds its contents in their place. During pregnancy and labour, this hammock can become stretched and weakened. At its most severe, sagging of the pelvic floor can lead to **prolapse**, when pelvic organs (the bladder, rectum or uterus) protrude into the vagina. Most women with children will have some degree of prolapse on close examination. However, very few will experience major problems as a result. But because diabetes is filling up the bladder rapidly, and increasing its volume, any symptoms of a weak pelvic floor are accentuated in women with type 2 diabetes.

WHAT CAN BE DONE ABOUT BLADDER PROBLEMS?

Although some decline in bladder function is inevitable, there is much that can be done to keep your bladder in good shape.

- Achieving and maintaining good glucose control will slow the flow of urine, especially at night, and reduce irritability in the bladder acquired from making so much urine.
- Weight control will reduce the risk and severity of incontinence in people with diabetes who are overweight.
- Some medications can increase the amount of urine made, including SGLT-2 inhibitors and diuretics. Sometimes, starting these agents can accentuate underlying bladder problems that you were otherwise not aware of.
- Keep an eye on the amount and timing of your fluid intake, drinking most fluid in the morning or early afternoon, rather than in the evening.
- Avoid things that irritate the bladder such as caffeine in tea and coffee.
- Limit alcohol intake in the evening.
- Empty your bladder and bowels as a routine before going to bed.
- Empty your bladder as fully as possible each time you go to the toilet. One way to do this is the **double voiding technique**. As the name suggests, double voiding means emptying the bladder twice, by urinating a second time 10 to 15 minutes after the first time. It is a very simple way to reduce the pooling of urine in the bladder.
- Rather than waiting for the uncontrollable urge, sometimes it is best to establish a pattern of going to the toilet frequently (every couple of hours through the day, regardless of any urge).

Rather than suffering in silence, it is important to seek help early as many options are available to improve bladder function and quality of life. These are generally more effective the earlier they are initiated. Some of these treatments include the following.

Pelvic floor exercises

Pelvic floor exercises are useful to strengthen the muscles of the pelvic floor which support the structures of the bladder and reduce the chance of leaking. These are also known as Kegel exercises. These exercises simply involve consciously trying to contract and relax the muscles of the pelvis, as though you want to stop a flow of urine. Hold onto the contraction for 5 seconds, then relax for 5 seconds, then repeat this ten times in a row, at least three times a day. Work your way up to keeping the muscles contracted for 10 seconds at a time, relaxing for 10 seconds between contractions. For best results, focus on tightening only your pelvic floor muscles and avoid holding your breath. Regular pelvic floor muscle training combined with bladder training can solve most bladder problems in many women. It can also be useful for men with bladder problems.

Medications for an irritable bladder

Some people with an overactive bladder can benefit from medications that reduce bladder irritability, the strength of sudden urges and the frequency of voiding. However, because of the way they work within the body, most have unwanted side effects such as dry mouth and eyes, blurred vision, sedation and constipation. Local oestrogen creams can also keep the tissues around the bladder and vagina healthy and reduce irritability in some cases.

It is often suggested that cranberry juice is good for bladder problems. However, rigorous studies do not back up these claims, and bacteria quickly become resistant to any potentially useful effects. Probiotics, such as lactobacillus in yoghurt and some supplements, are also widely touted for bladder problems, but again robust evidence for any beneficial effect is lacking.

A number of new techniques are also emerging, including electrical stimulation devices that can be used to help empty a sluggish bladder.

Surgery

Surgical treatment is sometimes necessary to fix bothersome bladder problems. This used to mean removal of the uterus, or womb (known as a hysterectomy). Although prolapse is currently the major reason for having a hysterectomy, many other options are available, especially if initiated at an early stage, including pessaries to support the pelvic floor. A number of non-destructive and less invasive surgical procedures are also now available, many with good success rates.

DIABETES AND THE PROSTATE

Men also have their own special burden, the prostate gland, which sits just under the bladder. The prostate gland slowly enlarges in all men as they age, sometimes enough to slow the flow of urine. This can result in a number of troublesome symptoms including an interrupted or dribbling stream, frequency, urgency and/or incontinence. It is still controversial whether diabetes makes prostate enlargement worse. Many of the factors that lead to the development of diabetes (such as obesity, lack of physical activity, smoking and a high fat diet) are also associated with a larger prostate gland. Diabetes also means more urine so that the bladder symptoms associated with prostate problems are often worse, including nocturia and urgency, which means that prostate enlargement is simply picked up more often in men with type 2 diabetes.

Again, it is not necessary to suffer in silence or consign your symptoms to your diabetes. There are now a number of effective treatments available to get the flow going again. These include medications to shrink the prostate or relax the neck of the bladder to improve urine flow. Minimally invasive surgical options are also now available. Diets rich in phytoestrogens (found in fresh fruit, vegetables, soy, lentils, flaxseed and chickpeas), lycopenes (in red fruit such as watermelon, tomatoes), onions and garlic are also associated with lower rates of prostate enlargement, although none can fix prostate problems once they occur. Supplements containing saw palmetto extract, zinc or beta-sitosterol are widely advertised as alternative therapies for prostate enlargement but have not been shown to be effective in rigorous trials. In contrast, regular exercise seems to help keep the prostate under control, as well as other parts of your diabetes management.

15

DIABETES ON MY MIND

Understand
- Strokes are more common in people with type 2 diabetes and their impact is greater.
- Good glucose, lipid and blood pressure control in someone with type 2 diabetes can reduce your risk of having a stroke by over two-thirds.
- Many people with type 2 diabetes will develop dementia during their lifetime. But the risk can also be reduced by good diabetes control.

Manage

- Become familiar with the warning signs of a stroke. Have an action plan for what to do in the event of a stroke and when to call for an ambulance.
- Achieve and maintain smooth control of your blood pressure.
- Monitor your blood pressure, not just when you see the doctor but at home, work and other times as well to ensure you are keeping control all of the time.

The brain is central to all the functions of the body. Through the nerves and other signals, it is connected to and regulates all aspects of your health. Looking after your brain and mind is as important for managing type 2 diabetes as any other aspect of diabetes care — some would say more so. While glucose, lipid and blood pressure control are all achievable, they can seem futile when the mind is not also on board.

WHAT ARE STROKES AND HOW DO YOU AVOID THEM?

One of the most devastating consequences of type 2 diabetes is its association with an increased risk of having a stroke. As detailed in Chapter 10, all parts of the body depend on the flow of blood for their survival. If this flow is stopped, even for a brief period, any parts downstream from the blockage suffer and may die. When a permanent blockage in blood flow to the brain occurs, it is called a **stroke** (also known as a **cerebrovascular accident** or **CVA**).

Type 2 diabetes is associated with an increased risk of stroke that is over twice that observed in people without diabetes. Approximately one in eight people with type 2 diabetes will have a stroke. The impact of having a stroke is also more serious, as the frequency of irreversible brain damage, recurrent strokes, disability and mortality are also higher in those with type 2 diabetes.

The most common cause of blockage to the blood vessels supplying your brain is atherosclerosis. This is the same process that leads to heart attacks (detailed in Chapter 10). In this process, increasing amounts of cholesterol are deposited in the walls of blood vessels, making them increasingly unstable and sensitive to the stresses of blood pressure. Then one fateful day there is an erosion or rupture of its protective surface and a blood vessel becomes clotted and obstructed. This can be the first (and last) sign there is anything wrong with your blood vessels.

Blockages may occur at the site of **atherosclerosis** or further downstream, as bits of clot fly off only to get stuck in blood vessels too small to let them pass. With so much blood going to our brain, this is often where they go. If these blockages can't be quickly cleared, then any parts of the brain that depended on the flow of blood coming from that blood vessel will die. Unlike damage to your skin, brain cells cannot grow back, so any significant loss of flow always means some permanent loss of function.

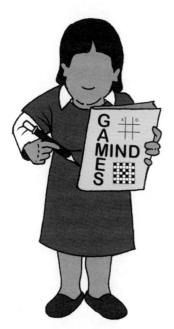

Looking after your mind is as important for managing diabetes as any other aspect of diabetes care. Some would say more so.

Age, high glucose, blood pressure and cholesterol levels, smoking and the presence of atherosclerosis elsewhere (in the heart or legs) are the major risk factors for having a stroke in a person with type 2 diabetes.

These are the same risk factors for heart disease; this is because it is essentially the same process, just in different blood vessels. Consequently, the same things that reduce the risk of heart attacks, detailed in Chapter 10, will also reduce your risk of having a stroke, including:

- reducing your systolic blood pressure and its variability
- reducing the bad (LDL) cholesterol levels in the blood
- raising the good (HDL) cholesterol in the blood
- improving your glucose control

- stopping smoking
- weight management
- increasing your physical activity
- managing your stress
- thinning your blood (with medications).

Clinical studies in people with type 2 diabetes suggest that if you do all of these things to the best of your ability, you can reduce your risk of having a stroke by over two-thirds.

Blockage of blood vessels supplying the brain may also occur if a clot accidentally forms in your heart, is dislodged and then pushed by the flow of the blood into your brain. This is known as an **embolic stroke** and is thought to account for about 10 per cent of all strokes. Clots can occur in the heart if heart valves are damaged or if the smooth flow of blood through the heart is disrupted. This can occur when some parts contract more forcefully than others or if the rhythm of the heart becomes erratic. The most common example of this is **atrial fibrillation** (or AF). Any lack of coordination of your heartbeat leads to turbulence and eddies of relatively stagnant blood flow where clotting can occur. AF is more common in patients with diabetes due to their heart being stiffer (see Chapter 10). The risk of embolic stroke can be reduced in people with AF by using medication to thin the blood and prevent clotting.

Some strokes occur when there is bleeding into the brain (known as a **haemorrhagic stroke**). They result from a weakened vessel that ruptures and bleeds into the surrounding brain. The blood then accumulates and compresses the surrounding brain tissue, starving it of oxygen in essentially the same way when a blood vessel supplying the brain is blocked with a clot. Type 2 diabetes does not increase the risk of this kind of stroke, although high blood pressure, kidney disease and increasing age that accompany diabetes mean that at least 10 per cent of all strokes in those with diabetes are associated with bleeding into the brain.

There are now many effective ways to treat a stroke, should it occur. These are most effective when delivered as close to the first moment of blockage as possible, and at the very least within three hours from the onset of symptoms. The longer any blockage is left, the greater the damage to the brain and the more limited any recovery. This is why planning and knowing what to do in the event of a stroke can be as important in saving your life as any medication you currently take.

As with a heart attack, all individuals with type 2 diabetes should be familiar with the warning signs of a stroke and have an action plan for what to do in the event of a stroke and when to call for an ambulance. Warning signs of a stroke may include:

- sudden weakness or heaviness of the face, arm or leg affecting only one side of the body
- sudden change in your vision, especially in one eye
- sudden change in or loss of speech, trouble talking or pronouncing words clearly or difficulty understanding them
- sudden onset of dizziness, unsteadiness or loss of balance.

There are now many different ways to rapidly restore blood flow along blocked arteries following a stroke. Again, these are most effective when delivered as close to the first moment of blockage as possible, and at the very least within three hours from the onset of symptoms. The longer arterial blockage is left, the greater the damage to the brain and the more limited any recovery. All those with type 2 diabetes should be proactive and report any sudden new symptoms rather than hope they will go away.

A stroke is diagnosed when someone experiences these persistent symptoms and is usually verified by a brain scan that shows reduced blood supply to one area of the brain.

Transient ischaemic attacks

Sometimes people experience only short-lived symptoms of stroke which last a few minutes but then fully resolve. This is known as a **transient ischaemic attack** or TIA. It is also sometimes also called a mini-stroke. These represent a warning that there is something wrong with the blood vessels supplying the brain and that more serious or long-lasting damage may be just around the corner. Approximately one-third of people who experience TIA go on to have a stroke within a year.

TIAs are thought to occur when a clot blocks a damaged blood vessel to the brain, but then is quickly dissolved or is broken up by the force of the blood pressure. Because TIAs can be a harbinger of more serious problems to come, such episodes are treated very seriously in people with diabetes, usually with your doctor prescribing blood thinners and aiming for more intensive lipid and blood pressure control. Surgery to clean out damaged and narrowed blood vessels (known as an **endarterectomy**) may also be appropriate for people with atherosclerosis in the blood vessels of the neck that supply the brain (known as the **carotid arteries**). Doctors sometimes also recommend a balloon to dilate blocked or damaged blood vessels (known as **angioplasty**) and implantable steel screens (known as **stents**) to hold open blood vessels.

WHAT IS DEMENTIA?

For many people, one of their greatest fears is that they will experience a decline in their ability to think, remember, calculate and learn (known as **cognitive function**). Sadly, in some people these deficits can be severe and widespread, and compromise their ability to function independently; this is known as dementia. At least one-quarter of those with type 2 diabetes aged over 60 will develop dementia during their lifetime. Many others will suffer lesser degrees of impairment of their cognitive functions. Such changes are not inevitable. To some extent, they can also be prevented.

Alzheimer's disease is widely recognized as the most common cause of dementia. Although it is more common in older people, Alzheimer's disease is not 'brain ageing'.

Like diabetes, it is an insidious disease which progresses slowly over five to ten years. However, its impact on your thinking can be quite variable and is influenced by a number of factors, including social support, mood and the presence or absence of other brain problems. Your brain can only take so much. For example, poor circulation to the brain makes it more likely that those with Alzheimer's disease will also develop dementia.

The same process of progressive damage to blood vessels that leads to heart attacks and strokes in people with type 2 diabetes may also lead to a much more piecemeal loss of brain function. This is known as **vascular dementia** and is second only to Alzheimer's disease as a major cause of impaired cognitive function. As your brain uses over half of the body's glucose and at least 20 per cent of its oxygen, it is critically dependent on good blood flow. If blood supply is reduced to the brain, it turns down its activities, partly as a way of prolonging its survival. However, this may also be at the expense of its thinking functions. So combined with Alzheimer's disease, poor brain circulation is a recipe for a more rapid decline.

All the things that reduce your risk of stroke (detailed above) will also reduce your risk of dementia. Blood pressure lowering, sustained weight loss, improved glucose and lipid control, smoking cessation and regular physical activity can all help you retain your marbles.

There is also some evidence that the composition of your diet may also influence your risk of cognitive decline through its effects on your weight, blood pressure, glucose and lipid levels.

Diets high in trans fats and saturated (animal) fats are associated with faster rates of cognitive decline. By contrast, diets naturally high in fish and a Mediterranean diet high in monounsaturated fat (see Chapter 9) are associated with a lower risk of dementia. Maintaining a moderate level of regular physical activity is also associated with better preservation of the brain's functions.

Finally, it is also clear that regular mental activity is good for the brain. Any kind of social isolation can lead to mental stress, depression and mental decline. By contrast, remaining mentally challenged has a number of rewards, including keeping the brain sharp. There is no single answer for everyone. Some people will prefer solving crosswords to playing chess, bridge or Sudoku. Crafts, reading, learning new languages or skills can all be stimulating activities. It is possible to join a club or society and stay socially as well as mentally active. The trick is to find something challenging that you can enjoy every day to keep your brain active. This will also help to keep it healthy.

16

DIABETES ON MY MOOD

Understand

- It is perfectly normal to feel angry, guilty, overwhelmed, despondent, fearful or in denial about aspects of your diabetes.
- It is sometimes important to acknowledge and explore these feelings as a way to move forward.
- Stress can be a killer and having diabetes is really stressful. This means that finding your own ways to deal with inevitable stresses is just as important as any other component of your diabetes care.

- Depression is a serious and common complication in people with type 2 diabetes.
- Depression is not a simple illness. It is sometimes difficult to see it for what it is against a background of other problems in people with type 2 diabetes.

Manage

- Cultivate your relationship with your diabetes care team. They will know what you are going through and have many resources available that can help.
- Don't shut off your emotions. They may be as much a determinant of your health as your diabetes is.
- Take the time to accent the positive and eliminate the negative in everything you do. Optimism is good for your health.
- Explore new ways to relax and unburden yourself.
- Recognize the symptoms of depression

in yourself and ask for help in getting
on top of them.

Effective management of diabetes is much more than biology and chemistry. It also means keeping your chin up and maintaining and optimizing your mental wellbeing. This is not always easy.

Having diabetes is confronting. There are complex treatments, targets and goals, successes and failures. Diabetes often results in a range of emotional responses that are as different as the people who experience them. Broadly, these responses can be classified into eight different reactions.

1. Anger and frustration

- 'Why me?'
- 'It's not fair!'
- 'How can this be happening to me?'
- 'I hate my diabetes.'

2. Denial/ridicule/rejection/disbelief

- 'I feel fine.'
- 'This can't be happening to me.'
- 'It's not that serious.'
- 'It's only a touch of ...'

3. Guilt/self-blame

- 'I caused this mess.'
- 'It's all my fault.'
- 'I deserved this.'

4. Bargaining

- 'I have to do this now.'
- 'If I do this, then ...'

- 'I'll do anything for ...'
- 'I don't care what it takes.'

5. Withdrawal/nihilism/feeling overwhelmed/ defeated/fatigued/resigned/hopelessness

- 'It's all too hard.'
- 'What's the point?'
- 'Why should I bother to keep taking these/doing this?'
- 'The harder I try the harder I fall.'
- 'Stop the world I want to get off!'
- 'I don't care anymore.'

6. Depression/negative thinking/low self-esteem

- 'I'm not worth the effort.'
- 'They should just let me die.'
- 'I'm stupid.'
- 'I'm a bad person.'

7. Stress/distress/anxiety/fear/dread

- 'What will happen now?'
- 'What will I do if ...?'

8. Acceptance

- 'I'm okay with my diabetes.'
- 'I have a plan.'
- 'It's just the way it is.'
- 'I'll just have to get on with it.'

These different emotional reactions are often called **defence or coping mechanisms**. They are perfectly normal. Part of coping with type 2 diabetes will inevitably involve experiencing some or all of these different emotional responses. They are not stages.

There is no particular order or requirement to experience

any of these reactions. But at the same time, it is sometimes important to acknowledge and express these feelings as a way to move forward. You can also use these emotions as a trigger for change.

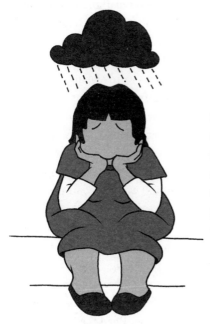

Having diabetes is challenging. This often results in a range of emotional responses that are as different as the people who experience them.

However, sometimes these emotions can get the better of you. This is often described as being 'stuck in a hole'. And this is when the stress of diabetes really begins to take a toll and when problems seem to magnify the longer you are stuck there. One of the most important differences between people who are able to survive their diabetes and those who succumb to its many challenges and complications lies in their ability to cope with illness and rebuild again and again.

Finding your way out is a personal journey, but one you shouldn't need to make alone. Your diabetes care team will know what you are going through and have many resources available that can help.

The best way to prevent stress from diabetes is to cultivate your relationship with your diabetes care team, and work with them to create and achieve common goals.

Some of the simple things they may get you to do include:

- Disclosure. Putting into words what you are feeling and letting others share your concerns can sometimes help you to know what you are really feeling. Talking to your diabetes management team, your family and friends will always make a difference. Even just communicating with yourself by keeping a personal diary can be a useful way to conceptualize your feelings.

- Self-awareness. Focus on the triggers that set you off. Find out what's making you angry or upset and when. Understand the things that make you feel good and find a way to go there when you're stuck.

- Exploration. Have a look at what other people with diabetes are experiencing. Read the blog or internet journal of someone else with type 2 diabetes. Attend group sessions where you hear about what other people are doing to keep control and how they are coping. Borrow new ideas or new recipes that might work for you.

- Goal realignment. Many of the challenges of diabetes come from unrealistic and unnecessary expectations. It is always important to realign your goals and aim to control what is in your control. This is where close contact with your diabetes management team will make a real difference and allow you to have a dynamic and evolving plan for coping with your diabetes.

- Planning. The best way to know where you should be going is to have a map. By establishing comprehensive plans and routines and following them closely, it is much easier to track your progress and never feel lost. Make your intentions clear to ensure you are in control of where your management is going. As you become more and more familiar with where you are, it also becomes easier to step off the map for brief periods and try new things, as you always know your way back.

- Accenting the positive. The impacts of any stress can be modified by changing the way it is perceived. If you think you are stressed, then you are. But when you think you have the resources to cope, then stress is no longer such a threat. Some of this 'stress resilience' comes from your confidence and coping skills. Some also comes from a positive outlook. All these can be cultivated and fostered. Stress-resilient people may have the same stressors (e.g. diabetes) but they expect everything will be okay, rather than a problem. They are better able to deal with stress because they know they can.

A number of studies have shown that simply learning to 'accentuate the positive' in everything you do is associated with reduced stress and less heart disease. Optimism can be learned with practice and become part of your life.

STRESS AND ITS EFFECT ON DIABETES

Every life is filled with many stresses. Your brain is the main driver of your response to stress, as well as its main target. It decides when there is a problem and acts automatically to gives the body the tools it needs to fight, survive or quickly run away (known as the 'fight or flight' response). The intensity of any stress response is determined not only by the perceived intensity of the threat, but also a host of other factors known cumulatively as your resilience. These include things like your genes, your gender, previous stressful experiences, coping skills and personality traits.

Having type 2 diabetes is a very stressful experience. Over and above your glucose control and any other aspect of your diabetes care, how you respond to this major stress in your life is also a major determinant of your subsequent health and wellbeing.

When stress gets the better of you it can cause many problems, including interfering with your ability to achieve and maintain control over them. In general, stressed people with type 2 diabetes have worse glucose control. This is not simply because they are too stressed to take their medication consistently or adhere to diet and lifestyle programs (although this doesn't help). The chemicals that are released by the body in response to stress also serve to directly drive up glucose levels while at the same time cause resistance to the actions of insulin. At the same time, if you take people with type 2 diabetes and teach them yoga, meditation, tai chi or other relaxation techniques, on average they will achieve improvements in their glucose control roughly equivalent to adding in an additional glucose-lowering medication.

Over and above its effect on your glucose control, chronic activation of the stress response can also increase your risk of complications from your diabetes, including:

- Heart attacks and strokes. Up to one-third of all heart attacks may be attributable to chronic stress. For example, people reporting stress at work or marital stress have twice the risk of having a heart attack or stroke. The increase in risk in those suffering from acute or chronic stress is about the same as having a high cholesterol level or being a smoker.
- High blood pressure. In susceptible people (especially those with diabetes), stress can drive the blood pressure higher. By contrast, effective stress management invariably lowers blood pressure and improves the function of blood vessels.
- Infections. When you are stressed you seem to pick up every bug that is going around. Stress also reduces the effectiveness of vaccination to diseases like the flu. These are just some examples of the effects that stress can have on your ability to fight off infections. Of course in diabetes, when your immunity is low anyway, stress is the last thing you need.
- Brain function. Any stress can make it difficult to concentrate, learn and focus. But prolonged stress will actually cause some areas of the brain to shrink.
- Depression and mental illness. In certain susceptible individuals, chronic stress can trigger depression (see below) and other mental illnesses.
- Sleep. Stress can interfere with you getting the sleep you need each night. This can lead to even more stress (see Chapter 17).
- Sexual function. Stress can also interfere with your sex life (see Chapter 18).

One important way to cope with having diabetes is to manage your (inevitable) stress better. Some people will need more help than others, based on their resilience and the size of their burden. But everyone will need some help sooner or later.

There are many different ways you can handle stress: some you can do yourself (also known as self-help programs) and others you perform with the help of different health practitioners. Some of the best-known and effective stress management techniques include yoga, relaxation, mind–body techniques, mindful breathing, biofeedback, hypnosis, tai chi, exercise, mindfulness meditation, guided imagery, conditioning and time out. When used routinely, each serves to build resilience to stress in some people. But it's not the same for everyone. Not everyone can do yoga. Not everyone likes exercise. The most effective strategies are the ones you can enjoy, the ones that put your mind at ease and the ones you want to do again and again.

There are many medicines that can also be useful in some people suffering from severe and chronic stress. Each one has its side effects and limitations. In addition, most lose their effectiveness in the long term, especially on their own. The combination with other stress management techniques better allows these medicines to be used just for short periods, when the stress is most acute, with other techniques coming into their own and taking over once control is achieved.

DEPRESSION AND DIABETES

Depression is a serious and common problem for people with type 2 diabetes. It is common for everyone to feel low at times during their life. But depression is a disproportionate and pervasive mood that interferes with your ability to function. It can affect your relationships, your work, your sleep and many other aspects of your health and wellbeing. Depression can also affect your diabetes control, the likelihood of complications and their impact.

Not everyone with diabetes will become depressed, no matter how bad their illness gets. Certainly, women are twice as likely to become depressed as men. Single people are more at risk than married ones. At the same time those people who stay socially connected with their family and friends have a lower risk of depression.

Depression is not a simple illness. It is sometimes difficult to see it for what it is against a background of other problems in people with type 2 diabetes. However, identifying and managing depression is an important and under-recognized part of diabetes care.

One way to identify those people who could be depressed is the Patient Health Questionnaire-2. It asks only two simple questions:

1. Have you often had little interest or pleasure in doing things over the past month?

2. Have you often been bothered by feeling down, depressed or hopeless over the past month?

Most people suffering from depression will answer yes to one or both of these questions. If this is you, then it is worth talking to your doctor or other members of your diabetes care team about the need for further evaluation. About half of those with positive responses will turn out not to be depressed, but it is still important to ask your doctor or specialist for their formal assessment.

Treating depression

Depression is not something you have to put up with. Like any other illness, depression can be treated. Not only will this make you feel and function better, the effective treatment of depression will also mean better diabetes control.

A number of different treatment options are available that will be suited to different people and different clinical situations. Most doctors will often first try to use treatments that don't involve taking pills. The most widely used of these is **psychotherapy** (also known as counselling). This can be very effective in many people with depression. The response rate is roughly similar to that of taking antidepressant pills, although when combined they may be even more effective than either alone.

There are many different forms of psychotherapy, but most involve structured weekly sessions delivered by trained therapists to retrain thinking and behaviour or develop new coping skills. Relaxation and stress management are also key components. These sessions can be delivered to you alone or as part of a group.

Participation in **physical exercise programs**, or increasing your physical activity in a social setting (such as walking the dog, golf, walking groups, tennis, etc.), can also significantly improve symptoms of depression in some people and have a range of other benefits for your overall health (see Chapter 5).

Many people with depression also need **antidepressant pills** to help them out. Each of these medications acts in a different way to balance disturbed chemistry in the depressed brain. Some common antidepressant medications include:

- Selective serotonin-reuptake inhibitors (SSRIs). These are often used as the first-line drug treatment for depression, especially in those over 60.

- Serotonin–norepinephrine reuptake inhibitors (SNRIs). These may be particularly useful for patients with chronic pain due to nerve damage associated with diabetes.
- Tricyclic antidepressants (TCAs). These agents are effective but may have significant side effects, especially in those with heart problems.
- Monoamine oxidase inhibitors (MAOIs). These older agents also work in some patients, but require close monitoring and a special diet to prevent side effects, so may be less suitable for those with type 2 diabetes.

Antidepressants do not blunt normal emotional reactions or turn you into a zombie. Antidepressants also do not lead to dependence or addiction. However, many of these medications do have significant side effects, so are used only where having depression is a worse alternative.

About half of those treated with any given antidepressant show a positive response, often within as little as a month of treatment, although it may take a few more months for a full response to occur. Once a remission is achieved, antidepressants are usually continued for a further six to twelve months, as stopping too soon can increase the risk of recurrence. In those who do not respond initially, a trial of an alternative antidepressant medication or combination of medicines, with or without psychotherapy, is often undertaken. Where needed, the actions of antidepressants can also sometimes be augmented by other medications.

There are a number of different supplements and over-the-counter herbal remedies that are advertised to help treat the symptoms of depression in some people. However, their effectiveness is variable, and most people with depression experience little or no benefit from them.

17

DIABETES IN MY SLEEP

Understand

- Good quality sleep in good quantities is important for daytime health and wellbeing.
- Sleep problems are a common complication of type 2 diabetes, yet often go unrecognized against a background of other issues.
- Cramps and restless legs are not something you simply have to put up with because you have type 2 diabetes.
- Obstructive sleep apnoea affects at least one-quarter of people with type 2 diabetes, especially men and those who are overweight.

Manage

- Ask your partner about how you are sleeping, whether you are snoring or waking often with a start.
- Make changes to your bedroom and night routines that will help you get the sleep you need.
- Aim to control your glucose levels during the night as well as the day.
- Don't let your bladder get in the way of a good night's sleep. There are a number of simple ways to retrain your bladder and make it less irritable.

A good night's sleep is an important part of a healthy life. The third of your life you spend asleep can significantly affect the two-thirds you spend awake. Everyone needs a good quantity of sleep and good quality sleep to keep their brain and body working in peak condition. This is especially true in those with type 2 diabetes.

Sleep serves a number of essential functions you simply can't do without. It does far more than just passively conserve your energy for daytime activities.

Without sleep you not only feel tired, but many other things don't work, including your attempts to successfully manage your diabetes.

There is good evidence to show that too little sleep, and in particular too little quality sleep, can contribute to a range of problems:

- Excessive weight gain. Those with habitually poor sleep tend to gain weight more easily and struggle to take it off. This is partly explained by the fact that tired bodies think they have too little energy and try to compensate by making you feel hungry, encouraging you to eat more. This is the last thing someone with type 2 diabetes really needs.
- Poor glucose control. Those with habitually poor sleep often have difficulty achieving and maintaining control of blood glucose levels. In fact, poor sleep is actually associated with an increased risk for developing type 2 diabetes.
- Higher blood pressure and cholesterol levels.
- Irregular heart rhythms, including atrial fibrillation, a risk factor for strokes (see Chapter 15).
- Increased risk of errors in judgement, loss of performance and accidents, especially from falling asleep while driving.
- Low mood, motivation and energy.
- Increased sensitivity to pain.
- More bacterial and viral infections.

Sleep also significantly affects the building of your memories. Your body may be resting when you're asleep, but this time off allows your brain to get on with the important task of processing your day. During deep sleep the brain rewires its circuits to make lasting connections between events, sensations and other information. Sleep ensures that all newly gained knowledge is consolidated, organized and stored for future use. Getting more quality sleep really does help you remember, process and understand things better. This is partly why the ability to think and process in the daytime declines the less sleep you get (not just because you feel tired). This is also why an active brain demands more sleep, like those of children and adolescents.

The most obvious and important consequence of too little night-time sleep is daytime sleepiness! You all know those days where you have difficulty concentrating, remembering and feel generally irritable and exhausted. It's easy to know what the problem is. You can't wait to just go home and go to bed! However, it's not just one really bad night that does this. Sometimes even small amounts of sleep debt can creep up on you. And after a period of missing too much sleep, stress takes over the show, increasing blood pressure and producing stress hormones, which also make it even harder for you to sleep.

WHAT IS SLEEP?

Most people think of sleep as a loss of consciousness that lasts continuously for 7 to 9 hours every night. In fact, the normal sleep pattern is more like a roller-coaster ride. After turning out the lights, you usually fall asleep within about 15 to 30 minutes. You spend a few minutes in very light sleep then slowly descend into deeper and deeper sleep. This deep sleep is thought to be the most important for rejuvenating you for the next day, and brain activity during this deep sleep is characterised by delta waves. This is the same activity induced by meditation.

After about an hour or so, you ascend into lighter sleep and about 10 minutes later enter the phase known as rapid eye movement (REM) sleep during which your brain is not asleep but is actually very active. This is when you have most of your dreams, and your eyes and brain are darting around as if watching an action movie. Maybe you are. After about 20 minutes of dream sleep, your brain falls asleep and the roller-coaster ride of sleep starts all over again.

The whole sleep cycle takes about an hour and a half. REM sleep accounts for 20 to 25 per cent of the time you are asleep, and deep (non-REM) sleep accounts for the other 75 to 80 per cent. The proportion of each sleep cycle spent in deep sleep tends to be greater in the first cycles of the night, while REM sleep tends to be longer in the later cycles, so that by the final sleep cycle of the night you spend approximately half your sleep cycle (dreaming) in REM sleep. This means the early morning dreams are generally longer and more vivid.

If one cycle is cut short in any component of your sleep (such as when you drink too much alcohol, which suppresses REM sleep), you tend to catch up in others (so that when the booze wears off the hangover dreams are even more vivid on the rebound).

Most people fit in about five up-and-down sleep cycles a night. It is quite normal to wake up in between your sleep cycles. In fact this becomes quite common as sleep becomes lighter as people get older. Being briefly awake at some time during the night is certainly not a sign of problems with your sleep and is not something to stay awake worrying about. Historical records suggest that our ancestors probably used to sleep in two parts: an initial sleep of around 4 to 5 hours (three sleep cycles) followed by 1 to 2 hours of being awake and then a second sleep period of another 3 hours (another two sleep cycles) before dawn.

HOW DO YOU KNOW YOU ARE GETTING ENOUGH?

The amount of quality sleep you need for good health is hard to define. There is no magic number of hours that suits everyone. Some people need 9 hours yet others function very well on 6 hours' sleep.

The amount of sleep needed varies from person to person as well as varying for the same person at different stages of their life.

The amount of sleep you need also varies through the seasons and even over the course of the working week. One simple way to tell if you're getting sufficient sleep is that you should feel refreshed and able to function throughout the day.

If you are waking up still tired and lethargic or if you habitually doze off or fall asleep through the day, it may be that you are not getting the sleep you need. Of course, there may be other reasons apart from poor sleep for not feeling your best through the day, so talk to your doctor about what the next step should be (and certainly before starting to treat yourself). To see if poor sleep is really your problem, your doctor will also often ask you to keep a sleep diary, to find out just how much sleep you are really getting and how it affects your life during the day.

Most people suffer from trouble sleeping at some time during their lives. But these periods of sleeplessness are usually short-lived and settle on their own with no lasting effects. However, it is clear that people who are habitually not getting the sleep they need night after night have an increased risk of problems with their health, including diabetes.

Interestingly, some studies suggest that those people who usually sleep more than 10 hours a night also have more health problems. This may reflect their broken sleep pattern, lack of quality sleep and desperate need to catch up, rather than any aspect of sleep being bad for you or getting too much of a good thing.

HOW MIGHT DIABETES AFFECT YOUR SLEEP?

Having diabetes can impact your nights as much as your days. It can stop you getting the sleep you need in a number of different ways.

Diabetes can indirectly affect your sleep pattern by causing you to need to get up and go to the toilet, often many times during the night. This is known as **nocturia**. Healthy kidneys are able to make more concentrated urine overnight. This means that most adults do not need to get up more than once, if at all. However, getting up more frequently at night is a common symptom of diabetes and a common cause of disrupted sleep.

Nocturia can sometimes be a sign of poor glucose control during the night. When glucose levels get too high, glucose spills over into your urine, which increases the amount of urine you will make (see Chapter 14). This is most noticeable at night, when you should normally be making less. Most people don't test their glucose levels at night (as they are asleep) so it can be hard to detect. But when glucose control is improved, this symptom can quickly go away. So it is always worthwhile pointing it out to your diabetes care team and asking their advice.

Damage to the kidneys or the bladder associated with diabetes may also cause you to get up frequently in the night. Many people with bladder problems benefit from bladder retraining and/or taking medications in the evening to reduce the irritability of their bladder. These are discussed in detail in Chapter 14.

Passing more urine at night can also be a sign of problems with your heart. Again, instead of making less urine during the night, some people with impaired heart function (known as heart failure) make more. This is to enable them to clear the extra fluid from their body that has accumulated in their legs during the day, but comes back into their system when they lie down. This is treated by diuretics — medication to increase the amount of fluid lost into the urine through the day, making less of a burden at night.

Sometimes, low glucose levels (hypoglycaemia) at night can also cause you to wake up. To protect against hypoglycaemia, the body has a number of defence mechanisms that trigger warning symptoms to alert you that things are awry. One of them is to wake you up and make it hard to go back to sleep until you have eaten. Again, hypos can't occur in the majority of people with type 2 diabetes because their body is able to make enough glucose in the event that levels fall. However, in some people with type 2 diabetes who take medications that increase their insulin levels (sulphonylureas and meglitinides) or are injecting insulin itself, hypos can occur at night. Techniques for avoiding and treating hypos are discussed in detail in Chapter 7.

Type 2 diabetes is also associated with increased levels of stress and mental illness, including depression and anxiety disorders. These can significantly affect the quantity and quality of your sleep. Their assessment and management are discussed in the previous chapter.

The health of your feet also affects how well you sleep. It is not unusual for people with type 2 diabetes to experience pain in their feet (due to ulcers, infection, nerve damage and/or vascular disease). Pain from these foot problems is often worse at night (or even limited to night-time) as the feet are elevated, warm and partly compressed by the bedclothes. These conditions are discussed in detail in Chapter 12. Each has a specific treatment that includes medication and/or surgery; in addition, simple things such as using a bed cradle can keep sheets and blankets from touching your sensitive feet and legs.

Some people with type 2 diabetes experience an unpleasant 'crawling' feeling in their legs at night, accompanied by a tremendous urge to move. This is known as restless legs syndrome. It is often dismissed as something due to your diabetes, back problems or 'just nerves'. However, a number of different medications are now available to tackle this real problem, once it is recognized for what it is.

Another problem that can keep you up at night is **leg cramps**, usually affecting the calves but also sometimes the thighs or the feet. These cramps can be intensely painful and last up to several minutes before subsiding. This is followed by a deep muscle ache that can last up to a few hours. Leg cramps are more common in people with type 2 diabetes, especially older people, those with kidney problems or poor circulation. Again, this is not a problem that should be simply put up with. In those with troubling or frequent cramping, symptoms can be reduced by using verapamil or diltiazem (commonly prescribed as blood pressure-lowering medications). Vitamin B complex may also be helpful in some people. Quinine, the active ingredient in tonic water, may also be useful in some people although its effects are quite variable.

Snoring and obstructive sleep apnoea

Some people with type 2 diabetes experience sudden episodes of shortness of breath and/or coughing at night which wake them from their sleep. These episodes can have a number of different causes, including heart and kidney problems (see chapters 10 and 13). However, one of the most common and important causes is a condition called obstructive sleep apnoea, in which the flow of air into your lungs becomes temporarily blocked while you are deeply asleep, causing you to choke for a brief moment before the act of waking up opens your airway and allows the air to flow freely again.

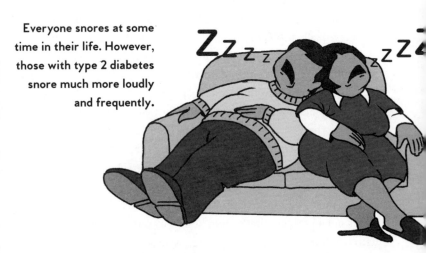

Everyone snores at some time in their life. However, those with type 2 diabetes snore much more loudly and frequently.

When you fall deeply asleep, your body normally goes into a floppy state of relaxation. This also happens in your airway. Like sucking through a straw, the 'suck' of air associated with breathing causes your (now floppy) airway to cave in a little bit when you are asleep. This happens in everyone when they sleep, but usually it has no significant effect. But if your airway is already narrowed or is excessively floppy, any further narrowing can make things very tight. When this happens the normally smooth flow of air into the lungs becomes turbulent. Like sucking air through a narrow straw, this is noisy and is heard by others as snoring.

Everyone snores at some time in their life, such as when you have a cold, when your throat is swollen, or when you (and your airways) are excessively relaxed when drunk or using sleeping pills. However, those with type 2 diabetes, especially those who are very overweight, snore much more frequently and loudly.

Sometimes, the cave-in of your airway during deep sleep can be so significant that it completely obstructs all air flow and stops your breathing (known as an apnoea). Like being strangled, this suddenly wakes you up (known as an arousal), allowing your muscles to open your airway and breathe freely again. **Obstructive sleep apnoea** is a condition that occurs when this cycle of obstruction, apnoea and arousal happens over and over again during every sleep (more than five times every hour). This results in a very fragmented sleep pattern with the associated serious consequences on daytime health. Obstructive sleep apnoea is thought to affect at least one-quarter of people with type 2 diabetes.

These sudden dramatic arousals through the night don't just break up your sleep. The release of stress hormones that occurs with each episode can also drive up glucose, blood pressure and lipid levels. This may contribute to an increased risk of heart disease and strokes in snorers.

It is hard to know yourself that you have obstructive sleep apnoea. You may just be feeling excessively tired or inattentive during the daytime. Often your sleep pattern just gets overlooked as a cause of daytime issues. However, partners or family members will very often complain about your loud snoring with periods of silence followed by gasps, choking episodes or sudden arousals. So it's worth asking them if they are just being nice by not telling you. There are also simple phone apps that can be used to check up on how well you are sleeping and whether you need some help. Once it is suspected, it is very easy to find out whether obstructive sleep apnoea is present by using a **sleep test**. During this simple test your breathing pattern is observed while you are sleeping in a special laboratory.

There are now a number of treatments for obstructive sleep apnoea that differ depending on the severity of the problem and the presence of other medical problems. For people with type 2 diabetes, the most important treatment is losing weight through diet, exercise and, if appropriate, bariatric surgery (see Chapter 4).

Simple manoeuvres such as avoiding too much alcohol and sleeping pills (which relax an already narrow airway), quitting smoking or sleeping on your side can also reduce snoring and apnoeas. Sleeping at a 30-degree angle, in a recliner chair or adjustable bed, can also be effective, especially in very overweight people. Special exercises to strengthen the muscles of the airways can also help. One of these useful exercises includes getting men to learn to play the didgeridoo (for cultural reasons it should not be played by women). Special dental splints can also be used to hold open the airway. These look similar to mouthguards used in sport to protect the teeth. When properly fitted, a dental splint will reduce snoring and help in mild to moderate cases of obstructive sleep apnoea.

For severe cases, the most effective way to reduce sleepiness and other daytime impacts is **continuous positive airway pressure** (CPAP). This means sleeping with a facemask that blows pressurised air into your airways to hold them open, just as the pressure of air in a balloon keeps it expanded. Not everyone can tolerate CPAP because of discomfort, noise, congestion or claustrophobia. But for those who can, it can lead to weight loss, improved mood and overall health.

GETTING A GOOD NIGHT'S SLEEP

Each of the ways in which diabetes disrupts your sleep can be effectively managed in conjunction with your diabetes care team. Treating the underlying condition may resolve some or many of your symptoms. However, it may not necessarily improve your sleep. While fixing these other problems increases the chances that your sleep will improve, treating both your sleep and other conditions that influence it can simultaneously improve the outcomes for each.

Just because sleep is an unconscious activity doesn't mean you have no control over it.

The things you do while you're awake can greatly influence the quality and quantity of your sleep.

There are a number of simple things you can do to make it easier to get the sleep you need. These are known collectively as **sleep hygiene**. In essence, these routine activities accent the positive triggers that help you to go to sleep while eliminating many of the negative barriers that serve to keep you awake.

- Darkness. Keep your bedroom dark. Block out the light from the street or the next room.
- Coolness. Falling body temperature is an important cue for bedtime and sleep. This can be enhanced by keeping your bedroom cooler than the rest of the house, or by having a bath or shower in the evening, allowing natural cooling to enhance your sleep.
- Quiet. Noise and stimulation are supposed to keep us awake. The bedroom should therefore be a quiet place.
- Routine. Most people establish a routine for their night-time activities. When this is disrupted, so is their sleep. For those with trouble sleeping it is

sometimes useful to establish a pattern of going to bed and waking at the same time every day, even on weekends. Go to bed when your body tells you you're sleepy and get up when you wake. Bright sunlight in the morning also helps to regulate your body clock.

- Comfort. Your bed should be a comfortable place. You spend more of your lifetime there than any other single place. But beds seldom receive as much attention as the car or the television. Simple things can help, such as replacing your worn out, uneven or uncomfortable mattress and pillows with those that allow you to maintain an anatomically neutral position. Keeping the pressure off your feet with a cradle or a short quilt can also be helpful for sleep.

- No stimulation. The brain is supposed to be winding down for sleep. Taking caffeine (in tea or coffee) any time after 2 p.m. can see the buzz staying around until bedtime. Similarly, late meals can keep the brain going; late-night snacks are not a long-term solution for hypoglycaemia (see Chapter 7). Also, keep the television and the computer out of the bedroom, as both of these keep the eyes and the mind active when you should be sleeping.

There are a number of short-term interventions for sleeplessness, including the use of sleeping pills (also known as **sedatives**). These are used to re-establish a pattern and restore confidence that a good night's sleep is achievable. However, using sleeping pills is at best a short-term solution and may be associated with side effects, including residual daytime sleepiness and dependence if used chronically. A number of psychological (training) techniques can also help sleep in the short term, with far fewer side effects.

18

DIABETES IN MY BED

Understand

- While diabetes does not prevent sex, it can sometimes reduce the ability to achieve satisfying and enjoyable sex.
- For women with type 2 diabetes the most common sexual problem is a low libido.
- Women with diabetes may also find it difficult to attain adequate vaginal lubrication, making intercourse uncomfortable and climax more difficult to reach.
- For men with type 2 diabetes, the most common problem is an inability to

get or maintain an erection. This may affect up to three-quarters of all men with type 2 diabetes.

Manage

- Be honest with yourself and your partner. Pretending that there is no problem is not a solution.
- Ask for help. There are many safe and effective medical treatments now available which, alongside psychological support, can help you to rediscover your sex life.
- Change the way you approach sex to be more in keeping with what your body can do. More foreplay, more stimulation and more lubrication are all practical and enjoyable additions that will help make sex work better for you.

The bed is not just for sleep. For many people, sex is a major part of their health, wellbeing, self-esteem and quality of life. It is often said that sex keeps you alive. This is more than just having the kind of relationship or youthful vigour that makes frequent sex possible. Satisfying sex is associated with better health. Sex also serves to enhance intimacy and reinforce relationships. By contrast, when sex becomes a let-down it can not only be frustrating but it can also be harmful for your health.

While diabetes does not prevent sex, it can sometimes reduce the ability to achieve satisfying and enjoyable sex. This is known as sexual dysfunction.

DEALING WITH A LOW LIBIDO

Desire for or interest in sex is known as **libido**. Having a low libido is a common sexual issue for many people with type 2 diabetes. A number of different factors may be involved. A low libido can be the result of complex changes in brain and body chemistry due to diabetes. Equally, psychological factors such as physical fatigue, body image, pain, poor sleep, low self-esteem and stress can make sex the last thing on your mind.

There is good evidence that keeping good control of your glucose levels will also help you keep your sex life going. But for those who are experiencing problems in bed, better glucose control is usually not enough. Helping you find your libido again usually involves working with your mind as well as your body. It cannot be fixed solely by taking medications such as Viagra, which only work on the penis.

There are many valuable practitioners who can discreetly assist couples and help to put them back on the right track. Some of the most successful treatments are delivered by sex therapists, who work on improving a couple's closeness and communication both in and out of the bedroom through guided discussion, getting rid of negative thoughts and unrealistic performance goals.

Type 2 diabetes can sometimes be the cause of reduced levels of sex hormones such as testosterone. This can contribute to a reduced desire for sex both in men and women. Low testosterone levels can also cause you to feel tired, reduce your capacity to concentrate and disturb your sleep. Note that not everyone with low testosterone levels will have problems with their health or their sex life. But in those people with low levels and who are also experiencing troublesome symptoms, taking hormone supplements can improve how they feel both in the bedroom and out of it.

For men, there are a range of different testosterone supplements that can be prescribed, including injections, patches and gels. The best one for you will be determined by specific blood tests, which will confirm that your levels are low and allow your doctor to develop an individualised treatment plan. In post-menopausal women with low testosterone levels, only small doses may be required to restore normal levels and improve energy and libido. This can often be simply achieved by taking chemicals such as DHEA, which are partly metabolised into testosterone.

In both men and women, these supplements only work when combined with psychological support and good diabetes management. Taking testosterone or DHEA is not enough on its own to bring sex back into your life.

A number of over-the-counter medications advertise their unique ability to increase sexual desire. This is largely because people think they do. But because sexual desire is mostly in the mind it probably doesn't matter. However, their safety and the consistency of their effects may be quite variable and should not be relied upon.

DIABETES AND THE VAGINA

Some women with type 2 diabetes may also find it difficult to attain adequate **vaginal lubrication**, making intercourse uncomfortable and climax more difficult to reach. Vaginal dryness is a common problem for all ageing women but particularly in women with type 2 diabetes, due to fluid losses that also cause the eyes, mouth and skin to feel dry. Each of these symptoms can be reduced with good glucose control. Diabetes can also cause hormonal changes and damage to the blood vessels and nerves of the pelvis that control vaginal fluid production. Some medications used to treat diabetes can also reduce vaginal lubrication.

Although it is a common problem, this need not be a barrier to sexual enjoyment. It just needs to be recognized for what it is and so incorporated into how you have sex. For example, all women with diabetes will benefit from sufficient stimulation/foreplay to ensure that lubrication is naturally enhanced before sex. The use of lubricants can also help and form a new fun part of sex. Oestrogen-containing creams can also improve the health of the vagina and its ability to make lubricating fluids during sex. However, hormone replacement pills are not appropriate for post-menopausal women with type 2 diabetes because of the increased risk of heart disease and clotting.

Women with type 2 diabetes are also prone to genital infections, especially thrush. This can be quite uncomfortable and distressing. Although thrush is easily treated, it is common for it to come back repeatedly and further courses of treatment are often needed. Fortunately, thrush is easy to recognize and rapidly treated using medicines available over the counter at a pharmacy. Many women will have ready supplies in their medicine cabinet for such eventualities. It is not necessary to wait to see a doctor before treating yourself. Achieving and maintaining good glucose control will reduce your chances of getting thrush and assist in its eradication. Other tricks to prevent thrush include oestrogen creams which help to build your resistance to infection. Probiotic bacteria, such as lactobacilli in yoghurt and some supplements, may also help to prevent infection in some cases. As discussed in Chapter 6, some medications used to treat diabetes known as -SGLT-2 inhibitors, can significantly increase the risk of thrush. So when starting these pills, special attention should be taken for early treatment should you become suddenly troubled by itch, pain or discharge.

NOT GETTING AN ERECTION

It's perfectly normal for men to have an occasional problem keeping an erection. But for some men, these difficulties are frequent and severe, making sex all but impossible.

A consistent inability to get or maintain an erection for sex is the most common sexual problem affecting men with type 2 diabetes.

This is known as erectile dysfunction and may affect at least three-quarters of men with type 2 diabetes. In fact of all the complications of diabetes, this is numerically the most common. But it is also probably the least talked about. An inability to maintain an erection can be the result of many factors. Coordinated function among nerves and blood vessels and the right mind-set are all required for the penis to become and stay erect. If any of these necessary components isn't functioning optimally, an erection will fail. Unfortunately, type 2 diabetes can affect all these different components, which is why erectile dysfunction is so common.

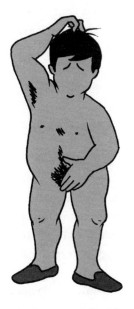

The consistent inability to get or maintain an erection may affect over three-quarters of men with type 2 diabetes. But this can be fixed!

The good news is that there are a number of very effective treatments now available. The most widely used treatments are the type 5 phosphodiesterase inhibitors, the first and best-known of these is **Viagra**. There are also now many others available that vary in how long they work for. This influences how long they need to be taken before sex and how long they last. Viagra is usually taken about an hour before sex and lasts for around 8 hours. Some other medications of this type can be taken many hours before and still work a day later.

These pills all work by increasing blood flow to the penis when it is stimulated, enhancing the chances of an erection. These medications have no direct effect on the penis in the absence of sexual stimulation, so won't cause an erection unless you want one. However, they work in only about 60 per cent of men with type 2 diabetes.

Viagra also has no direct effect on your mind so it won't make you suddenly sex crazed. However, it does have a profound psychological effect that comes from the anticipation of sex. Viagra and other medications of the same class are generally safe in men with diabetes. Some men experience headaches, flushing or nasal stuffiness. However, they shouldn't be used in people with heart problems requiring nitroglycerine as part of their treatment.

Unfortunately, this strategy will work in only about 60 per cent of men with type 2 diabetes. But there are other alternatives for those in whom it doesn't work. Two alternatives to pills are penis injections or tiny suppositories placed inside the penis. These act to trigger an erection within 10 to 15 minutes whenever they are used. Unlike Viagra, they produce erections without any stimulation so are helpful in men who have nerve damage due to diabetes. Because these medications only act in your groin they have few side effects elsewhere. The erection usually subsides within an hour. Other options include vacuum erection devices and penile prostheses. When used in the right setting, each can improve sex and your quality of life.

ALWAYS ASK FOR HELP

While dissatisfaction with sex is more common in both men and women with type 2 diabetes, it is not the first thing you hear people complain about when they see their diabetes care team. Just focusing on glucose control in diabetes sometimes means that you are not focusing on your total health and wellbeing. Ignoring problems with sex does not make them go away and can sometimes make them worse. Your doctor won't usually ask. So it's up to you.

The biggest barrier is usually a reluctance to share your feelings, and reticence in asking for help from your partner or your health specialist. Sex and sexuality are often kept too private. It is not that you don't know there is a problem. Rather, most people are understandably uncomfortable disclosing or discussing sexual matters. Yet there are many effective resources now available to prevent diabetes coming in the way of a healthy and fulfilling sex life. This always means first asking for help.

ACKNOWLEDGMENTS

Baker IDI would like to thank Professor Don Chisholm AO, Garvan Institute of Medical Research; Dr Pat Phillips, Endocrinologist, The QE Specialist Centre, Woodville, South Australia; and Professor Trisha Dunning AM, Chair in Nursing and Director Centre for Nursing and Allied Health Research Deakin University and Barwon Health, who provided insightful and independent reviews of the early draft text of the first edition of this book.

We would also like to acknowledge the following Baker IDI staff: Professor Mark Cooper, Associate Professor Jonathan Shaw, Ms Michele Mack and Ms Rebecca Stiegler, who provided their time and expertise in reviewing the book.

The generosity of these reviewers has helped to create a text that is accurate, useful and understandable to readers.

RESOURCES

There are many pages on the internet to help you learn more about type 2 diabetes. Here are some good sites to get you started. There are many more you'll be able to discover as you continue to explore your diabetes and its treatment. Just be careful, as some make claims that cannot be supported. Always discuss possible changes in your management with your diabetes care team before embarking on them and never use them to the exclusion of your recommended treatment.

By the author

www.bakeridi.edu.au/research/biochemistry_of_diabetic_complications/

www.slowageingbook.com

www.penguin.com.au/products/9780143202264/csiro-and-baker-idi-diabetes-diet-and-lifestyle-plan

Diabetes organizations

www.cdc.gov/diabetes/consumer/index.htm

www.diabetesaustralia.com.au

www.diabetes.ca/

www.diabeteschannel.com.au

www.diabetes.co.uk/

www.diabetes.org

www.diabetes.org.nz/resources/pamphlets

www.iddt.org/

www.idf.org/

www./ndep.nih.gov/i-have-diabetes/index.aspx

Diet

www.diabetes-book.com/index.shtml

www.diabetes-diet.org.uk/

https://diabeticmediterraneandiet.com/

www.dsolve.com/

www.glycemicindex.com

www.gofor2and5.com.au

www.lowcarbdiabetic.co.uk/

www.myphotodiet.com/

www.nhs.uk/Change4Life

Exercise

www.10000steps.org.au

www.diabeticlifestyle.com/exercise/diabetes-beginning-exercise-plan

www.getwalking.org/

www.liftforlife.com.au

www.runsweet.com/

Complications

www.beyondblue.org.au

diabetespeptalk.ca/en/

www.hearthub.org/

www.heartfoundation.org.au

www.kidney.org

www.kidney.org.au

www.limbs4life.com/

www.nei.nih.gov/health/diabetic/retinopathy.asp

Other useful diabetes resources and blogs

www.battlediabetes.com/

www.bbc.co.uk/health/physical_health/conditions/in_depth/
diabetes/index.shtml

www.diabetesandrelatedhealthissues.com/

www.diabetes.boomja.com/

www.diabetescare.net/

www.diabetesdigest.com/

www.DiabetesEveryDay.com

www.diabetesforum.com/

www.diabeteshealth.com/

www.diabeteslocal.org/

www.diabetesmine.com/

www.diabetesmonitor.com/

www.diabeteswellbeing.com/

www.irunoninsulin.com/

www.mydiabetesmyway.scot.nhs.uk/default.asp

www.patient.co.uk/education/diabetes

www.thediabetesresource.com/

INDEX

U

unsaturated fats 175
urge incontinence 256
urinary retention 256
urinary tract infections 257
urination
    bladder control 254–57
    frequent 242
urine, albumin in 244, 247–48

V

vaginal lubrication 303
vascular dementia 269–270
vegetables
    fibre-rich 51
    peels 51
Viagra 305–6
visceral fat 23
visual impairment *see* sight
vitreal haemorrhage 221
vitrectomy 221
VLDL cholesterol 181
VO$_2$ fitness test 88–89
voiding 258

W

waist
    healthy circumference 23
    toxic waist 24–25
waist management *see* weight control
walking program 87
water pills/tablets 160–61
weight control
    heart benefits 197
    physical activity 81–82
    systolic blood pressure 154
weight gain, sulphonylureas 108
weight loss
    blood pressure 153
    cholesterol levels 179–180
    goals 73
    management 55
    non-dietary options 74–76
    understanding 54–55

weight loss diets 58–68
    categories 58–59
    low calorie 60–65
    low fat 65–66, 174–76
    see also low carbohydrate diets
white-coat hypertension 147
wholegrain foods, fibre content
    49–51
wholemeal flour 49–50

Z

Zone Diet 67

PENGUIN MODERN CLASSICS

Understanding a Photograph

John Berger was born in London in 1926. His acclaimed works of fiction and non-fiction include the seminal *Ways of Seeing* and the novel *G.*, which won the Booker Prize in 1972. In 1962 he left Britain permanently, and he now lives in a small village in the French Alps.

Geoff Dyer is the author of four novels and many non-fiction books. He is a winner of the Somerset Maugham Prize, the International Center of Photography's 2006 Infinity Award for *The Ongoing Moment* and a 2012 National Book Critics Circle Award for the essay collection *Otherwise Known as the Human Condition*.

JOHN BERGER

Understanding a Photograph

Edited and Introduced by GEOFF DYER

PENGUIN BOOKS

PENGUIN CLASSICS

Published by the Penguin Group
Penguin Books Ltd, 80 Strand, London WC2R ORL, England
Penguin Group (USA) Inc., 375 Hudson Street, New York, New York 10014, USA
Penguin Group (Canada), 90 Eglinton Avenue East, Suite 700, Toronto, Ontario, Canada M4P 2Y3
 (a division of Pearson Penguin Canada Inc.)
Penguin Ireland, 25 St Stephen's Green, Dublin 2, Ireland (a division of Penguin Books Ltd)
Penguin Group (Australia), 707 Collins Street, Melbourne, Victoria 3008, Australia
 (a division of Pearson Australia Group Pty Ltd)
Penguin Books India Pvt Ltd, 11 Community Centre, Panchsheel Park, New Delhi – 110 017, India
Penguin Group (NZ), 67 Apollo Drive, Rosedale, Auckland 0632, New Zealand
 (a division of Pearson New Zealand Ltd)
Penguin Books (South Africa) (Pty) Ltd, Block D, Rosebank Office Park, 181 Jan Smuts Avenue,
Parktown North, Gauteng 2193, South Africa
Penguin Books Ltd, Registered Offices: 80 Strand, London WC2R ORL, England
www. penguin. com
First published in Penguin Classics 2013
006

Copyright © John Berger, 1967, 1968, 1969, 1972, 1978, 1979, 1980, 1982, 1985, 1988, 1991, 1992, 1996, 1998,
1999, 2001, 2002, 2004, 2005, 2007, 2013
Introduction and editorial material © Geoff Dyer, 2013
All rights reserved

The moral right of the author and of the editor and introducer has been asserted

The first-time publication details on pp. 217–19 constitute an extension of this page

Set in Monotype Dante
Typeset by Dinah Drazin
Printed in Great Britain by Clays Ltd, St Ives plc

Except in the United States of America, this book is sold subject
to the condition that it shall not, by way of trade or otherwise, be lent,
re-sold, hired out, or otherwise circulated without the publisher's
prior consent in any form of binding or cover other than that in
which it is published and without a similar condition including this
condition being imposed on the subsequent purchaser

ISBN: 978-0-141-39202-8

www.greenpenguin.co.uk

MIX
Paper from
responsible sources
FSC
www.fsc.org   FSC® C018179

Penguin Books is committed to a sustainable
future for our business, our readers and our planet.
This book is made from Forest Stewardship
Council™ certified paper.

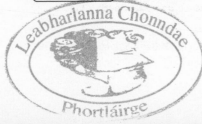

Contents

Contents

List of Illustrations

Rwandan Tutsi and Hutu refugees, Tanzania, 1994, by Sebastião Salgado. (© Sebastião Salgado/Amazonas images/NB pictures; image courtesy of NB pictures)

p. 178 Photograph from 'The Reality Beneath'/*Nearly Invisible*, 2001, by Moyra Peralta. (Courtesy of the artist; © Moyra Peralta)

p. 190 Untitled, 1989, by Marc Trivier. (Courtesy of the artist; © The Estate of Alberto Giacometti (Fondation Giacometti, Paris, and ADAGP, Paris), licensed in the UK by ACS and DACS, London 2012)

p. 194 *Annette*, Basel, 1989, by Marc Trivier. (Courtesy of the artist; © The Estate of Alberto Giacometti (Fondation Giacometti, Paris, and ADAGP, Paris), licensed in the UK by ACS and DACS, London 2012)

p. 202 Untitled, from the series 'Forest', 2000–2005, by Jitka Hanzlová. (Courtesy of Jitka Hanzlová and Mai 36 Galerie Zurich; © 2013 Artists Rights Society (ARS), New York/VG Bild-Kunst, Bonn)

p. 208 Untitled (*Trackers* no. 57), Lakhish Army Base, Beit Gubrin, Israel/Palestine, 2005, by Ahlam Shibli. Chromogenic print, 37 x 55.5cm. (Courtesy of the artist; © Ahlam Shibli)

to Beverly

Introduction

I became interested in photography not by taking or looking at photographs but by reading about them. The names of the three writers who served as guides will come as no surprise: Roland Barthes, Susan Sontag and John Berger. I read Sontag on Diane Arbus before I'd seen any photographs by Arbus (there are no pictures in *On Photography*), and Barthes on André Kertész, and Berger on August Sander without knowing any photographs other than the few reproduced in *Camera Lucida* and *About Looking*. (The fact that the photo on the cover of *About Looking* was credited to someone called Garry Winogrand meant nothing to me.)

Berger was indebted to both of the others. Dedicated to Sontag, the 1978 essay 'Uses of Photography' is offered as a series of 'responses' to *On Photography*, published the previous year: 'The thoughts are sometimes my own, but all originate in the experience of reading her book' (p. 49). Writing about *The Pleasure of the Text* (1973), Berger described Barthes as 'the only living critic or theorist of literature and language whom I, as a writer, recognise'.[1]

For his part, Barthes included Sontag's *On Photography* in the list of books – omitted from the English edition – at the end of *Camera Lucida* (1980). Sontag, in turn, had been profoundly shaped by her reading of Barthes. All three had been influenced by Walter Benjamin whose 'A Small History of Photography' (1931) reads like the oldest surviving part of a map this later trio tried – in their different ways, using customized projections – to extend, enhance and improve. Benjamin is a constantly flickering presence in much of Barthes' writing. The anthology of quotations at the end of *On Photography* is dedicated – with the kind of intimate relation to greatness that Sontag cultivated, adored and believed to be her due – 'to W. B.' At the end of the first part of *Ways of Seeing* Berger acknowledges that 'many of the ideas' had been taken from an essay of Benjamin's titled 'The Work of Art in the Age of Mechanical Reproduction'. (This was 1972, remember, before Benjamin's essay became one of the most mechanically reproduced and quoted ever written.)

Photography, for all four, was an area of special interest, but not a specialism. They approached photography not with the authority of curators or historians of the medium but as essayists, writers. Their writings on the subject were less the product of accumulated knowledge than active records of how knowledge and understanding had been acquired or was in the process of being acquired.

This is particularly evident in the case of Berger, who did not devote an entire book to the subject until *Another Way of Telling* in 1982. In a sense, though, he was the one whose training and career led most directly to photography. Sontag had followed a fairly established path of academic study before becoming a freelance writer, and Barthes remained in academia for his entire career. Berger's creative life, however, was rooted in the visual arts. Leaving school possessed by a single idea – 'I wanted to draw naked women. All day long'[2] – he attended the Chelsea and Central Schools of Art. In the early 1950s he began writing about art and became a regular critic – iconoclastic, Marxist, much admired, often derided – for the *New Statesman*. His first novel, *A Painter of Our Time* (1958), was a direct result of his immersion in the world of art and the politics of the left. By the mid-1960s he had widened his scope far beyond art *and* the novel to become a writer unhindered by category and genre. Crucially, for the current discussion, he had begun collaborating with a photographer, Jean Mohr. Their first book, *A Fortunate Man* (1967), made a significant step beyond the pioneering work of Walker Evans and James Agee in *Let Us Now Praise Famous Men* (1941), on rural poverty in the Great Depression. (*A Fortunate Man* is subtitled 'The Story of a Country Doctor', in homage, presumably, to the great photo essay by W. Eugene Smith, 'Country Doctor', published in *Life* in 1948.) This was followed by their study of migrant labour, *A Seventh Man* (1975), and, eventually, *Another Way of Telling*. The important thing, in all three books, is that the photographs are not there to illustrate the text, and, conversely, the text is not intended to serve as any kind of extended caption for the images. Rejecting what Berger regards as a kind of 'tautology', words and image exist, instead, in an integrated, mutually enhancing relationship. A new form was being forged and refined.

A side-effect of this ongoing relationship with Mohr was that Berger had, for many years, not only observed Mohr at work; he had also been the subject of that work. Lacking the training as a photographer that he'd enjoyed as an artist he became very familiar with the other side of the experience, of being photographed. With the exception of one picture, by another friend – Henri Cartier-Bresson! – the author photographs on his books have almost always been by Mohr; they constitute Mohr's visual biography of his friend. (The essay on Mohr included here records Berger's attempt to reciprocate, to make a sketch of the photographer.) His writings on drawing speak with the authority of the drawer; his writings on photography often concentrate on the experience, the depicted lives, of those photographed. Barthes expressed the initial impetus for *Camera Lucida* as photography '*against* film';[3] Berger's writing on photography hinges on its relationship to painting and drawing. As Berger has grown older, his early training – in drawing – rather than fading in importance has become a more and more trusted tool of investigation and inquiry. (Tellingly, his latest book, published in 2011 and inspired in part by Spinoza, is called *Bento's*

Sketchbook.) A representative passage in 'My Beautiful' records how, in a museum in Florence, he came across the porcelain head of an angel by Luca della Robbia: 'I did a drawing to try to understand better the expression of her face' (p. 200). Could this be part of the fascination of photography for Berger? Not just that it is a wholly different form of image production, but that it is immune to explication by drawing? A photograph *can* be drawn, obviously, but how can its meaning best be *drawn out*?

This was the goal Barthes and Berger shared: to articulate the essence of photography – or, as Alfred Stieglitz had expressed it in 1914, 'the *idea* photography'.[4] While this ambition fed, naturally enough, into photographic theory, Berger's method was always too personal, the habits of the autodidact too ingrained, to succumb to the kind of discourse- and semiotics-mania that seized cultural studies in the 1970s and '80s. Victor Burgin – to take a representative figure of the time – had much to learn from Berger; Berger comparatively little from Burgin. After all, by the time of *About Looking* (1980), the collection that contained some of his most important essays on photography, Berger had been living in the Haute-Savoie for the best part of a decade. His researches – I let the word stand in spite of being so thoroughly inappropriate – into photography proceeded in tandem with the struggle to gain a different kind of knowledge and understanding: of the peasants he had been living among and was writing about in the trilogy *Into Their Labours*. Except, of course, the knowledge and methods were not so distinct after all. Writing the fictional lives of Lucie Cabrol or Boris – in *Pig Earth* (1979) and *Once in Europa* (1987), the first two volumes of the trilogy – or about Paul Strand's photograph of Mr Bennett (p. 46), both required the kind of attentiveness celebrated by D. H. Lawrence in his poem 'Thought':

> Thought is gazing on to the face of life, and reading what can be read,

Thought is pondering over experience, and coming to a
    conclusion.
Thought is not a trick, or an exercise, or a set of dodges,
Thought is a man in his wholeness wholly attending.[5]

In Berger's case, the habit of thought is like a sustained and disciplined version of something that had come instinctively to him
as a boy. In *Here is Where We Meet* the author's mother remembers
him as a child on a tram in Croydon: 'I never saw anyone look as
hard as you did, sitting on the edge of the seat.'[6] If the boy ended
up becoming a 'theorist', then it is by adherence to the method
described by Goethe, quoted by Benjamin (in 'A Small History') and
re-quoted by Berger in 'The Suit and the Photograph': 'There is a
delicate form of the empirical which identifies itself so intimately
with its object that it thereby becomes theory' (p. 36).[7]

This is what makes Berger such a wonderful practical critic and
reader of individual photographs ('gazing on to the face of life,
and reading what can be read'), questioning them with his signa-
ture intensity of attention – and, often, tenderness. (See, for example, the analysis of Kertész's picture 'A Red Hussar Leaving, June
1919, Budapest', p. 74.) To that extent his writing on photography
continues the interrogation of the visible that characterized his
writing on painting. As he explains at the beginning of the conversation with Sebastião Salgado: 'I try to put into words what I
see' (p. 169).

In 1960 Berger had defined his aesthetic criteria simply and con-
fidently: 'does this work help or encourage men to know and claim
their social rights?'[8] Consistent with this, his writing on photography was from the start – from the essay on Che Guevara of
1967, 'Image of Imperialism' – avowedly and unavoidably political.
(Which meant, in 'Photographs of Agony', of 1972, he could argue
that pictures of war and famine which *seemed* political often served
to remove the suffering depicted from the political decisions that

brought it about into an unchangeable and apparently permanent realm of the human condition.) Naturally, he has gravitated
towards political, documentary or 'campaigning' photographers,
but the range is wide and the notion of political never reducible
to what the Indian photographer Raghubir Singh called 'the abject
as subject'.[9] In 'The Suit and the Photograph' Sander's image of
three peasants going to a dance becomes the starting point for the
history of the suit as an idealization of 'purely *sedentary* power'
(p. 41) and an illustration of Gramsci's notion of hegemony. (As
with Benjamin's 'Work of Art', remember that this was the 1970s,
almost twenty years before Gore Vidal informed Michael Foot
that 'the young, even in America, are reading Gramsci'.[10]) Lee
Friedlander, the least theory-driven of photographers, once com-
mented on how much stuff – how much unintended information
– accidentally ended up in his pictures. 'It's a generous medium,
photography,' he concluded drily.[11] 'The Suit and the Photograph'
is an object lesson in how much information is there to be discovered and revealed even in photographs lacking the visual density
of Friedlander's. It's also exemplary, reminding us that many of the
best essays are also journeys, epistemological journeys that take
us beyond the moment depicted, often beyond photography – and
sometimes back again. In 'Between Here and Then', written for
an exhibition by Marc Trivier in 2005, Berger mentions the photographs only briefly before telling a story about an old and beloved
clock, how the sound of its ticking makes the kitchen where he
lives breathe. The clock breaks (is actually broken by the author
in what must have been a furious moment of temporal slapstick),
Berger takes it to a mender only to find . . . Well, that would spoil
the story but, at the end, as well as a literal return there is also a
coming together, a tacit exchange of greetings between Berger
and Barthes, who wrote, in one of the most beautiful passages of
Camera Lucida:

For me the noise of Time is not sad: I love bells, clocks, watches – and I recall that at first photographic implements were related to techniques of cabinetmaking and the machinery of precision: cameras, in short, were clocks for seeing, and perhaps in me someone very old still hears in the photographic mechanism the living sound of the wood.[12]

This is a glimpse of Barthes the novelist in exquisite miniature. Berger's critical writing, meanwhile, has gone hand in hand with the creation of a substantial body of fiction. As Berger examines and coaxes out a photograph's stories – both the ones it reveals and those that lie concealed – so the task of the critic and interrogator of images gives way to the vocation and embrace of the storyteller. And it does not stop there, since, as he reminds us in *And Our Faces, My Heart, Brief as Photos*, 'the traffic between storytelling and metaphysics is continuous'.[13]

The essays in this book are arranged more or less chronologically. They comprise selections from books by Berger and previously uncollected pieces written for exhibitions or as introductions and afterwords to catalogues. A few very minor mistakes have been silently corrected and some other very small changes have been made to eliminate discrepancies resulting from the pieces having gone through the different wash cycles of previous house styles. All of the pieces would benefit from being more comprehensively illustrated. This is more of a problem, obviously, than it was when a given piece appeared in a book filled with large, high-quality reproductions. It is less of a problem now than it was back in the time of Sontag's *On Photography* since so many of the pictures can be found instantly online, can even be viewed on the same device on which this book may be read. Having said that, it bears repeating that *Another Way of Telling* was conceived as a collaboration. The images are as important as the words. In the essays included here ('Appearances' and

'Stories'), we have only Berger's words which, in this context, serve as signposts, directing you back to the book, where they can be reunited with Mohr's pictures.

Geoff Dyer
Iowa City, August 2012

Notes

1 John Berger, *New Society*, 26 February 1976, p. 445.

2 John Berger, *Selected Essays* (London: Bloomsbury, 2001), p. 559.

3 Roland Barthes, *The Grain of the Voice* (London: Jonathan Cape, 1985), p. 359.

4 Alfred Stieglitz, *Photographs and Writings*, ed. Sarah Greenough (Washington, DC: National Gallery of Art/Bulfinch Press, 1999), p. 13.

5 D. H. Lawrence, *Complete Poems* (Harmondsworth: Penguin, 1994), p. 673.

6 John Berger, *Here is Where We Meet* (London: Bloomsbury, 2005), p. 8.

7 For a different translation of the passage on p. 36, see Walter Benjamin, *One Way Street and Other Writings*, trans. Edmund Jephcott and Kingsley Shorter (London: New Left Books, 1979), p. 252.

8 John Berger, *Selected Essays*, p. 7.

9 Raghubir Singh, *River of Colour* (London: Phaidon, 1998), p. 12.

10 Gore Vidal, *The Last Empire* (New York: Doubleday, 2001), p. 304.

11 Peter Galassi, *Friedlander* (New York: Museum of Modern Art, 2005), p. 14.

12 Roland Barthes, *Camera Lucida*, trans. Richard Howard (New York: Hill and Wang, 1981) p. 15.

13 John Berger, *And Our Faces, My Heart, Brief as Photos* (New York: Pantheon, 1984), p. 30.

Understanding
a Photograph

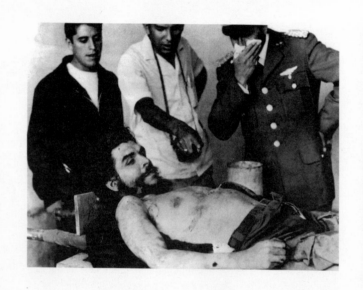

Image of Imperialism

On Tuesday 10 October 1967, a photograph was transmitted to the world to prove that Guevara had been killed the previous Sunday in a clash between two companies of the Bolivian army and a guerrilla force on the north side of the Rio Grande River near a jungle village called Higueras. (Later this village received the proclaimed reward for the capture of Guevara.) The photograph of the corpse was taken in a stable in the small town of Vallegrande. The body was placed on a stretcher and the stretcher was placed on top of a cement trough.

During the preceding two years 'Che' Guevara had become legendary. Nobody knew for certain where he was. There was no incontestable evidence of anyone having seen him. But his presence was constantly assumed and invoked. At the head of his last statement – sent from a guerrilla base 'somewhere in the world' to the Tricontinental Solidarity Organization in Havana – he quoted a line from the nineteenth-century revolutionary poet José Martí: 'Now is the time of the furnaces, and only light should be seen.' It was as though in his own declared light Guevara had become invisible and ubiquitous.

Now he is dead. The chances of his survival were in inverse ratio to the force of the legend. The legend had to be nailed. 'If,' said *The New York Times*, 'Ernesto Che Guevara was really killed in Bolivia, as now seems probable, a myth as well as a man has been laid to rest.'

We do not know the circumstances of his death. One can gain some idea of the mentality of those into whose hands he fell by their treatment of his body after his death. First they hid it. Then they displayed it. Then they buried it in an anonymous grave in an unknown place. Then they disinterred it. Then they burnt it. But before burning it, they cut off the fingers for later identification. This might suggest that they had serious doubts whether it was really Guevara whom they had killed. Equally it can suggest that they had no doubts but feared the corpse. I tend to believe the latter.

The purpose of the photograph of 10 October was to put an end to a legend. Yet on many who saw it its effect may have been very different. What is its meaning? What, precisely and unmysteriously, does this photograph mean now? I can but cautiously analyse it as regards myself.

There is a resemblance between the photograph and Rembrandt's painting of *The Anatomy Lesson of Doctor Nicolaes Tulp.* The immaculately dressed Bolivian colonel with a handkerchief to his nose has

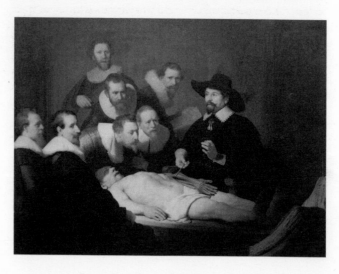

taken the doctor's place. The two figures on his right stare at the cadaver with the same intense but impersonal interest as the two nearest doctors to the left of Doctor Tulp. It is true that there are more figures in the Rembrandt – as there were certainly more men, unphotographed, in the stable at Vallegrande. But the placing of the corpse in relation to the figures above it, and in the corpse the sense of global stillness – these are very similar.

Nor should this be surprising, for the function of the two pictures is similar: both are concerned with showing a corpse being formally and objectively examined. More than that, both are concerned with *making an example of the dead*: one for the advancement of medicine, the other as a political warning. Thousands of photographs are taken of the dead and the massacred. But the occasions are seldom formal ones of demonstration. Doctor Tulp is demonstrating the ligaments of the arm, and what he says applies to the normal arm of every man. The colonel with the handkerchief is demonstrating the final fate – as decreed by 'divine providence' – of a notorious guerrilla leader, and what he says is meant to apply to every guerrillero on the continent.

I was also reminded of another image: Mantegna's painting of the dead Christ, now in the Brera at Milan. The body is seen from the same height, but from the feet instead of from the side. The hands are in identical positions, the fingers curving in the same gesture. The drapery over the lower part of the body is creased and formed in the same manner as the blood-sodden, unbuttoned, olive-green trousers on Guevara. The head is raised at the same angle. The mouth is slack of expression in the same way. Christ's eyes have been shut, for there are two mourners beside him. Guevara's eyes are open, for there are no mourners: only the colonel with the handkerchief, a US intelligence agent, a number of Bolivian soldiers and the journalists. Once again, the similarity need not surprise. There are not so many ways of laying out the criminal dead.

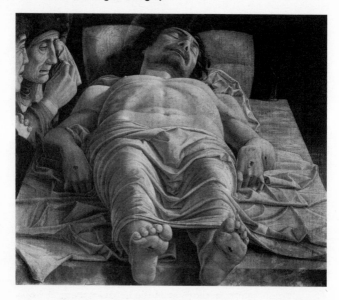

Yet this time the similarity was more than gestural or functional. The emotions with which I came upon that photograph on the front page of the evening paper were very close to what, with the help of historical imagination, I had previously assumed the reaction of a contemporary believer might have been to Mantegna's painting. The power of a photograph is comparatively short-lived. When I look at the photograph now, I can only reconstruct my first incoherent emotions. Guevara was no Christ. If I see the Mantegna again in Milan, I shall see in it the body of Guevara. But this is only because in certain rare cases the tragedy of a man's death completes and exemplifies the meaning of his whole life. I am acutely aware of that about Guevara, and certain painters were once aware of it about Christ. That is the degree of emotional correspondence.

The mistake of many commentators on Guevara's death has been to suppose that he represented only military skill or a certain revolutionary strategy. Thus they talk of a setback or a defeat. I am in no position to assess the loss which Guevara's death may mean to the revolutionary movement of South America. But it is certain that Guevara represented and will represent more than the details of his plans. He represented a decision, a conclusion.

Guevara found the condition of the world as it is intolerable. It had only recently become so. Previously, the conditions under which two-thirds of the people of the world lived were approximately the same as now. The degree of exploitation and enslavement was as great. The suffering involved was as intense and as widespread. The waste was as colossal. But it was not intolerable because the full measure of the truth about these conditions was unknown – even by those who suffered it. Truths are not constantly evident in the circumstances to which they refer. They are born – sometimes late. This truth was born with the struggles and wars of national liberation. In the light of the newborn truth, the significance of imperialism changed. Its demands were seen to be different. Previously it had demanded cheap raw materials, exploited labour and a controlled world market. Today it demands a mankind that counts for nothing.

Guevara envisaged his own death in the revolutionary fight against this imperialism.

Wherever death may surprise us, let it be welcome, provided that this, our battle-cry, may have reached some receptive ear and another hand may be extended to wield our weapons and other men be ready to intone the funeral dirge with the staccato chant of the machine-gun and new battle-cries of war and victory.[1]

1 'Vietnam Must Not Stand Alone', *New Left Review*, London, no. 43, 1967.

His envisaged death offered him the measure of how intolerable his life would be if he accepted the intolerable condition of the world as it is. His envisaged death offered him the measure of the necessity of changing the world. It was by the licence granted by his envisaged death that he was able to live with the necessary pride that becomes a man.

At the news of Guevara's death, I heard someone say: 'He was the world symbol of the possibilities of one man.' Why is this true? Because he recognized what was intolerable for man and acted accordingly.

The measure by which Guevara had lived suddenly became a unit which filled the world and obliterated his life. His envisaged death became actual. The photograph is about this actuality. The possibilities have gone. Instead there is blood, the smell of formol, the untended wounds on the unwashed body, flies, the shambling trousers: the small private details of the body rendered in dying as public and impersonal and broken as a razed city.

Guevara died surrounded by his enemies. What they did to him while he was alive was probably consistent with what they did to him after he was dead. In his extremity he had nothing to support him but his own previous decisions. Thus the cycle was closed. It would be the vulgarest impertinence to claim any knowledge of his experience during that instant or that eternity. His lifeless body, as seen in the photograph, is the only report we have. But we are entitled to deduce the logic of what happens when the cycle closes. Truth flows in the obverse direction. His envisaged death is no more the measure of the necessity for changing the intolerable condition of the world. Aware now of his actual death, he finds in his life the measure of his justification, and the world-as-his-experience becomes tolerable to him.

The foreseeing of this final logic is part of what enables a man or a people to fight against overwhelming odds. It is part of the secret of the moral factor which counts as three to one against weapon power.

The photograph shows an instant: that instant at which Guevara's body, artificially preserved, has become a mere object of demonstration. In this lies its initial horror. But what is it intended to demonstrate? Such horror? No. It is to demonstrate, at the instant of horror, the identity of Guevara and, allegedly, the absurdity of revolution. Yet by virtue of this very purpose, the instant is transcended. The life of Guevara and the idea or fact of revolution immediately invoke processes which preceded that instant and which continue now. Hypothetically, the only way in which the purpose of those who arranged for and authorized the photograph could have been achieved would have been to preserve artificially at that instant the whole state of the world as it was: to stop life. Only in such a way could the content of Guevara's living example have been denied. As it is, either the photograph means nothing because the spectator has no inkling of what is involved, or else its meaning denies or qualifies its demonstration.

I have compared it with two paintings because paintings, before the invention of photography, are the only visual evidence we have of how people saw what they saw. But in its effect it is profoundly different from a painting. A painting, or a successful one at least, comes to terms with the processes invoked by its subject matter. It even suggests an attitude towards those processes. We can regard a painting as almost complete in itself.

In face of this photograph we must either dismiss it or complete its meaning for ourselves. It is an image which, as much as any mute image ever can, calls for decision.

October 1967

Prompted by another recent newspaper photograph, I continue to consider the death of 'Che' Guevara.

Until the end of the eighteenth century, for a man to envisage his death as the possibly direct consequence of his choice of a certain course of action is the measure of his *loyalty* as a servant. This is true whatever the social station or privilege of the man. Inserted between himself and his own meaning there is always a power to which his only possible relationship is one of service or servitude. The power may be considered abstractly as Fate. More usually it is personified in God, King or the Master.

Thus the choice which the man makes (the choice whose foreseen consequence may be his own death) is curiously incomplete. It is a choice submitted to a superior power for acknowledgement. The man himself can only judge *sub judice*: finally it is he who will be judged. In exchange for this limited responsibility he receives benefits. The benefits can range from a master's recognition of his courage to eternal bliss in heaven. But in all cases the ultimate decision and the ultimate benefit are located as exterior to his own self and life. Consequently death, which would seem to be so definitive an *end*, is for him a *means*, a treatment to which he submits for the sake of some aftermath. Death is like the eye of a needle through which he is threaded. Such is the mode of his heroism.

The French Revolution changed the nature of heroism. (Let it be clear that I do not refer to specific courages: the endurance of pain or torture, the will to attack under fire, the speed and lightness of movement and decision in battle, the spontaneity of mutual aid under danger – these courages must be largely defined by physical experience and have perhaps changed very little. I refer only to the choice which may precede these other courages.) The French Revolution brings the King to judgement and condemns him.

Saint-Just, aged twenty-five, in his first speech to the Convention argues that monarchy is crime, because the King usurps the sovereignty of the people.

It is impossible to reign innocently: the madness of it is too clear.
Every king is a rebel and a usurper.[2]

It is true that Saint-Just serves – in his own mind – the General Will
of the people, but he has freely chosen to do so because he believes
that the people, if allowed to be true to their own nature, embody
Reason and that their Republic represents Virtue.

> In the world there are three kinds of infamy with which Republican
> virtue can reach no compromise: the first are kings: the second is the
> serving of kings: the third is the laying down of arms while there
> still exists anywhere a master and a slave.[3]

It is now less likely that a man envisages his own death as the measure of his loyalty as a servant to a master. His envisaged death is
likely to be the measure of his love of Freedom: a proof of the
principle of his own liberty.

Twenty months after his first speech Saint-Just spends the night
preceding his own execution writing at his desk. He makes no active
attempt to save himself. He has already written:

> Circumstances are only difficult for those who draw back from the
> grave . . . I despise the dust of which I am composed, the dust which
> is speaking to you: anyone can pursue and put an end to this dust.
> But I defy anybody to snatch from me what I have given myself,
> an independent life in the sky of the centuries.[4]

'What I have given myself'. The ultimate decision is now located
within the self. But not categorically and entirely; there is a certain

2 Saint-Just, *Discours et rapports* (Paris: Éditions Sociales, 1957), p. 66 (translation
by the author).
3 Ibid., p. 90.
4 Ibid.

ambiguity. God no longer exists, but Rousseau's Supreme Being is there to confuse the issue by way of a metaphor. The metaphor allows one to believe that the self will share in the historical judgement of one's own life. 'An independent life in the sky' of historical judgement. There is still the ghost of a pre-existent order.

Even when Saint-Just is declaring the opposite – in his defiant last speech of defence for Robespierre and himself – the ambiguity remains:

> Fame is an empty noise. Let us put our ears to the centuries that have gone: we no longer hear anything; those who, at another time, shall walk among our urns, shall hear no more. The good – that is what we must pursue, whatever the price, preferring the title of a dead hero to that of a living coward.[5]

But in life, as opposed to the theatre, the dead hero never hears himself so called. The political stage of a revolution often has a theatrical, because exemplary, tendency. The world watches to learn.

> Tyrants everywhere looked upon us because we were judging one of theirs; today when, by a happier destiny, you are deliberating on the liberty of the world, the people of the earth who are the truly great of the earth will, in their turn, watch you.[6]

Yet, notwithstanding the truth of this, there is, philosophically, a sense in which Saint-Just dies triumphantly trapped within his 'stage' role. (To say this in no way detracts from his courage.)

Since the French Revolution, the bourgeois age. Among those few who envisage their own death (and not their own fortunes) as the direct consequence of their principled decisions, such marginal ambiguity disappears.

5 Ibid.
6 Ibid. Saint-Just to the Convention, on the Constitution.

The confrontation between the living man and the world as he finds it becomes total. There is nothing exterior to it, not even a principle. A man's envisaged death is the measure of his refusal to accept what confronts him. There is nothing beyond that refusal.

The Russian anarchist Voinarovsky, who was killed throwing a bomb at Admiral Dubassov, wrote:

> Without a single muscle on my face twitching, without saying a word, I shall climb on the scaffold – and this will not be an act of violence perpetrated on myself, it will be the perfectly natural result of all that I have lived through.[7]

He envisages his own death on the scaffold – and a number of Russian terrorists at that time died exactly as he describes – as though it were the peaceful death of an old man. Why is he able to do this? Psychological explanations are not enough. It is because he finds the world of Russia, which is comprehensive enough to seem like the whole world, intolerable. Not intolerable to him personally, as a suicide finds the world, but intolerable *per se*. His foreseen death 'will be the perfectly natural result' of all that he has lived through in his attempt to change the world, because the foreseeing of anything less would have meant that he found the 'intolerable' tolerable.

In many ways the situation (but not the political theory) of the Russian anarchists at the turn of the century prefigures the contemporary situation. A small difference lies in 'the world of Russia' *seeming* like the whole world. There was, strictly speaking, an alternative beyond the borders of Russia. Thus, in order to destroy this alternative and make Russia a world unto itself, many of the anarchists were drawn towards a somewhat mystical patriotism.

7 Quoted in Albert Camus, *The Rebel* (Harmondsworth: Penguin Books, 1963), p. 140.

Today there is no alternative. The world is a single unit, and it has become intolerable.

Was it ever more tolerable? you may ask. Was there ever less suffering, less injustice, less exploitation? There can be no such audits. It is necessary to recognize that the intolerability of the world is, in a certain sense, an historical achievement. The world was not intolerable so long as God existed, so long as there was the ghost of a pre-existent order, so long as large tracts of the world were unknown, so long as one believed in the distinction between the spiritual and the material (it is there that many people still find their justification in finding the world tolerable), so long as one believed in the natural inequality of man.

The photograph shows a South Vietnamese peasant being interrogated by an American soldier. Shoved against her temple is the muzzle of a gun, and, behind it, a hand grasps her hair. The gun, pressed against her, puckers the prematurely old and loose skin of her face.

In wars there have always been massacres. Interrogation under threat or torture has been practised for centuries. Yet the meaning to be found – even via a photograph – in this woman's life (and by now her probable death) is new.

It will include every personal particular, visible or imaginable: the way her hair is parted, her bruised cheek, her slightly swollen lower lip, her name and all the different significations it has acquired according to who is addressing her, memories of her own childhood, the individual quality of her hatred of her interrogator, the gifts she was born with, every detail of the circumstances under which she has so far escaped death, the intonation she gives to the name of each person she loves, the diagnosis of whatever medical weakness she may have and their social and economic causes, everything that she opposes in her subtle mind to the muzzle of the gun jammed against her temple. But it will also include global truths: no violence has been so intense, so widespread or has continued for so long as that inflicted by the imperialist countries upon the majority of the world: the war in Vietnam is being waged to destroy the example of a united people who resisted this violence and proclaimed their independence: the fact that the Vietnamese are proving themselves invincible against the greatest imperialist power on earth is a proof of the extraordinary resources of a nation of 32 million: elsewhere in the world the resources (such resources include not only materials and labour but the possibilities of each life lived) of our 2,000 millions are being squandered and abused.

It is said that exploitation must end in the world. It is known that exploitation increases, extends, prospers and becomes ever more ruthless in defence of its right to exploit.

Let us be clear: it is not the war in Vietnam that is intolerable: Vietnam confirms the intolerability of the present condition of the world. This condition is such that the example of the Vietnamese people offers hope.

Guevara recognized this and acted accordingly. The world is not intolerable until the possibility of transforming it exists but is denied. The social forces historically capable of bringing about the transformation are – at least in general terms – defined. Guevara chose to identify himself with these forces. In doing so he was not submitting to so-called 'laws' of history but to the historical nature of his own existence.

His envisaged death is no longer the measure of a servant's loyalty, nor the inevitable end of an heroic tragedy. The eye of death's needle has been closed – there is nothing to thread through it, not even a future (unknown) historical judgement. Provided that he makes no transcendental appeal and provided that he acts out of the maximum possible consciousness of what is knowable to him, his envisaged death has become the measure of the parity which can now exist between the self and the world: it is the measure of his total commitment and his total independence.

It is reasonable to suppose that after a man such as Guevara has made his decision, there are moments when he is aware of this freedom which is qualitatively different from any freedom previously experienced.

This should be remembered as well as the pain, the sacrifice and the prodigious effort involved. In a letter to his parents when he left Cuba, Guevara wrote:

> Now a will-power that I have polished with an artist's attention will support my feeble legs and tired-out lungs. I will make it.[8]

January 1968

---

8 E. 'Che' Guevara, *Le Socialisme et l'homme* (Paris: Maspero, 1967), p. 113 (translation by the author).

Understanding a Photograph

For over a century, photographers and their apologists have argued that photography deserves to be considered a fine art. It is hard to know how far the apologetics have succeeded. Certainly the vast majority of people do not consider photography an art, even while they practise, enjoy, use and value it. The argument of apologists (and I myself have been among them) has been a little academic.

It now seems clear that photography deserves to be considered as though it were not a fine art. It looks as though photography (whatever kind of activity it may be) is going to outlive painting and sculpture as we have thought of them since the Renaissance. It now seems fortunate that few museums have had sufficient initiative to open photographic departments, for it means that few photographs have been preserved in sacred isolation, it means that the public have not come to think of any photographs as being *beyond* them. (Museums function like homes of the nobility to which the public at certain hours are admitted as visitors. The class nature of the 'nobility' may vary, but as soon as a work is placed in a museum it acquires the *mystery* of a way of life which excludes the mass.)

Let me be clear. Painting and sculpture as we know them are not dying of any stylistic disease, of anything diagnosed by the professionally horrified as cultural decadence; they are dying because, in the world as it is, no work of art can survive and not become a valuable property. And this implies the death of painting and sculpture because property, as once it was not, is now inevitably opposed to all other values. People believe in property, but in essence they only believe in the illusion of protection which property gives. All works of fine art, whatever their content, whatever the sensibility of an individual spectator, must now be reckoned as no more than props for the confidence of the world spirit of conservatism.

By their nature, photographs have little or no property value because they have no rarity value. The very principle of photography is that the resulting image is not unique, but on the contrary infinitely reproducible. Thus, in twentieth-century terms, photographs are records of things seen. Let us consider them no closer to works of art than cardiograms. We shall then be freer of illusions. Our mistake has been to categorize things as art by considering certain phases of the process of creation. But logically this can make all man-made objects art. It is more useful to categorize art by what has become its social function. It functions as property. Accordingly, photographs are mostly outside the category.

Photographs bear witness to a human choice being exercised in a given situation. A photograph is a result of the photographer's decision that it is worth recording that this particular event or this particular object has been seen. If everything that existed were continually being photographed, every photograph would become meaningless. A photograph celebrates neither the event itself nor the faculty of sight in itself. A photograph is already a message about the event it records. The urgency of this message is not entirely dependent on the urgency of the event, but neither can it be entirely independent from it. At its simplest, the message, decoded, means: *I have decided that seeing this is worth recording.*

This is equally true of very memorable photographs and the most banal snapshots. What distinguishes the one from the other is the degree to which the photograph explains the message, the degree to which the photograph makes the photographer's decision transparent and comprehensible. Thus we come to the little-understood paradox of the photograph. The photograph is an automatic record through the mediation of light of a given event: yet it uses the *given* event to *explain* its recording. Photography is the process of rendering observation self-conscious.

We must rid ourselves of a confusion brought about by continually comparing photography with the fine arts. Every handbook on photography talks about composition. The good photograph is the well-composed one. Yet this is true only in so far as we think of photographic images imitating painted ones. Painting is an art of arrangement: therefore it is reasonable to demand that there is some kind of order in what is arranged. Every relation between forms in a painting is to some degree adaptable to the painter's purpose. This is not the case with photography. (Unless we include those absurd studio works in which the photographer arranges every detail of his subject before he takes the picture.) Composition in the profound, formative sense of the word cannot enter into photography.

The formal arrangement of a photograph explains nothing. The events portrayed are in themselves mysterious or explicable according to the spectator's knowledge of them prior to his seeing the photograph. What then gives the photograph as photograph meaning? What makes its minimal message – *I have decided that seeing this is worth recording* – large and vibrant?

The true content of a photograph is invisible, for it derives from a play, not with form, but with time. One might argue that photography is as close to music as to painting. I have said that a photograph bears witness to a human choice being exercised. This choice is not between photographing X and Y: but between photographing at X moment or at Y moment. The objects recorded in any photograph (from the most effective to the most commonplace) carry approximately the same weight, the same conviction. What varies is the intensity with which we are made aware of the poles of absence and presence. Between these two poles photography finds its proper meaning. (The most popular use of the photograph is as a memento of the absent.)

A photograph, while recording what has been seen, always and by its nature refers to what is not seen. It isolates, preserves and presents a moment taken from a continuum. The power of a painting depends upon its internal references. Its reference to the natural world beyond the limits of the painted surface is never direct; it deals in equivalents. Or, to put it another way: painting interprets the world, translating it into its own language. But photography has no language of its own. One learns to read photographs as one learns to read footprints or cardiograms. The language in which photography deals is the language of events. All its references are external to itself. Hence the continuum.

A movie director can manipulate time as a painter can manipulate the confluence of the events he depicts. Not so the still photographer. The only decision he can take is as regards the moment he chooses to isolate. Yet this apparent limitation gives the photograph its unique power. *What it shows invokes what is not shown.* One can look at any photograph to appreciate the truth of this. The immediate relation between what is present and what is absent is particular to each photograph: it may be that of ice to sun, of grief to a tragedy, of a smile to a pleasure, of a body to love, of a winning race-horse to the race it has run.

A photograph is effective when the chosen moment which it records contains a quantum of truth which is generally applicable, which is as revealing about what is absent from the photograph as about what is present in it. The nature of this quantum of truth, and the ways in which it can be discerned, vary greatly. It may be found in an expression, an action, a juxtaposition, a visual ambiguity, a configuration. Nor can this truth ever be independent of the spectator. For the man with a Polyfoto of his girl in his pocket, the quantum of truth in an 'impersonal' photograph must still depend upon the general categories already in the spectator's mind.

All this may seem close to the old principle of art transforming the particular into the universal. But photography does not deal in constructs. There is no transforming in photography. There is only decision, only focus. The minimal message of a photograph may be less simple than we first thought. Instead of it being: *I have decided that seeing this is worth recording*, we may now decode it as: *The degree to which I believe this is worth looking at can be judged by all that I am willingly not showing because it is contained within it.*

Why complicate in this way an experience which we have many times every day – the experience of looking at a photograph? Because the simplicity with which we usually treat the experience is wasteful and confusing. We think of photographs as works of art, as evidence of a particular truth, as likenesses, as news items. Every photograph is in fact a means of testing, confirming and constructing a total view of reality. Hence the crucial role of photography in ideological struggle. Hence the necessity of our understanding a weapon which we can use and which can be used against us.

October 1968

A-I-Z

ERSCHEINT WÖCHENTLICH EINMAL • PREIS 20 PFG., Kc. 1,60
30 GR., 30 SCHWEIZER RP. • V. b. b. • NEUER DEUTSCHER
VERLAG, BERLIN W8 • JAHRGANG XI • NR. 42 • 16.10.1932

DER SINN DES HITLERGRUSSES:

Motto:
**MILLIONEN
STEHEN
HINTER MIR!**

Kleiner Mann bittet um große Gaben

Political Uses of Photo-Montage

John Heartfield, whose real name was Helmut Herzfelde, was born in Berlin in 1891. His father was an unsuccessful poet and anarchist. Threatened with prison for public sacrilege, the father fled from Germany and settled in Austria. Both parents died when Helmut was eight. He was brought up by the peasant mayor of the village on the outskirts of which the Herzfelde family had been living in a forest hut. He had no more than a primary education.

As a youth he got a job in a relative's bookshop and from there worked his way to art school in Munich, where he quickly came to the conclusion that the fine arts were an anachronism. He adopted the English name Heartfield in defiance of German wartime patriotism. In 1916 he started with his brother Wieland a dissenting left-wing magazine, and, with George Grosz, invented the technique of photo-montage. (Raoul Hausmann claims to have invented it elsewhere at the same time.) In 1918 Heartfield became a founder member of the German Communist Party. In 1920 he played a leading role in the Berlin Dada Fair. Until 1924 he worked in films and for the theatre. Thereafter he worked as a graphic propagandist for the German communist press and between about 1927 and 1937 became internationally famous for the wit and force of his photo-montage posters and cartoons.

He remained a communist, living after the war in East Berlin, until his death in 1968. During the second half of his life, none of his published work was in any way comparable in originality or passion to the best of his work done in the decade 1927–37. The latter offers a rare example outside the Soviet Union during the revolutionary years of an artist committing his imagination wholly to the service of a mass political struggle.

What are the qualities of this work? What conclusions may we draw from them? First, a general quality.

There is a Heartfield cartoon of Streicher standing on a pavement beside the inert body of a beaten-up Jew. The caption reads: 'A Pan-German'. Streicher stands in his Nazi uniform, hands behind his back, eyes looking straight ahead, with an expression that neither denies nor affirms what has happened at his feet. It is literally and metaphorically beneath his notice. On his jacket are a few slight traces of dirt or blood. They are scarcely enough to incriminate him – in different circumstances they would seem insignificant. All that they do is slightly to soil his tunic.

In Heartfield's best critical works there is a sense of everything having been soiled – even though it is not possible, as it is in the Streicher cartoon, to explain exactly why or how. The greyness, the very tonality of the photographic print suggest it, as do the folds of the grey clothes, the outlines of the frozen gestures, the half-shadows on the pale faces, the textures of the street walls, of the medical overalls, of the black silk hats. Apart from what they depict, the images themselves are sordid: or, more precisely, they express disgust at their own sordidness.

One finds a comparable physical disgust suggested in nearly all modern political cartoons which have survived their immediate purpose. It does not require a Nazi Germany to provoke such disgust. One sees this quality at its clearest and simplest in the great political portrait caricatures of Daumier. It represents the deepest universal reaction to the stuff of modern politics. And we should understand why.

It is disgust at that particular kind of sordidness which exudes from those who now wield individual political power. This sordidness is not a confirmation of the abstract moral belief that all power corrupts. It is a specific historical and political phenomenon. It could not occur in a theocracy or a secure feudal society. It must await the principle of modern democracy and then the cynical manipulating of that principle. It is endemic in, but by no means exclusive to, latter-day bourgeois politics and advanced capitalism. It is nurtured from the gulf between the aims a politician claims and the actions he has in fact already decided upon.

It is not born of personal deception or hypocrisy as such. Rather, it is born of the manipulator's assurance, of his own indifference to the flagrant contradiction which he himself displays between words and actions, between noble sentiments and routine practice. It resides in his complacent trust in the hidden undemocratic power of the state. Before each public appearance he knows that his words are only for those whom they can persuade, and that with those whom they do not there are other ways of dealing. Note this sordidness when watching the next party political broadcast.

What is the particular quality of Heartfield's best work? It stems from the originality and aptness of his use of photo-montage. In Heartfield's hands the technique becomes a subtle but vivid means of political education, and more precisely of Marxist education.

With his scissors he cuts out events and objects from the scenes to which they originally belonged. He then arranges them in a new, unexpected, discontinuous scene to make a political point – for example, parliament is being placed in a wooden coffin. But this much might be achieved by a drawing or even a verbal slogan. The peculiar advantage of photo-montage lies in the fact that everything which has been cut out keeps its familiar photographic appearance. We are still looking first at *things* and only afterwards at symbols.

But because these things have been shifted, because the natural continuities within which they normally exist have been broken, and because they have now been arranged to transmit an unexpected message, we are made conscious of the arbitrariness of their continuous normal message. Their ideological covering or disguise, which fits them so well when they are in their proper place that it becomes indistinguishable from their appearances, is abruptly revealed for what it is. Appearances themselves are suddenly showing us how they deceive us.

Two simple examples. (There are many more complex ones.) A photograph of Hitler returning the Nazi salute at a mass meeting (which we do not see). Behind him, and much larger than he is, the faceless figure of a man. This man is discreetly passing a wad of banknotes into Hitler's open hand raised above his head. The message of the cartoon (October 1932) is that Hitler is being supported and financed by the big industrialists. But, more subtly, Hitler's charismatic gesture is being divested of its accepted current meaning.

A cartoon of one month later. Two broken skeletons lying in a crater of mud on the Western Front, photographed from above. Everything has disintegrated except for the nailed boots which are still on their feet, and, although muddy, are in wearable condition. The caption reads: 'And again?' Underneath there is a dialogue between the two dead soldiers about how other men are already lining up to take their place. What is being visually contested here is the power and virility normally accorded by Germans to the sight of jackboots.

Those interested in the future didactic use of photo-montage for social and political comment should, I am sure, experiment further with this ability of the technique to *demystify things*. Heartfield's genius lay in his discovery of this possibility.

Photo-montage is at its weakest when it is purely symbolic, when it uses its own means to further rhetorical mystification. Heartfield's work is not always free from this. The weakness reflects deep political contradictions.

For several years before 1933, communist policy towards the

Nazis on the one hand and the German social democrats on the other was both confused and arbitrary. In 1928, after the fall of Bukharin and under Stalin's pressure, the Comintern decided to designate all social democrats as 'social fascists' – there is a Heartfield cartoon of 1931 in which he shows an SPD leader with the face of a snarling tiger. As a result of this arbitrary scheme of simplified moral clairvoyance being imposed from Moscow on local contradictory facts, any chance of the German communists influencing or collaborating with the nine million SPD voters who were mostly workers and potential anti-Nazis was forfeited. It is possible that with a different strategy the German working class might have prevented the rise of Hitler.

Heartfield accepted the party line, apparently without any misgivings. But among his works there is a clear distinction between those which demystify and those which exhort with simplified moral rhetoric. Those which demystify treat of the rise of Nazism in Germany – a social-historical phenomenon with which Heartfield was tragically and intimately familiar; those which exhort are concerned with global generalizations which he inherited ready-made from elsewhere.

Again, two examples. A cartoon of 1935 shows a minuscule Goebbels standing on a copy of *Mein Kampf*, putting out his hand in a gesture of dismissal. 'Away with these degenerate subhumans,' he says – a quotation from a speech he made at Nuremberg. Towering above him as giants, making his gesture pathetically absurd, is a line of impassive Red Army soldiers with rifles at the ready. The effect of such a cartoon on all but loyal communists could only have been to confirm the Nazi lie that the USSR represented a threat to Germany. In ideological contrasts, as distinct from reality, there is only a paper-thin division between thesis and antithesis; a single reflex can turn black into white.

A poster for the First of May 1937 celebrating the Popular Front in France. An arm holding a red flag and sprigs of cherry blossom;

a vague background of clouds (?), sea waves (?), mountains (?). A caption from the *Marseillaise*: 'Liberté, liberté chérie, combats avec tes défenseurs!' Everything about this poster is as symbolic as it is soon to be demonstrated politically false.

I doubt whether we are in a position to make moral judgements about Heartfield's integrity. We would need to know and to feel the pressures, both from within and without, under which he worked during that decade of increasing menace and terrible betrayals. But, thanks to his example, and that of other artists such as Mayakovsky or Tatlin, there is one issue which we should be able to see more clearly than was possible earlier.

It concerns the principal type of moral leverage applied to committed artists and propagandists in order to persuade them to suppress or distort their own original imaginative impulses. I am not speaking now of intimidation but of moral and political argument. Often such arguments were advanced by the artist himself against his own imagination.

The moral leverage was gained through asking questions concerning utility and effectiveness. Am I being useful enough? Is my work effective enough? These questions were closely connected with the belief that a work of art or a work of propaganda (the distinction is of little importance here) was a *weapon* of political struggle. Works of imagination can exert great political and social influence. Politically revolutionary artists hope to integrate their work into a mass struggle. But the influence of their work cannot be determined, either by the artist or by a political commissar, in advance. And it is here that we can see that to compare a work of imagination with a weapon is to resort to a dangerous and far-fetched metaphor.

The effectiveness of a weapon can be estimated quantitatively. Its performance is isolable and repeatable. One chooses a weapon for a situation. The effectiveness of a work of imagination cannot be estimated quantitatively. Its performance is not isolable or repeatable. It changes with circumstances. It creates its own situation. There is no *foreseeable* quantitative correlation between the quality of a work of imagination and its effectiveness. And this is part of its nature because it is intended to operate within a field of subjective interactions which are interminable and immeasurable. This is not to grant to art an ineffable value; it is only to emphasize that the imagination, when true to its impulse, is continually and inevitably questioning the existing category of usefulness. It is ahead of that part of the social self which asks the question. It must deny itself in order to answer the question in its own terms. By way of this denial revolutionary artists have been persuaded to compromise, and to do so in vain – as I have indicated in the case of John Heartfield.

It is lies that can be qualified as useful or useless; the lie is surrounded by what has not been said and its usefulness or not can be gauged according to what has been hidden. The truth is always first discovered in open space.

October 1969

Photographs of Agony

The news from Vietnam did not make big headlines in the papers this morning. It was simply reported that the American air force is systematically pursuing its policy of bombing the north. Yesterday there were 270 raids.

Behind this report there is an accumulation of other information. The day before yesterday the American air force launched the heaviest raids of this month. So far more bombs have been dropped this month than during any other comparable period. Among the bombs being dropped are the seven-ton superbombs, each of which flattens an area of approximately 8,000 square metres. Along with the large bombs, various kinds of small antipersonnel bombs are being dropped. One kind is full of plastic barbs which, having ripped through the flesh and embedded themselves in the body, cannot be located by X-ray. Another is called the Spider: a small bomb like a grenade with almost invisible 30-centimetre-long antennae, which, if touched, act as detonators. These bombs, distributed over the ground where larger explosions have taken place, are designed to blow up survivors who run to put out the fires already burning, or go to help those already wounded.

There are no pictures from Vietnam in the papers today. But there is a photograph taken by Donald McCullin in Hue in 1968 which could have been printed with the reports this morning.[9] It

9 See Donald McCullin, *The Destruction Business* (London: Open Gate Books, 1972).

shows an old man squatting with a child in his arms; both of them are bleeding profusely with the black blood of black-and-white photographs.

In the last year or so, it has become normal for certain mass-circulation newspapers to publish war photographs which earlier would have been suppressed as being too shocking. One might explain this development by arguing that these newspapers have come to realize that a large section of their readers are now aware of the horrors of war and want to be shown the truth. Alternatively, one might argue that these newspapers believe that their readers have become inured to violent images and so now compete in terms of ever more violent sensationalism.

The first argument is too idealistic and the second too transparently cynical. Newspapers now carry violent war photographs because their effect, except in rare cases, is not what it was once presumed to be. A paper like the *Sunday Times* continues to publish shocking photographs about Vietnam or about Northern Ireland while politically supporting the policies responsible for the violence. This is why we have to ask: what effect do such photographs have?

Many people would argue that such photographs remind us shockingly of the reality, the lived reality, behind the abstractions of political theory, casualty statistics or news bulletins. Such photographs, they might go on to say, are printed on the black curtain which is drawn across what we choose to forget or refuse to know. According to them, McCullin serves as an eye we cannot shut. Yet what is it that they make us see?

They bring us up short. The most literal adjective that could be applied to them is *arresting*. We are seized by them. (I am aware that there are people who pass them over, but about them there is nothing to say.) As we look at them, the moment of the other's suffering engulfs us. We are filled with either despair or indignation. Despair takes on some of the other's suffering to no purpose.

Indignation demands action. We try to emerge from the moment of the photograph back into our lives. As we do so, the contrast is such that the resumption of our lives appears to be a hopelessly inadequate response to what we have just seen.

McCullin's most typical photographs record sudden moments of agony – a terror, a wounding, a death, a cry of grief. These moments are in reality utterly discontinuous with normal time. It is the knowledge that such moments are probable and the anticipation of them that makes 'time' in the front line unlike all other experiences of time. The camera which isolates a moment of agony isolates no more violently than the experience of that moment isolates itself. The word *trigger*, applied to rifle and camera, reflects a correspondence which does not stop at the purely mechanical. The image seized by the camera is doubly violent and both violences reinforce the same contrast: the contrast between the photographed moment and all others.

As we emerge from the photographed moment back into our lives, we do not realize this; we assume that the discontinuity is our responsibility. The truth is that any response to that photographed moment is bound to be felt as inadequate. Those who are there in the situation being photographed, those who hold the hand of the dying or staunch a wound, are not seeing the moment as we have and their responses are of an altogether different order. It is not possible for anyone to look pensively at such a moment and to emerge stronger. McCullin, whose 'contemplation' is both dangerous and active, writes bitterly underneath a photograph: 'I only use the camera like I use a toothbrush. It does the job.'

The possible contradictions of the war photograph now become apparent. It is generally assumed that its purpose is to awaken concern. The most extreme examples – as in most of McCullin's work – show moments of agony in order to extort the maximum concern. Such moments, whether photographed or not, are discontinuous with all other moments. They exist by themselves. But the reader who has been arrested by the photograph may tend to feel this discontinuity as his own personal moral inadequacy. *And as soon as this happens even his sense of shock is dispersed*: his own moral inadequacy may now shock him as much as the crimes being committed in the war. Either he shrugs off this sense of inadequacy as being only too familiar, or else he thinks of performing a kind of penance – of which the purest example would be to make a contribution to OXFAM or to UNICEF.

In both cases, the issue of the war which has caused that moment is effectively depoliticized. The picture becomes evidence of the general human condition. It accuses nobody and everybody.

Confrontation with a photographed moment of agony can mask a far more extensive and urgent confrontation. Usually the wars which we are shown are being fought directly or indirectly in 'our' name. What we are shown horrifies us. The next step should be for us to confront our own lack of political freedom. In the political systems as they exist, we have no legal opportunity of effectively influencing the conduct of wars waged in our name. To realize this and to act accordingly is the only effective way of responding to what the photograph shows. Yet the double violence of the photographed moment actually works against this realization. That is why they can be published with impunity.

July 1972

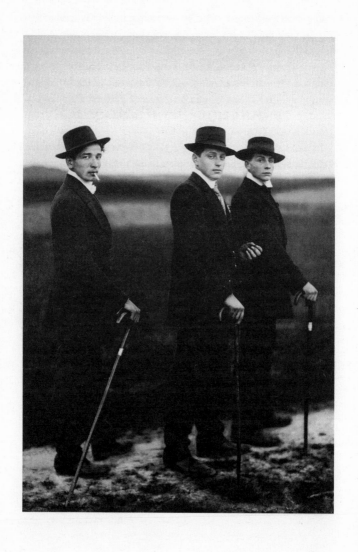

The Suit and the Photograph

What did August Sander (1876–1964) tell his sitters before he took their pictures? And how did he say it so that they all believed him in the same way?

They each look at the camera with the same expression in their eyes. In so far as there are differences, these are the results of the sitter's experience and character – the priest has lived a different life from the paper-hanger; but to all of them Sander's camera represents the same thing.

Did he simply say that their photographs were going to be a recorded part of history? And did he refer to history in such a way that their vanity and shyness dropped away, so that they looked into the lens telling themselves, using a strange historical tense: *I looked like this*. We cannot know. We simply have to recognize the uniqueness of his work, which he planned with the overall title of 'People of the Twentieth Century'.

His full aim was to find, in the area around Cologne, archetypes to represent every possible type, social class, sub-class, job, vocation, privilege. He hoped to take, in all, 600 portraits. His project was cut short by Hitler's Third Reich.

His son Erich, a socialist and anti-Nazi, was sent to jail for his beliefs, where he died. The father hid his archives in the countryside. What remains today is an extraordinary social and human document. No other photographer, taking portraits of his own countrymen, has ever been so translucently documentary.

Understanding a Photograph

Walter Benjamin wrote in 1931 about Sander's work:

It was not as a scholar, advised by race theorists or social research-ers, that the author [Sander] undertook his enormous task, but, in the publisher's words, 'as the result of immediate observation'. It is indeed unprejudiced observation, bold and at the same time delicate, very much in the spirit of Goethe's remark: 'There is a delicate form of the empirical which identifies itself so intimately with its object that it thereby becomes theory.' Accordingly it is quite proper that an observer like Döblin should light upon pre-cisely the scientific aspects of this opus and point out: 'Just as there is a comparative anatomy which enables one to understand the nature and history of organs, so here the photographer has produced a comparative photography, thereby gaining a scientific standpoint which places him beyond the photographer of detail.' It would be lamentable if economic circumstances prevented the further publication of this extraordinary corpus . . . Sander's work is more than a picture book, it is an atlas of instruction.

In the inquiring spirit of Benjamin's remarks I want to examine Sander's well-known photograph of three young peasants on the road in the evening, going to a dance. There is as much descriptive information in this image as in pages by a descriptive master like Zola. Yet I only want to consider one thing: their suits.

The date is 1914. The three young men belong, at the very most, to the second generation who ever wore such suits in the Euro-pean countryside. Twenty or thirty years earlier, such clothes did not exist at a price which peasants could afford. Among the young today, formal dark suits have become rare in the villages of at least Western Europe. But for most of this century most peasants – and most workers – wore dark three-piece suits on ceremonial occa-sions, Sundays and fêtes.

When I go to a funeral in the village where I live, the men of my age and older are still wearing them. Of course there have been modifications of fashion: the width of trousers and lapels, the length of jackets change. Yet the physical character of the suit and its message does not change.

Let us first consider its physical character. Or, more precisely, its physical character when worn by village peasants. And to make generalization more convincing, let us look at a second photograph of a village band (see p. 38).

Sander took this group portrait in 1913, yet it could well have been the band at the dance for which the three with their walking sticks are setting out along the road. Now make an experiment. Block out the faces of the band with a piece of paper, and consider only their clothed bodies.

By no stretch of the imagination can you believe that these bodies belong to the middle or ruling class. They might belong to workers, rather than peasants; but otherwise there is no doubt. Nor is the clue their hands – as it would be if you could touch them. Then why is their class so apparent?

Is it a question of fashion and the quality of the cloth of their suits? In real life such details would be telling. In a small black-and-white photograph they are not very evident. Yet the static photograph shows, perhaps more vividly than in life, the fundamental reason why the suits, far from disguising the social class of those who wore them, underlined and emphasized it.

Their suits deform them. Wearing them, they look as though they were physically misshapen. A past style in clothes often looks absurd until it is reincorporated into fashion. Indeed the economic logic of fashion depends on making the old-fashioned look absurd. But here we are not faced primarily with that kind of absurdity; here the clothes look less absurd, less 'abnormal' than the men's bodies which are in them.

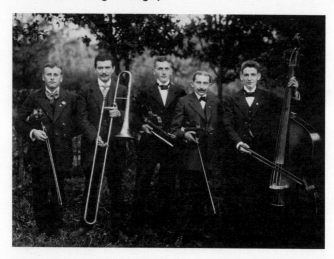

The musicians give the impression of being uncoordinated, bandy-legged, barrel-chested, low-arsed, twisted or scalene. The violinist on the right is made to look almost like a dwarf. None of their abnormalities is extreme. They do not provoke pity. They are just sufficient to undermine physical dignity. We look at bodies which appear coarse, clumsy, brute-like. And incorrigibly so.

Now make the experiment the other way round. Cover the bodies of the band and look only at their faces. They are country faces. Nobody could suppose that they are a group of barristers or managing directors. They are five men from a village who like to make music and do so with a certain self-respect. As we look at the faces we can imagine what the bodies would look like. And what we imagine is quite different from what we have just seen. In imagination we see them as their parents might remember them when absent. We accord them the normal dignity they have.

To make the point clearer, let us now consider an image where tailored clothes, instead of deforming, *preserve* the physical identity and therefore the natural authority of those wearing them. I have deliberately chosen a Sander photograph which looks old-fashioned and could easily lend itself to parody: the photograph of four Protestant missionaries in 1931 (see p. 40).

Despite the portentousness, it is not even necessary to make the experiment of blocking out the faces. It is clear that here the suits actually confirm and enhance the physical presence of those wearing them. The clothes convey the same message as the faces and as the history of the bodies they hide. Suits, experience, social formation and function coincide.

Look back now at the three on the road to the dance. Their hands look too big, their bodies too thin, their legs too short. (They use their walking sticks as though they were driving cattle.) We can make the same experiment with the faces and the effect is exactly the same as with the band. They can wear only their hats as if they suited them.

Where does this lead us? Simply to the conclusion that peasants can't buy good suits and don't know how to wear them? No, what is at issue here is a graphic, if small, example (perhaps one of the most graphic which exists) of what Gramsci called class hegemony. Let us look at the contradictions involved more closely.

Most peasants, if not suffering from malnutrition, are physically strong and well developed. Well developed because of the very varied hard physical work they do. It would be too simple to make a list of physical characteristics – broad hands through working with them from a very early age, broad shoulders relative to the body through the habit of carrying and so on. In fact many variations and exceptions also exist. One can, however, speak of a characteristic physical rhythm which most peasants, both women and men, acquire.

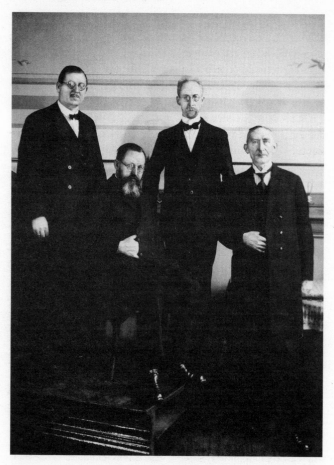

This rhythm is directly related to the energy demanded by the amount of work which has to be done in a day, and is reflected in typical physical movements and stance. It is an extended sweeping rhythm. Not necessarily slow. The traditional acts of scything or sawing may exemplify it. The way peasants ride horses makes it distinctive, as also the way they walk, as if testing the earth with each stride. In addition peasants possess a special physical dignity: this is determined by a kind of functionalism, a way of being *fully at home in effort*.

The suit, as we know it today, developed in Europe as a professional ruling-class costume in the last third of the nineteenth century. Almost anonymous as a uniform, it was the first ruling-class costume to idealize purely *sedentary* power. The power of the administrator and conference table. Essentially the suit was made for the gestures of talking and calculating abstractly. (As distinct, compared to previous upper-class costumes, from the gestures of riding, hunting, dancing, duelling.)

It was the English *gentleman*, with all the apparent restraint which that new stereotype implied, who launched the suit. It was a costume which inhibited vigorous action, and which action ruffled, uncreased and spoilt. 'Horses sweat, men perspire and women glow.' By the turn of the century, and increasingly after the First World War, the suit was mass-produced for mass urban and rural markets.

The physical contradiction is obvious. Bodies which are fully at home in effort, bodies which are used to extended sweeping movement: clothes idealizing the sedentary, the discrete, the effortless. I would be the last to argue for a return to traditional peasant costumes. Any such return is bound to be escapist, for these costumes were a form of capital handed down through generations, and in the world today, in which every corner is dominated by the market, such a principle is anachronistic.

We can note, however, how traditional peasant working or ceremonial clothes respected the specific character of the bodies they were clothing. They were in general loose, and only tight in places where they were gathered to allow for freer movement.

They were the antithesis of tailored clothes, clothes cut to follow the idealized shape of a more or less stationary body and then to hang from it!

Yet nobody forced peasants to buy suits, and the three on their way to the dance are clearly proud of them. They wear them with a kind of panache. This is exactly why the suit might become a classic and easily taught example of class hegemony.

Villagers – and, in a different way, city workers – were persuaded to choose suits. By publicity. By pictures. By the new mass media. By salesmen. By example. By the sight of new kinds of travellers. And also by political developments of accommodation and state central organization. For example: in 1900, on the occasion of the great Universal Exhibition, all the mayors of France were, for the first time ever, invited to a banquet in Paris. Most of them were the peasant mayors of village communes. Nearly thirty thousand came! And, naturally, for the occasion the vast majority wore suits.

The working classes – but peasants were simpler and more naïve about it than workers – came to accept as *their own* certain standards of the class that ruled over them – in this case standards of the chic and sartorial worthiness. At the same time their very acceptance of these standards, their very conforming to these norms which had nothing to do with either their own inheritance or their daily experience, condemned them, within the system of those standards, to being always, and recognizably to the classes above them, second-rate, clumsy, uncouth, defensive. That indeed is to succumb to a cultural hegemony.

Perhaps one can nevertheless propose that when the three arrived and had drunk a beer or two, and had eyed the girls (whose clothes had not yet changed so drastically), they hung up their jackets, took off their ties and danced, maybe wearing their hats, until the morning and the next day's work.

March 1979

Paul Strand

There is a widespread assumption that if one is interested in the visual, one's interest must be limited to a technique of somehow *treating* the visual. Thus the visual is divided into categories of special interest: painting, photography, real appearances, dreams and so on. And what is forgotten – like all essential questions in a positivist culture – is the meaning and enigma of visibility itself.

I think of this now because I want to describe what I can see in two books which are in front of me. They are two volumes of a retrospective monograph on the work of Paul Strand. The first photographs date from 1915, when Strand was a sort of pupil of Alfred Stieglitz; the most recent ones were taken in 1968.

The earliest works deal mostly with people and sites in New York. The first of them shows a half-blind beggar woman. One of her eyes is opaque, the other sharp and wary. Round her neck she wears a label with BLIND printed on it. It is an image with a clear social message. But it is something else, too. We shall see later that in all Strand's best photographs of people, he presents us with the visible evidence, not just of their presence, but of their *life*. At one level, such evidence of a life is social comment – Strand has consistently taken a left political position – but, at a different level, such evidence serves to suggest visually the totality of another lived life, from within which we ourselves are no more than a sight. This is why the black letters B-L-I-N-D on a white label do more than spell the word. While the picture remains in front of us, we can never take them as read. The earliest image in the book forces us to reflect on the significance of seeing itself.

The next section of photographs, from the 1920s, includes photographs of machine parts and close-ups of various natural forms – roots, rocks and grasses. Already Strand's technical perfectionism and strong aesthetic interests are apparent. But equally his obstinate, resolute respect for the thing-in-itself is also apparent. And the result is often disconcerting. Some would say that these photographs fail, for they remain details of what they have been taken from: they never become independent images. Nature, in these photographs, is intransigent to art, and the machine-details mock the stillness of their perfectly rendered images.

From the 1930s onwards, the photographs fall typically into groups associated with journeys that Strand made: to Mexico, New England, France, Italy, the Hebrides, Egypt, Ghana, Rumania. These are the photographs for which Strand has become well known, and it is on the evidence of these photographs that he should be considered a great photographer. With these black-and-white photographs, with these records which are distributable anywhere, he offers us the sight of a number of places and people in such a way that our view of the world can be qualitatively extended.

The social approach of Strand's photography to reality might be called documentary or neo-realist in so far as its obvious cinematic equivalent is to be found in the pre-war films of Flaherty or the immediate postwar Italian films of de Sica or Rossellini. This means that on his travels Strand avoids the picturesque, the panoramic, and tries to find a city in a street, the way of life of a nation in the corner of a kitchen. In one or two pictures of power dams and some 'heroic' portraits he gives way to the romanticism of Soviet socialist realism. But mostly his approach lets him choose ordinary subjects which in their ordinariness are extraordinarily representative.

He has an infallible eye for the quintessential: whether it is to be found on a Mexican doorstep, or in the way that an Italian village schoolgirl in a black pinafore holds her straw hat. Such photographs enter so deeply into the particular that they reveal to us the stream of a culture or a history which is flowing through that particular subject like blood. The images of these photographs, once seen, subsist in our mind until some actual incident, which we witness or live, refers to one of them as though to a more solid reality. But it is not this which makes Strand as a photographer unique.

His method as a photographer is more unusual. One could say that it was the antithesis to Henri Cartier-Bresson's. The photographic moment for Cartier-Bresson is an instant, a fraction of a second, and he stalks that instant as though it were a wild animal. The photographic moment for Strand is a biographical or historic moment, whose duration is ideally measured not by seconds but by its relation to a lifetime. Strand does not pursue an instant, but encourages a moment to arise as one might encourage a story to be told.

In practical terms this means that he decides what he wants before he takes the picture, never plays with the accidental, works slowly, hardly ever crops a picture, often still uses a plate camera, formally asks people to pose for him. His pictures are all remarkable for their intentionality. His portraits are very frontal. The subject is looking at us; we are looking at the subject; it has been arranged like that. But there is a similar sense of frontality in many of his other pictures of landscapes or objects or buildings. His camera is not free-roving. He chooses where to place it.

Where he has chosen to place it is not where something is about to happen, but where a number of happenings will be related. Thus, without any use of anecdote, he turns his subjects into narrators. The river narrates itself. The field where the horses are grazing recounts itself. The wife tells the story of her marriage. In each case Strand, the photographer, has chosen the place to put his camera as listener.

The approach: neo-realist. The method: deliberate, frontal, formal, with every surface thoroughly scanned. What is the result?

His best photographs are unusually dense – not in the sense of being over-burdened or obscure, but in the sense of being filled with an unusual amount of substance per square inch. And all this substance becomes the stuff of the life of the subject. Take the famous portrait of Mr Bennett from Vermont, New England. His jacket, his shirt, the stubble on his chin, the timber of the house behind, the air around him become in this image the face of his life, of which his actual facial expression is the concentrated spirit. It is the whole photograph, frowning, which surveys us.

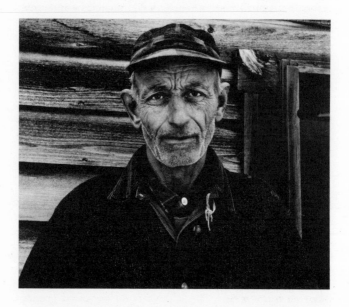

A Mexican woman sits against a wall. She has a woollen shawl over her head and shoulders and a broken plaited basket on her lap. Her skirt is patched and the wall behind her very shabby. The only fresh surface in the picture is that of her face. Once again, the surfaces we read with our eyes become the actual chafing texture of her daily life; once again the photograph is a panel of her being. At first sight the image is soberly materialist, but just as her body wears through her clothes and the load in the basket wears away the basket, and passers-by have rubbed off the surface of the wall, so her being as a woman (her own existence for herself) begins, as one goes on looking at the picture, to rub through the materialism of the image.

A young Rumanian peasant and his wife lean against a wooden fence. Above and behind them, diffused in the light, is a field and, above that, a small modern house, totally insignificant as architecture, and the grey silhouette of a nondescript tree beside it. Here it is not the substantiality of surfaces which fills every square inch but a Slav sense of distance, a sense of plains or hills that continue indefinitely. And, once more, it is impossible to separate this quality from the presence of the two figures; it is there in the angle of his hat, the long extended movement of his arms, the flowers embroidered on her waistcoat, the way her hair is tied up; it is there across the width of their wide faces and mouths. What informs the whole photograph – space – is part of the skin of their lives.

These photographs depend upon Strand's technical skill, his ability to select, his knowledge of the places he visits, his eye, his sense of timing, his use of the camera; but he might have all these talents and still not be capable of producing such pictures. What has finally determined his success in his photographs of people and in his landscapes – which are only extensions of people who happen to be invisible – is his ability to invite the narrative: to present himself to his subject in such a way that the subject is willing to say: *I am as you see me.*

This is more complicated than it may seem. The present tense of the verb *to be* refers only to the present; but nevertheless, with the first-person singular in front of it, it absorbs the past which is inseparable from the pronoun. *I am* includes all that has made me so. It is more than a statement of immediate fact: it is already an explanation, a justification, a demand – it is already autobiographical. Strand's photographs suggest his sitters trust him to *see* their life story. And it is for this reason that, although the portraits are formal and posed, there is no need, either on the part of photographer or photograph, for the disguise of a borrowed role.

Photography, because it preserves the appearance of an event or a person, has always been closely associated with the idea of the historical. The ideal of photography, aesthetics apart, is to seize an 'historic' moment. But Paul Strand's relation as a photographer to the historic is a unique one. His photographs convey a unique sense of duration. The *I am* is given its time in which to reflect on the past and to anticipate its future: the exposure time does no violence to the time of the *I am*: on the contrary, one has the strange impression that the exposure time *is* the lifetime.

March 1972

Uses of Photography

For Susan Sontag

I want to write down some of my responses to Susan Sontag's book *On Photography*. All the quotations I will use are from her text. The thoughts are sometimes my own, but all originate in the experience of reading her book.

The camera was invented by Fox Talbot in 1839. Within a mere thirty years of its invention as a gadget for an elite, photography was being used for police filing, war reporting, military reconnaissance, pornography, encyclopedic documentation, family albums, postcards, anthropological records (often, as with the Indians in the United States, accompanied by genocide), sentimental moralizing, inquisitive probing (the wrongly named 'candid camera'), aesthetic effects, news reporting and formal portraiture. The first cheap popular camera was put on the market, a little later, in 1888. The speed with which the possible uses of photography were seized upon is surely an indication of photography's profound, central applicability to industrial capitalism. Marx came of age the year of the camera's invention.

It was not, however, until the twentieth century and the period between the two world wars that the photograph became the dominant and most 'natural' way of referring to appearances. It was then that it replaced the word as immediate testimony. It was the period when photography was thought of as being most transparent, offering direct access to the real: the period of the great witnessing masters of the medium like Paul Strand and Walker Evans. It was, in the capitalist countries, the freest moment of photography: it had been liberated from the limitations of fine art, and it had become a public medium which could be used democratically.

Yet the moment was brief. The very 'truthfulness' of the new medium encouraged its deliberate use as a means of propaganda. The Nazis were among the first to use systematic photographic propaganda.

Photographs are perhaps the most mysterious of all the objects that make up, and thicken, the environment we recognize as modern. Photographs really are experience captured, and the camera is the ideal arm of consciousness in its acquisitive mood.

In the first period of its existence photography offered a new technical opportunity; it was an implement. Now, instead of offering new choices, its usage and its 'reading' were becoming habitual, an unexamined part of modern perception itself. Many developments contributed to this transformation. The new film industry. The invention of the lightweight camera – so that the taking of a photograph ceased to be a ritual and became a 'reflex'. The discovery of photojournalism – whereby the text follows the pictures instead of vice versa. The emergence of advertising as a crucial economic force.

Through photographs, the world becomes a series of unrelated, free-standing particles; and history, past and present, a set of anecdotes and *faits divers*. The camera makes reality atomic, manageable, and opaque. It is a view of the world which denies interconnectedness, continuity, but which confers on each moment the character of a mystery.

The first mass-media magazine was started in the United States in 1936. At least two things were prophetic about the launching of *Life*, the prophecies to be fully realized in the postwar television age. The new picture magazine was financed not by its sales, but by the advertising it carried. A third of its images were devoted to publicity. The second prophecy lay in its title. This is ambiguous. It may mean that the pictures inside are about life. Yet it seems to promise more: that these pictures *are* life. The first photograph in the first number played on this ambiguity. It showed a newborn baby. The caption underneath read: 'Life begins . . . '

What served in place of the photograph, before the camera's invention? The expected answer is the engraving, the drawing, the painting. The more revealing answer might be: memory. What photographs do out there in space was previously done within reflection.

> Proust somewhat misconstrues what photographs are: not so much
> an instrument of memory as an invention of it or a replacement.

Unlike any other visual image, a photograph is not a rendering, an imitation or an interpretation of its subject, but actually a trace of it. No painting or drawing, however naturalist, *belongs* to its subject in the way that a photograph does.

> A photograph is not only an image (as a painting is an image), an
> interpretation of the real; it is also a trace, something directly sten-
> cilled off the real, like a footprint or a death mask.

Human visual perception is a far more complex and selective process than that by which a film records. Nevertheless the camera lens and the eye both register images – because of their sensitivity to light – at great speed and in the face of an immediate event. What the camera does, however, and what the eye in itself can never do, is to *fix* the appearance of that event. It removes its appearance from the flow of appearances and it preserves it, not perhaps for ever but for as long as the film exists. The essential character of this preservation is not dependent upon the image being static; unedited film rushes preserve in essentially the same way. The camera saves a set of appearances from the otherwise inevitable supersession of further appearances. It holds them unchanging. And before the invention of the camera nothing could do this, except, in the mind's eye, the faculty of memory.

I am not saying that memory is a kind of film. That is a banal simile. From the comparison film/memory we learn nothing about the latter. What we learn is how strange and unprecedented was the procedure of photography.

Yet, unlike memory, photographs do not in themselves preserve meaning. They offer appearances – with all the credibility and gravity we normally lend to appearances – prised away from their meaning. Meaning is the result of understanding functions.

And functioning takes place in time, and must be explained in time. Only that which narrates can make us understand.

Photographs in themselves do not narrate. Photographs preserve instant appearances. Habit now protects us against the shock involved in such preservation. Compare the exposure time for a film with the life of the print made, and let us assume that the print only lasts ten years: the ratio for an average modern photograph would be approximately 20,000,000,000:1. Perhaps that can serve as a reminder of the violence of the fission whereby appearances are separated by the camera from their function.

We must now distinguish between two quite distinct uses of photography. There are photographs which belong to private experience and there are those which are used publicly. The private photograph – the portrait of a mother, a picture of a daughter, a group photo of one's own team – is appreciated and read in a context which is continuous with that from which the camera removed it. (The violence of the removal is sometimes felt as incredulousness: 'Was that really Dad?') Nevertheless such a photograph remains surrounded by the meaning from which it was severed. A mechanical device, the camera has been used as an instrument to contribute to a living memory. The photograph is a memento from a life being lived.

The contemporary public photograph usually presents an event, a seized set of appearances, which has nothing to do with us, its readers, or with the original meaning of the event. It offers information, but information severed from all lived experience. If the public photograph contributes to a memory, it is to the memory of an unknowable and total stranger. The violence is expressed in that strangeness. It records an instant sight about which this stranger has shouted: Look!

Who is the stranger? One might answer: the photographer. Yet if one considers the entire use-system of photographed images, the answer of 'the photographer' is clearly inadequate. Nor can one reply: those who use the photographs. It is because the photographs carry no certain meaning in themselves, because they are like images in the memory of a total stranger, that they lend themselves to any use.

Daumier's famous cartoon of Nadar in his balloon suggests an answer. Nadar is travelling through the sky above Paris – the wind has blown off his hat – and he is photographing with his camera the city and its people below.

Has the camera replaced the eye of God? The decline of religion corresponds with the rise of the photograph. Has the culture of capitalism telescoped God into photography? The transformation would not be as surprising as it may at first seem.

The faculty of memory led men everywhere to ask whether, just as they themselves could preserve certain events from oblivion, there might not be other eyes noting and recording otherwise unwitnessed events. Such eyes they then accredited to their ancestors, to spirits, to gods or to their single deity. What was seen by this supernatural eye was inseparably linked with the principle of justice. It was possible to escape the justice of men, but not this higher justice from which nothing or little could be hidden.

Memory implies a certain act of redemption. What is remembered has been saved from nothingness. What is forgotten has been abandoned. If all events are seen, instantaneously, outside time, by a supernatural eye, the distinction between remembering and forgetting is transformed into an act of judgement, into the rendering of justice, whereby recognition is close to *being remembered*, and condemnation is close to *being forgotten*. Such a presentiment, extracted from man's long, painful experience of time, is to be found in varying forms in almost every culture and religion, and, very clearly, in Christianity.

At first, the secularization of the capitalist world during the nineteenth century elided the judgement of God into the judgement of History in the name of Progress. Democracy and Science became the agents of such a judgement. And for a brief moment, photography, as we have seen, was considered to be an aid to these agents. It is still to this historical moment that photography owes its ethical reputation as Truth.

During the second half of the twentieth century the judgement of history has been abandoned by all except the underprivileged and dispossessed. The industrialized, 'developed' world, terrified of the past, blind to the future, lives within an opportunism which has emptied the principle of justice of all credibility. Such opportunism turns everything – nature, history, suffering, other people, catastrophes, sport, sex, politics – into spectacle. And the implement used to do this – until the act becomes so habitual that the conditioned imagination may do it alone – is the camera.

Our very sense of situation is now articulated by the camera's interventions. The omnipresence of cameras persuasively suggests that time consists of interesting events, events worth photographing. This, in turn, makes it easy to feel that any event, once underway, and whatever its moral character, should be allowed to complete itself – so that something else can be brought into the world, the photograph.

The spectacle creates an eternal present of immediate expectation: memory ceases to be necessary or desirable. With the loss of memory the continuities of meaning and judgement are also lost to us. The camera relieves us of the burden of memory. It surveys us like God, and it surveys for us. Yet no other god has been so cynical, for the camera records in order to forget.

Susan Sontag locates this god very clearly in history. He is the god of monopoly capitalism.

A capitalist society requires a culture based on images. It needs to furnish vast amounts of entertainment in order to stimulate buying and anaesthetize the injuries of class, race, and sex. And it needs to gather unlimited amounts of information, the better to exploit the natural resources, increase productivity, keep order, make war, give jobs to bureaucrats. The camera's twin capacities, to subjectivize reality and to objectify it, ideally serve these needs and strengthen them. Cameras define reality in the two ways essential to the workings of an advanced industrial society: as a spectacle (for masses) and as an object of surveillance (for rulers). The production of images also furnishes a ruling ideology. Social change is replaced by a change in images.

Her theory of the current use of photographs leads one to ask whether photography might serve a different function. Is there an alternative photographic practice? The question should not be answered naïvely. Today no alternative professional practice (if one thinks of the profession of photographer) is possible. The system can accommodate any photograph. Yet it may be possible to begin to use photographs according to a practice addressed to an alternative future. This future is a hope which we need now, if we are to maintain a struggle, a resistance, against the societies and culture of capitalism.

Photographs have often been used as a radical weapon in posters, newspapers, pamphlets and so on. I do not wish to belittle the value of such agitational publishing. Yet the current systematic public use of photography needs to be challenged, not simply by turning it round like a cannon and aiming it at different targets, but by changing its practice. How?

We need to return to the distinction I made between the private and public uses of photography. In the private use of photography, the context of the instant recorded is preserved so that the photograph lives in an ongoing continuity. (If you have a photograph of Peter on your wall, you are not likely to forget what Peter means to you.) The public photograph, by contrast, is torn from its context, and becomes a dead object which, exactly because it is dead, lends itself to any arbitrary use.

In the most famous photographic exhibition ever organized, *The Family of Man* (put together by Edward Steichen in 1955), photographs from all over the world were presented as though they formed a universal family album. Steichen's intuition was absolutely correct: the private use of photographs can be exemplary for their public use. Unfortunately the shortcut he took in treating the existing class-divided world as if it were a family inevitably made the whole exhibition, not necessarily each picture, sentimental and complacent. The truth is that most photographs taken of people are about suffering, and most of that suffering is man-made.

One's first encounter [writes Susan Sontag] with the photographic inventory of ultimate horror is a kind of revelation, the prototypically modern revelation: a negative epiphany. For me, it was photographs of Bergen-Belsen and Dachau which I came across by chance in a bookstore in Santa Monica in July 1945. Nothing I have seen – in photographs or in real life – ever cut me as sharply, deeply, instantaneously. Indeed, it seems plausible to me to divide my life into two parts, before I saw those photographs (I was twelve) and after, though it was several years before I understood fully what they were about.

Photographs are relics of the past, traces of what has happened. If the living take that past upon themselves, if the past becomes an integral part of the process of people making their own history, then all photographs would reacquire a living context, they would continue to exist in time, instead of being arrested moments. It is just possible that photography is the prophecy of a human memory yet to be socially and politically achieved. Such a memory would encompass any image of the past, however tragic, however guilty, within its own continuity. The distinction between the private and public uses of photography would be transcended. The Family of Man would exist.

Meanwhile we live today in the world as it is. Yet this possible prophecy of photography indicates the direction in which any alternative use of photography needs to develop. The task of an alternative photography is to incorporate photography into social and political memory, instead of using it as a substitute which encourages the atrophy of any such memory.

The task will determine both the kinds of pictures taken and the way they are used. There can of course be no formulae, no prescribed practice. Yet in recognizing how photography has come to be used by capitalism, we can define at least some of the principles of an alternative practice.

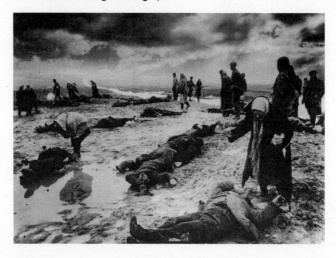

For the photographer this means thinking of her- or himself not so much as a reporter to the rest of the world but, rather, as a recorder for those involved in the events photographed. The distinction is crucial.

What makes photographs like these so tragic and extraordinary is that, looking at them, one is convinced that they were not taken to please generals, to boost the morale of a civilian public, to glorify heroic soldiers or to shock the world press: they were images addressed to those suffering what they depict. And given this integrity towards and with their subject matter, such photographs later became a memorial, to the 20 million Russians killed in the war, for those who mourn them. The unifying horror of a total people's war made such an attitude on the part of the war photographers (and even the censors) a natural one. Photographers, however, can work with a similar attitude in less extreme circumstances.

The alternative use of photographs which already exist leads us back once more to the phenomenon and faculty of memory.

The aim must be to construct a context for a photograph, to construct it with words, to construct it with other photographs, to construct it by its place in an ongoing text of photographs and images. How? Normally photographs are used in a very unilinear way – they are used to illustrate an argument, or to demonstrate a thought which goes like this:

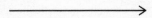

Very frequently also they are used tautologically so that the photograph merely repeats what is being said in words. Memory is not unilinear at all. Memory works radially, that is to say with an enormous number of associations all leading to the same event. The diagram is like this:

If we want to put a photograph back into the context of experience, social experience, social memory, we have to respect the laws of memory. We have to situate the printed photograph so that it acquires something of the surprising conclusiveness of that which *was* and *is*.

What Brecht wrote about acting in one of his poems is applicable to such a practice. For *instant* one can read photography, for *acting* the recreating of context:

> So you should simply make the instant
> Stand out, without in the process hiding
> What you are making it stand out from. Give your acting
> That progression of one-thing-after-another, that attitude of
> Working up what you have taken on. In this way
> You will show the flow of events and also the course
> Of your work, permitting the spectator

59

Understanding a Photograph

To experience this Now on many levels, coming from Previously
    and
Merging into Afterwards, also having much else Now
Alongside it. He is sitting not only
In your theatre but also
In the world.

There are a few great photographs which practically achieve this by
themselves. But any photograph may become such a 'Now' if an
adequate context is created for it. In general the better the photograph, the fuller the context which can be created.

Such a context re-places the photograph in time – not its own
original time for that is impossible – but in narrated time. Narrated
time becomes historic time when it is assumed by social memory
and social action. The constructed narrated time needs to respect
the process of memory which it hopes to stimulate.

There is never a single approach to something remembered. The
remembered is not like a terminus at the end of a line. Numerous
approaches or stimuli converge upon it and lead to it. Words, com-
parisons, signs need to create a context for a printed photograph
in a comparable way; that is to say, they must mark and leave open
diverse approaches. A radial system has to be constructed around
the photograph so that it may be seen in terms which are simultaneously personal, political, economic, dramatic, everyday and
historic.

August 1978

Editor's note

Quotations from Susan Sontag, *On Photography* (Harmondsworth: Penguin, 1977), in order of citation, are from pp. 3–4,
23, 165, 154, 23, 11, 178 and 19–20.

Appearances

The Ambiguity of the Photograph

What makes photography a strange invention – with unforeseeable consequences – is that its primary raw materials are light and time.

Yet let us begin with something more tangible. A few days ago a friend of mine found this photograph and showed it to me.

I know nothing about it. The best way of dating it is probably by its photographic technique. Between 1900 and 1920? I do not know whether it was taken in Canada, the Alps, South Africa. All one can see is that it shows a smiling middle-aged man with his horse (see p. 62). Why was it taken? What meaning did it have for the photographer? Would it have had the same meaning for the man with the horse?

One can play a game of inventing meanings. The Last Mountie. (His smile becomes nostalgic.) The Man Who Set Fire to Farms. (His smile becomes sinister.) Before the Trek of Two Thousand Miles. (His smile becomes a little apprehensive.) After the Trek of Two Thousand Miles. (His smile becomes modest.) . . .

The most definite information this photograph gives is about the type of bridle the horse is wearing, and this is certainly not the reason why it was taken. Looking at the photograph alone it is even hard to know to what category it belonged. Was it a family-album picture, a newspaper picture, a traveller's snap?

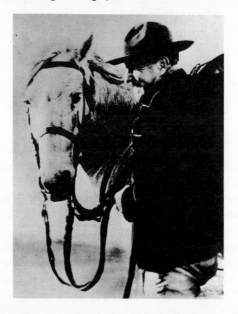

Could it have been taken, not for the sake of the man, but of the horse? Was the man acting as a groom, just holding the horse? Was he a horse-dealer? Or was it a still photograph taken during the filming of one of the early Westerns?

The photograph offers irrefutable evidence that this man, this horse and this bridle existed. Yet it tells us nothing of the significance of their existence.

A photograph arrests the flow of time in which the event photographed once existed. All photographs are of the past, yet in them an instant of the past is arrested so that, unlike a lived past, it can never lead to the present. Every photograph presents us with two messages: a message concerning the event photographed and another concerning a shock of discontinuity.

Between the moment recorded and the present moment of looking at the photograph, there is an abyss. We are so used to photography that we no longer consciously register the second of these twin messages – except in special circumstances: when, for example, the person photographed was familiar to us and is now far away or dead. In such circumstances the photograph is more traumatic than most memories or mementos because it seems to confirm, prophetically, the later discontinuity created by the absence or death. Imagine for a moment that you were once in love with the man with the horse and that he has now disappeared.

If, however, he is a total stranger, one thinks only of the first message, which here is so ambiguous that the event escapes one. What the photograph shows goes with any story one chooses to invent.

Nevertheless the mystery of this photograph does not quite end there. No invented story, no explanation offered will be quite as *present* as the banal appearances preserved in this photograph. These appearances may tell us very little, but they are unquestionable.

The first photographs were thought of as marvels because, far more directly than any other form of visual image, they presented the appearance of what was absent. They preserved the look of things and they allowed the look of things to be carried away. The marvel in this was not only technical.

Our response to appearances is a very deep one, and it includes elements which are instinctive and atavistic. For example, appearances alone – regardless of all conscious considerations – can sexually arouse. For example, the stimulus to action – however tentative it remains – can be provoked by the colour red. More widely, the look of the world is the widest possible confirmation of the *thereness* of the world, and thus the look of the world continually proposes and confirms our relation to that thereness, which nourishes our sense of Being.

Before you tried to read the photograph of the man with the horse, before you placed it or named it, the simple act of looking at it confirmed, however briefly, your sense of being in the world, with its men, hats, horses, bridles . . .

The ambiguity of a photograph does not reside within the instant of the event photographed: there the photographic evidence is less ambiguous than any eye-witness account. The photo-finish of a race is rightly decided by what the camera has recorded. The ambiguity arises out of that discontinuity which gives rise to the second of the photograph's twin messages. (The abyss between the moment recorded and the moment of looking.)

A photograph preserves a moment of time and prevents it being effaced by the supersession of further moments. In this respect photographs might be compared to images stored in the memory. Yet there is a fundamental difference: whereas remembered images are the *residue* of continuous experience, a photograph isolates the appearances of a disconnected instant.

And in life, meaning is not instantaneous. Meaning is discovered in what connects, and cannot exist without development. Without a story, without an unfolding, there is no meaning. Facts, information, do not in themselves constitute meaning. Facts can be fed into a computer and become factors in a calculation. No meaning, however, comes out of computers, for when we give meaning to an event, that meaning is a response, not only to the known, but also to the unknown: meaning and mystery are inseparable, and neither can exist without the passing of time. Certainty may be instantaneous; doubt requires duration; meaning is born of the two. An instant photographed can only acquire meaning in so far as the viewer can read into it a duration extending beyond itself. When we find a photograph meaningful, we are lending it a past and a future.

The professional photographer tries, when taking a photograph, to choose an instant which will persuade the public viewer to lend it an *appropriate* past and future. The photographer's intelligence or his empathy with the subject defines for him what is appropriate. Yet unlike the storyteller or painter or actor, the photographer only makes, in any one photograph, *a single constitutive choice*: the choice of the instant to be photographed. The photograph, compared with other means of communication, is therefore weak in intentionality.

A dramatic photograph may be as ambiguous as an undramatic one.

What is happening? It requires a caption for us to understand the significance of the event. 'Nazis Burning Books'. And the significance of the caption again depends upon a sense of history that we cannot necessarily take for granted.

All photographs are ambiguous. All photographs have been taken out of a continuity. If the event is a public event, this continuity is history; if it is personal, the continuity, which has been broken, is a life story. Even a pure landscape breaks a continuity: that of the light and the weather. Discontinuity always produces

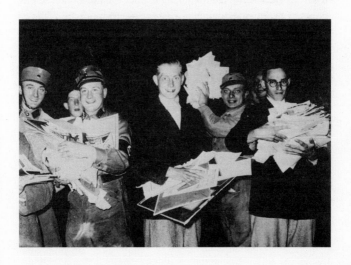

ambiguity. Yet often this ambiguity is not obvious, for as soon as photographs are used with words, they produce together an effect of certainty, even of dogmatic assertion.

In the relation between a photograph and words, the photograph begs for an interpretation, and the words usually supply it. The photograph, irrefutable as evidence but weak in meaning, is given a meaning by the words. And the words, which by themselves remain at the level of generalization, are given specific authenticity by the irrefutability of the photograph. Together the two then become very powerful; an open question appears to have been fully answered.

Yet it might be that the photographic ambiguity, if recognized and accepted as such, could offer to photography a unique means of expression. Could this ambiguity suggest another way of telling? This is a question I want to raise now and return to later.

Cameras are boxes for transporting appearances. The principle by which cameras work has not changed since their invention. Light, from the object photographed, passes through a hole and falls on to a photographic plate or film. The latter, because of its chemical preparation, preserves these traces of light. From these traces, through other slightly more complicated chemical processes, prints are made. Technically, by the standards of our century, it is a simple process. Just as the historically comparable invention of the printing press was, in its time, simple. What is still not so simple is to grasp the nature of the appearances which the camera transports.

Are the appearances which a camera transports a construction, a man-made cultural artefact, or are they, like a footprint in the sand, a trace *naturally* left by something that has passed? The answer is, both.

The photographer chooses the event he photographs. This choice can be thought of as a cultural construction. The space for this construction is, as it were, cleared by his rejection of what he did not choose to photograph. The construction is his reading of the event which is in front of his eyes. It is this reading, often intuitive and very fast, which decides his choice of the instant to be photographed.

Likewise, the photographed image of the event, when shown as a photograph, is also part of a cultural construction. It belongs to a specific social situation, the life of the photographer, an argument, an experiment, a way of explaining the world, a book, a newspaper, an exhibition.

Yet at the same time, the material relation between the image and what it represents (between the marks on the printing paper and the tree these marks represent) is an immediate and unconstructed one. And is indeed like a *trace*.

The photographer chooses the tree, the view of it he wants, the kind of film, the focus, the filter, the time exposure, the strength of the developing solution, the sort of paper to print on, the darkness or lightness of the print, the framing of the print – all this and more. But where he does not intervene – and cannot intervene without changing the fundamental character of photography – is between the light, emanating from that tree as it passes through the lens, and the imprint it makes on the film.

It may clarify what we mean by a *trace* if we ask how a drawing differs from a photograph. A drawing is a translation. That is to say each mark on the paper is consciously related, not only to the real or imagined 'model', but also to every mark and space already set out on the paper. Thus a drawn or painted image is woven together by the energy (or the lassitude, when the drawing is weak) of countless judgements. Every time a figuration is evoked in a drawing, everything about it has been mediated by consciousness, either intuitively or systematically. In a drawing an apple is *made* round and spherical; in a photograph, the roundness and the light and shade of the apple are received as a given.

This difference between making and receiving also implies a very different relation to time. A drawing contains the time of its own making, and this means that it possesses its own time, independent of the living time of what it portrays. The photograph, by contrast, receives almost instantaneously – usually today at a speed which cannot be perceived by the human eye. The only time contained in a photograph is the isolated instant of what it shows.

There is another important difference within the times contained by the two kinds of images. The time which exists within a drawing is not uniform. The artist gives more time to what she or he considers important. A face is likely to contain more time than the sky above it. Time in a drawing accrues according to human value. In a photograph time is uniform: every part of the image has been subjected to a chemical process of uniform duration. In the process of revelation all parts were equal.

These differences between a drawing and a photograph relating to time lead us to the most fundamental distinction between the two means of communication. The countless judgements and decisions which constitute a drawing are systematic. That is to say that they are grounded in an existent language. The teaching of this language and its specific usages at any given time are historically variable. A master-painter's apprentice during the Renaissance learnt a different practice and grammar of drawing from a Chinese apprentice during the Sung period. But every drawing, in order to recreate appearances, has recourse to a language.

Photography, unlike drawing, does not possess a language. The photographic image is produced instantaneously by the reflection of light; its figuration is *not* impregnated by experience or consciousness.

Barthes, writing about photography, talked of 'humanity encountering for the first time in its history *messages without a code*. Hence the photograph is not the last (improved) term of the great family of images; it corresponds to a decisive mutation of informational economies.'[10] The mutation being that photographs supply information without having a language of their own.

Photographs do not translate from appearances. They quote from them.

It is because photography has no language of its own, because it quotes rather than translates, that it is said that the camera cannot lie. It cannot lie because it prints directly.

(The fact that there were and are faked photographs is, paradoxically, a proof of this. You can only make a photograph tell an explicit lie by elaborate tampering, collage and re-photographing. You have in fact ceased to practise photography. Photography in itself has no language which can be *turned*.) And yet photographs can be, and are, massively used to deceive and misinform.

We are surrounded by photographic images which constitute a global system of misinformation: the system known as publicity, proliferating consumerist lies. The role of photography in this system is revealing. The lie is constructed before the camera. A 'tableau' of objects and figures is assembled. This 'tableau' uses a language of symbols (often inherited, as I have pointed out elsewhere,[11] from the iconography of oil painting), an implied narrative and, frequently, some kind of performance by models with a sexual content. This 'tableau' is then photographed. It is photographed precisely because the camera can bestow authenticity upon any set of appearances, however false. The camera does not lie even when it is used to quote a lie. And so, this makes the lie *appear* more truthful.

The photographic quotation is, within its limits, incontrovertible. Yet the quotation, placed like a fact in an explicit or implicit argument, can misinform. Sometimes the misinforming is deliberate, as in

---

10 Roland Barthes, *Image-Music-Text* (London: Fontana, 1977), p. 45.

11 John Berger, *Ways of Seeing* (London: British Broadcasting Corporation and Penguin Books, 1972), pp. 134, 141.

the case of publicity; often it is the result of an unquestioned ideological assumption.

For example, all over the world during the nineteenth century, European travellers, soldiers, colonial administrators, adventurers, took photographs of 'the natives', their customs, their architecture, their richness, their poverty, their women's breasts, their headdresses; and these images, besides provoking amazement, were presented and read as proof of the justice of the imperial division of the world. The division between those who organized and rationalized and surveyed, and those who *were* surveyed.

In itself the photograph cannot lie, but, by the same token, it cannot tell the truth; or rather, the truth it does tell, the truth it can by itself defend, is a limited one.

The idealistic early press photographers – in the twenties and thirties of this century – believed that their mission was to bring home the truth to the world.

> Sometimes I come away from what I am photographing sick at heart, with the faces of people in pain etched as sharply in my mind as on my negatives. But I go back because I feel it is my place to make such pictures. Utter truth is essential, and that is what stirs me when I look through the camera.
>
> Margaret Bourke-White

I admire the work of Margaret Bourke-White. And photographers, under certain political circumstances, have indeed helped to alert public opinion to the truth of what was happening elsewhere. For example: the degree of rural poverty in the United States in the 1930s; the treatment of Jews in the streets of Nazi Germany; the effects of US napalm bombing in Vietnam. Yet to believe that what one sees, as one looks through a camera on to the experience of others, is the 'utter truth' risks confusing very different levels of the truth. And this confusion is endemic to the present public use of photographs.

Photographs are used for scientific investigation: in medicine, physics, meteorology, astronomy, biology. Photographic information is also fed into systems of social and political control – dossiers, passports, military intelligence. Other photographs are used in the media as a means of public communication. The three contexts are different, and yet it has been generally assumed that the truthfulness of the photograph – or the way that this truth functions – is the same in all three.

In fact, when a photograph is used scientifically, its unquestionable evidence is an aid in coming to a conclusion: it supplies information *within the conceptual framework* of an investigation. It supplies a missing detail. When photographs are used in a control system, their evidence is more or less limited to establishing identity and presence. But as soon as a photograph is used as a means of communication, the nature of lived experience is involved, and then the truth becomes more complex.

An X-ray photograph of a wounded leg can tell the 'utter truth' about whether the bones are fractured or not. But how does a photograph tell the 'utter truth' about a man's experience of hunger or, for that matter, his experience of a feast?

At one level there are no photographs which can be denied. All photographs have the status of fact. What has to be examined is in what way photography can and cannot give meaning to facts.

Let us recall how and when photography was born, how, as it were, it was christened, and how it grew up.

The camera was invented in 1839. Auguste Comte was just finishing his *Cours de philosophie positive*. Positivism and the camera and sociology grew up together. What sustained them all as practices was the belief that observable quantifiable facts, recorded

71

by scientists and experts, would one day offer man such a total knowledge about nature and society that he would be able to order them both. Precision would replace metaphysics, planning would resolve social conflicts, truth would replace subjectivity, and all that was dark and hidden in the soul would be illuminated by empirical knowledge. Comte wrote that theoretically nothing need remain unknown to man except, perhaps, the origin of the stars! Since then cameras have photographed even the formation of stars! And photographers now supply us with more facts every month than the eighteenth-century Encylopedists dreamt of in their whole project.

Yet the positivist utopia was not achieved. And the world today is less controllable by experts, who have mastered what they believe to be its mechanisms, than it was in the nineteenth century.

What *was* achieved was unprecedented scientific and technical progress and, eventually, the subordination of all other values to those of a world market which treats everything, including people and their labour and their lives and their deaths, as a commodity. The unachieved positivist utopia became, instead, the global system of late capitalism wherein all that exists becomes quantifiable – not simply because it *can be* reduced to a statistical fact, but also because it *has been* reduced to a commodity.

In such a system there is no space for experience. Each person's experience remains an individual problem. Personal psychology replaces philosophy as an explanation of the world.

Nor is there space for the social function of subjectivity. All subjectivity is treated as private, and the only (false) form of it which is socially allowed is that of the individual consumer's dream.

From this primary suppression of the social function of subjectivity, other suppressions follow: of meaningful democracy (replaced by opinion polls and market-research techniques), of social conscience (replaced by self-interest), of history (replaced by racist and other myths), of hope – the most subjective and social of all energies (replaced by the sacralization of Progress as Comfort).

The way photography is used today both derives from and confirms the suppression of the social function of subjectivity. Photographs, it is said, tell the truth. From this simplification, which reduces the truth to the instantaneous, it follows that what a photograph tells about a door or a volcano belongs to the same order of truth as what it tells about a man weeping or a woman's body.

If no theoretical distinction has been made between the photograph as scientific evidence and the photograph as a means of communication, *this has been not so much an oversight as a proposal.*

The proposal was (and is) that when something is visible, it is a fact, and that facts contain the only truth.

Public photography has remained the child of the hopes of positivism. Orphaned – because these hopes are now dead – it has been adopted by the opportunism of corporate capitalism. It seems likely that the denial of the innate ambiguity of the photograph is closely connected with the denial of the social function of subjectivity.

A Popular Use of Photography

'In our age there is no work of art that is looked at so closely as a photograph of oneself, one's closest relatives and friends, one's sweetheart,' wrote Lichtwark back in 1907, thereby moving the inquiry out of the realm of aesthetic distinctions into that of social functions. Only from this vantage point can it be carried further.

Walter Benjamin, *A Small History of Photography* (1931)

A mother with her child is staring intently at a soldier. Perhaps they are speaking. We cannot hear their words. Perhaps they are saying nothing and everything is being said by the way they are looking at each other. Certainly a drama is being enacted between them.

The caption reads: 'A Red Hussar Leaving, June 1919, Budapest.' The photograph is by André Kertész.

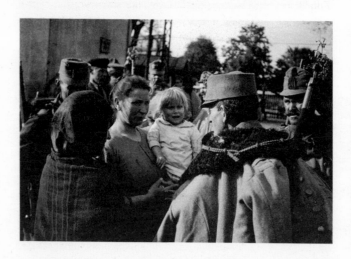

So, the woman has just walked out of their home and will shortly go back alone with the child. The drama of the moment is expressed in the difference between the clothes they are wearing. His for travelling, for sleeping out, for fighting; hers for staying at home.

The caption can also entail other thoughts. The Hapsburg monarchy had fallen the previous autumn. The winter had been one of extreme shortages (especially of fuel in Budapest) and economic distintegration. Three months before, in March, the socialist Republic of Councils had been declared. The Western allies in Paris, fearful lest the Russian and now the Hungarian example of revolution should spread throughout Eastern Europe and the Balkans, were planning to dismantle the new republic. A blockade was already imposed. General Foch himself was planning the military invasion being carried out by Rumanian and Czech troops. On 8 June Clemenceau telegraphed an ultimatum to Béla Kun demanding a Hungarian military withdrawal which would have left the Rumanians occupying the eastern third of their country. For another six weeks the Hungarian Red Army fought on, but it was finally overwhelmed. By August, Budapest was occupied and very soon after, the first European fascist regime under Horthy was established.

If we are looking at an image from the past and we want to relate it to ourselves, we need to know something of the history of that past. And so the foregoing paragraph – and much more than that might be said – is relevant to the reading of Kertész's photograph. Which is presumably why he gave it the caption he did and not just the title 'Parting'. Yet the photograph – or rather, the way this photograph demands to be read – cannot be limited to the historical.

Everything in it is historical: the uniforms, the rifles, the corner by the Budapest railway station, the identity and biographies of all the people who are (or were) recognizable – even the size of the trees on the other side of the fence. And yet it also concerns a resistance to history: an opposition.

This opposition is not the consequence of the photographer having said: Stop! It is not that the resultant static image is like a fixed post in a flowing river. We know that in a moment the soldier will turn his back and leave; we presume that he is the father of the child in the woman's arms. The significance of the instant photographed is already claiming minutes, weeks, years.

The opposition exists in the parting look between the man and the woman. This look is not directed towards the viewer. We witness it as the older soldier with the moustache and the woman with the shawl (perhaps a sister) do. The exclusivity of this look is further emphasized by the boy in the mother's arms; he is watching his father, and yet he is excluded from their look.

This look, which crosses before our eyes, is holding in place what *is*, not specifically what is there around them outside the station, but what *is* their life, what *are* their lives. The woman and the soldier are looking at each other so that the image of what *is* now shall remain for them. In this look their being *is* opposed to their history, even if we assume that this history is one they accept or have chosen.

How can one be opposed to history? Conservatives may oppose with force changes in history. But there is another kind of opposition. Who can read Marx and not feel his hatred towards the historical processes he discovered and his impatience for the end of history when, he believed, the realm of necessity would be transformed into the realm of freedom?

An opposition to history may be partly an opposition to what happens in it. But not only that. Every revolutionary protest is also a protest against people being the objects of history. And as soon as people feel, as the result of their desperate protest, that they are no longer such objects, *history ceases to have the monopoly of time.*

Imagine the blade of a giant guillotine as long as the diameter of the city. Imagine the blade descending and cutting a section through everything that is there – walls, railway lines, wagons, workshops, churches, crates of fruit, trees, sky, cobblestones. Such a blade has fallen a few yards in front of the face of everyone who is determined to fight. Each finds himself a few yards from the precipitous edge of an infinitely deep fissure which only he can see. The fissure, like a deep cut into the flesh, is unmistakably itself; there can be no doubting what has happened. But there is no pain at first.

The pain is the thought of one's own death probably being very near. It occurs to the men and women building the barricades that

what they are handling, and what they are thinking, are probably
being handled and thought by them for the last time. As they build
the defences, the pain increases.

. . . At the barricades the pain is over. The transformation is complete. It is completed by a shout from the rooftops that the soldiers
are advancing. Suddenly there is nothing to regret. The barricades
are between their defenders and the violence done to them throughout their lives. There is nothing to regret because it is the quintes-
sence of their past which is now advancing against them. On their
side of the barricades it is already the future.[12]

Revolutionary actions are rare. Feelings of opposition to history,
however, are constant, even if unarticulated. They often find their
expression in what is called private life. A home has become not
only a physical shelter but also a teleological shelter, however frail,
against the remorselessness of history; a remorselessness which
should be distinguished from the brutality, injustice and misery
the same history often contains.

People's opposition to history is a reaction (even a protest, but
a protest so intimate that it has no direct social expression and the
indirect ones are often mystified and dangerous: both fascism and
racism feed upon such protests) against a violence done to them.
The violence consists in conflating time and history so that the
two become indivisible, so that people can no longer read their
experience of either of them separately.

This conflation began in Europe in the nineteenth century, and
has become more complete and more extensive as the rate of
historical change has increased and become global. All popular
religious movements – such as the present mounting Islamic one
against the materialism of the West – are a form of resistance to
the violence of this conflation.

12 John Berger, G. (London: Weidenfeld & Nicolson, 1972), pp. 71–2.

What does this violence consist in? The human imagination which grasps and unifies time (before imagination existed, each time scale – cosmic, geological, biological – was disparate) has always had the capacity of undoing time. This capacity is closely connected with the faculty of memory. Yet time is undone not only by being remembered but also by the living of certain moments which defy the passing of time, not so much by becoming unforgettable but because, within the experience of such moments there is an imperviousness to time. They are experiences which provoke the words *for ever, toujours, siempre, immer*. Moments of achievement, trance, dream, passion, crucial ethical decision, prowess, near-death, sacrifice, mourning, music, the visitation of *duende*. To name some of them.

Such moments have continually occurred in human experience. Although not frequent in any one lifetime, they are common. They are the material of *all* lyrical expression (from pop music to Heine and Sappho). Nobody has lived without experiencing such moments. Where people differ is in the confidence with which they credit importance to them. I say confidence since I believe that intimately, if not publicly, no one fails to allow them some importance. They are summit moments and they are intrinsic to the relation imagination / time.

Before time and history were conflated, the rate of historical change was slow enough for an individual's awareness of time passing to remain quite distinct from her or his awareness of historical change. The sequences of an individual life were surrounded by the relatively changeless, and the relatively changeless (history) was in its turn surrounded by the timeless.

History used to pay its respects to mortality: the enduring honoured the value of what was brief. Graves were a mark of such respect. Moments which defied time in the individual life were like glimpses through a window; these windows, let into the life, looked *across* history, which changed slowly, towards the timeless which would never change.

When in the eighteenth century the rate of historical change began to accelerate, causing the principle of historical progress to be born, the timeless or unchanging was claimed by and gradually incorporated into historical time. Astronomy arranged the stars historically. Renan historicized Christianity. Darwin made every origin historical. Meanwhile, actively, through imperialism and proletarianization, other cultures and ways of life and work, which embodied different traditions concerning time, were being destroyed. The factory which works all night is a sign of the victory of a ceaseless, uniform and remorseless time. The factory continues even during the time of dreams.

The principle of historical progress insisted that the elimination of all other views of history save its own was part of that progress. Superstition, embedded conservatism, so-called eternal laws, fatalism, social passivity, the fear of eternity so skilfully used by churches to intimidate, repetition and ignorance: all these had to be swept away and replaced by the proposal that man could make his own history. And indeed this did – and does – represent progress, in that social justice cannot be fully achieved without such an awareness of the historical possibility, and this awareness depends upon historical explanations being given.

Nevertheless a deep violence was done to subjective experience. And to argue that this is unimportant in comparison with the objective historical possibilities created is to miss the point because, precisely, the modern anguished form of the distinction subjective/ objective begins and develops with this violence.

Today what surrounds the individual life can change more quickly than the brief sequences of that life itself. The timeless has been abolished, and history itself has become ephemerality. History no longer pays its respects to the dead: the dead are simply what it has passed through. (A study of the comparative number of public monuments erected during the last hundred years in the West would show a startling decline during the last twenty-five.) There is no longer any generally acknowledged value longer than that of a life, and most are shorter. The worldwide phenomenon of inflation is symptomatic in this respect: an unprecedented modern form of economic transience.

Consequently the common experience of those moments which defy time is now denied by everything which surrounds them. Such moments have ceased to be like windows looking across history towards the timeless. Experiences which prompt the term *for ever* have now to be assumed alone and privately. Their role has been changed: instead of transcending, they isolate. The period in which photography has developed corresponds to the period in which this uniquely modern anguish has become commonplace.

Yet fortunately people are never only the passive objects of history. And apart from popular heroism, there is also popular ingenuity. In this case such ingenuity uses whatever little there is at hand, to preserve experience, to recreate an area of 'timelessness', to insist upon the permanent. And so, hundreds of millions of photographs, fragile images, often carried next to the heart or placed by the side of the bed, are used to refer to that which historical time has no right to destroy.

The private photograph is treated and valued today as if it were the materialization of that glimpse through the window which looked across history towards that which was outside time.

The photograph of the woman and the Red Hussar represents an idea. The idea was not Kertész's. It was being lived in front of his eyes and he was receptive to it.

What did he see?

Summer sunlight.

The contrast between her dress and the heavy greatcoats of the soldiers who will have to sleep out.

The men waiting with a certain heaviness.

Her concentration – she looks at him as if already into the distance which will claim him.

Her scowl, which will not give way to weeping.

His modesty – one reads it by his ear and the way he holds his head because at this moment she is stronger than he.

Her acceptance, in the stance of her body.

The boy, surprised by the father's uniform, aware of the unusual occasion.

Her hair arranged before coming out, her worn dress.

The limits of their wardrobe.

It is only possible to itemize the things seen, for if they touch the heart, they do so essentially through the eye. For example, the appearance of the woman's hands clasped over her stomach tells how she might peel potatoes, how one of her hands might lie when asleep, how she would put up her hair.

The woman and the soldier are recognizing one another. How close a parting is to a meeting! And through that act of recognition, such as perhaps they have never experienced before, each hopes to take away an image of the other which will withstand anything that may happen. An image that nothing can efface. This is the idea being lived before Kertész's camera. And this is what makes this photograph paradigmatic. It shows a moment which is explicitly about what is implicit in all photographs that are not simply enjoyed but loved.

All photographs are possible contributions to history, and any photograph, under certain circumstances, can be used in order to break the monopoly which history today has over time.

The Enigma of Appearances

To read what has never been written.

Hofmannsthal

We have looked at two different uses of photography. An ideological use, which treats the positivist evidence of a photograph as if it represented the ultimate and only truth. And in contrast, a popular but private use, which cherishes a photograph to substantiate a subjective feeling.

I have not considered photography as an art. Paul Strand, who was a great photographer, thought of himself as an artist. In recent years art museums have begun to collect and show photographs. Man Ray said: 'I photograph what I do not wish to paint, and I paint what I cannot photograph.' Other equally serious photographers, like Bruce Davidson, claim it as a virtue that their pictures do not 'pose as art'.

The arguments, put forward from the nineteenth century onwards, about photography sometimes being an art have confused rather than clarified the issue because they have always led to some kind of comparison with the art of painting. And an art of translation cannot usefully be compared to an art of quotation. Their resemblances, their influence one upon the other, are purely formal; functionally they have nothing in common.

Yet however true this may be, a crucial question remains: why can photographs of unknown subjects move us? If photographs do not function like paintings, how do they function? I have argued that photographs quote from appearances. This may suggest that appearances themselves constitute a language.

What sense does it make to say this?

Let me first try to avoid a possible misunderstanding. In his last book Barthes wrote: 'Each time when having gone a little way with a language, I have felt that its system consists in, and in that way is slipping towards, a kind of reductionism and disapproval, I have quietly left and looked elsewhere.'

Unlike their late master, some of Barthes' structuralist followers love closed systems. They would maintain that in my reading of Kertész's photograph, I relied upon a number of semiological systems, each one being a social/cultural construct: the sign language of clothes, of facial expressions, of bodily gestures, of social manners, of photographic framing, etc. Such semiological systems do indeed exist and are continually being used in the making and reading of images. Nevertheless the sum total of these systems cannot exhaust, does not begin to cover, all that can be read in appearances. Barthes himself was of this opinion. The problem of appearances constituting something like a language cannot be resolved simply by reference to these semiological systems.

So we are left with the question: what sense does it make to say that appearances may constitute a language?

Appearances cohere. At the first degree they cohere because of common laws of structure and growth which establish visual affinities. A chip of rock can resemble a mountain; grass grows like hair; waves have the form of valleys; snow is crystalline; the growth of walnuts is constrained in their shells somewhat like the growth of brains in their skulls; all supporting legs and feet, whether static or mobile, visually refer to one another; etc., etc.

At the second degree, appearances cohere because as soon as a fairly developed eye exists, visual imitation begins. All natural camouflage, much natural colouring and a wide range of animal behaviour derive from the principle of appearances fusing or being suggestive of other appearances. On the underside of the wings of the Brassolinae, there are markings which imitate, with great accuracy, the eyes of an owl or another large bird. When attacked, these butterflies flick their wings and their attackers are intimidated by the flashing eyes.

Appearances both distinguish *and* join events.

During the second half of the nineteenth century, when the coherence of appearances had been largely forgotten, one man understood and insisted upon the significance of such a coherence.

> Objects interpenetrate each other. They never cease to live. Imperceptibly they spread intimate reflections around them.
>
> Cézanne

Appearances also cohere within the mind as perceptions. The sight of any single thing or event entrains the sight of other things and events. To recognize an appearance requires the memory of other appearances. And these memories, often projected as expectations, continue to qualify the seen long after the stage of primary recognition. Here for example, we recognize a baby at the breast, but neither our visual memory nor our visual expectations stop there. One image interpenetrates another.

As soon as we say that appearances *cohere* this *coherence* proposes a unity not unlike that of a language.

Seeing and organic life are both dependent upon light, and appearances are the face of this mutuality. And so appearances can be said to be doubly systematic. They belong to a natural affinitive system which exists as such because of certain universal structural and dynamic laws. This is why, as already noted, all legs resemble one another. Secondly, they belong to a perceptive system which organizes the mind's experience of the visible.

The primary energy of the first system is natural reproduction, always thrusting towards the future; the primary energy of the second system is memory, continually retaining the past. In all perceived appearances there is the double traffic of both systems.

We now know that it is the right hemisphere of the human brain which 'reads' and stores our visual experience. This is significant because the areas and centres where this takes place are structurally identical with those in the left hemisphere which process our experience of words. The apparatus with which we deal with appearances is identical with that with which we deal with verbal language. Furthermore, appearances in their unmediated state – that is to say, before they have been interpreted or perceived – lend themselves to reference systems (so that they may be stored at a certain level in the memory) which are comparable to those used for words. And this again prompts one to conclude that appearances possess some of the qualities of a code.

All cultures previous to our own treated appearances as signs addressed to the living. All was *legend*: all was there to be *read* by the eye. Appearances revealed resemblances, analogies, sympathies, antipathies, and each of these conveyed a message. The sum total of these messages explained the universe.

The Cartesian revolution overthrew the basis for any such explanation. It was no longer the relation between the look of things which mattered. What mattered was measurement and difference, rather than visual correspondences. The purely physical could no longer in itself reveal meaning; it could do so only if investigated by reason, which was the probe of the spiritual. Appearances ceased to be double-faced like the words of a dialogue. They became dense and opaque, requiring dissection.

Modern science became possible. The visible, however, deprived of any ontological function, was philosophically reduced to the area of aesthetics. Aesthetics was the study of sensuous perceptions as they affected an individual's feelings. Thus, the reading of appearances became fragmented; they were no longer treated as a signifying whole. Appearances were reduced to contingency, whose meaning was purely personal.

The development may help to explain the fitfulness and erratic history of nineteenth-century and twentieth-century visual art. For the first time ever, visual art was severed from the belief that it was in the very nature of appearances to be meaningful.

If, however, I persist in maintaining that appearances resemble a language, considerable difficulties arise. Where, for example, are its *universals*? A language of appearance implies an encoder; if appearances are there to be read, who wrote them?

It was a rationalist illusion to believe that in dispensing with religion, mysteries would be reduced. What has happened, on the contrary, is that mysteries multiply. Merleau-Ponty wrote:

> We must take literally what vision teaches us, namely that through it we come in contact with the sun and the stars, that we are every-where all at once, and that even our power to imagine ourselves elsewhere . . . borrows from vision and employs means we owe to it. Vision alone makes us learn that beings that are different, 'exterior', foreign to one another, are yet absolutely *together*, are 'simul-taneity'; this is a mystery psychologists handle the way a child handles explosives.[13]

There is no need to disinter ancient religious and magical beliefs which held that the visible is *nothing except a coded message*. These beliefs, being ahistorical, ignored the coincidence of the historical development of eye *and* brain. They also ignored the coincidence that both seeing and organic life are dependent upon light. Yet the enigma of appearances remains, whatever our historical explanations. Philosophically, we can evade the enigma. But we cannot *look* away from it.

One looks at one's surroundings (and one is always surrounded by the visible, even in dreams) and one reads what is there, according to circumstances, in different ways. Driving a car draws out one kind of reading; cutting down a tree another; waiting for a friend

13 Maurice Merleau-Ponty, *The Primacy of Perception* (Evanston, Ill.: Northwestern University Press, 1964), p. 187.

another. Each activity motivates its own reading.

At other times the reading, or the choices which make a reading, instead of being directed towards a goal, are the consequence of an event that has already occurred. Emotion or mood motivates the reading, and the appearances, thus read, become *expressive*. Such moments have often been described in literature, but they do not belong to literature, they belong to the visible.

Ghassan Kanafani, the Palestinian writer, describes a moment when everything he was looking at became expressive of the same pain and determination:

Never shall I forget Nadia's leg, amputated from the top of the thigh. No! Nor shall I forget the grief which had moulded her face and merged into its traits for ever. I went out of the hospital in Gaza that day, my hand clutched in silent derision on the two pounds I had brought with me to give Nadia. The blazing sun filled the streets with the colour of blood. And Gaza was brand new, Mustafa! You and I never saw it like this. The stones piled up at the beginning of the Shajiya quarter where we lived had a meaning, and they seemed to have been put there for no other reason but to explain it. This Gaza in which we had lived and with whose good people we had spent seven years of defeat was something new. It seemed to me just a beginning. I don't know why I thought it was just a beginning. I imagined that the main street that I walked along on the way back home was only the beginning of a long, long road leading to Safad. Everything in this Gaza throbbed with sadness which was not confined to weeping. It was a challenge; more than that, it was something like reclamation of the amputated leg.[14]

*

14 G. Kanafani, *Men in the Sun* (London: Heinemann Educational Books, 1978), p. 79.

In every act of looking there is an expectation of meaning. This expectation should be distinguished from a desire for an explanation. The one who looks may explain *afterwards*; but, prior to any explanation, there is the expectation of what appearances themselves may be about to reveal.

Revelations do not usually come easily. Appearances are so complex that only the search which is inherent in the act of looking can draw a reading out of their underlying coherence. If, for the sake of a temporary clarification, one artificially separates appearances from vision (and we have seen that in fact this is impossible), one might say that in appearances everything that can be read is already there, but undifferentiated. It is the search, with its choices, which differentiates. And *the seen*, the revealed, is the child of both appearances and the search.

Another way of making this relation clearer would be to say that appearances in themselves are oracular. Like oracles they go beyond, they insinuate further than the discrete phenomena they present, and yet their insinuations are rarely sufficient to make any more comprehensive reading indisputable. The precise meaning of an oracular statement depends upon the quest or need of the one who listens to it. Everyone listens to an oracle alone, even when in company.

The one who looks is essential to the meaning found, *and yet can be surpassed by it*. And this surpassing is what is hoped for. Revelation was a visual category before it was a religious one. The hope of revelation – and this is particularly obvious in every childhood – is the stimulus to the *will* to all looking which does not have a precise functional aim.

Revelation, when what we see does surpass us, is perhaps less rare than is generally assumed. By its nature, revelation does not easily lend itself to verbalization. The words used remain aesthetic exclamations! Yet whatever its frequency, our expectation of revelation is, I would suggest, a human constant. The form of this expectation may historically change, but in itself, it is a constituent of *the relation between the human capacity to perceive and the coherence of appearances.*

The totality of this relationship is perhaps best indicated by saying that appearances constitute a half-language. Such a formulation, suggesting both a resemblance to and a difference from a full language, is both clumsy and imprecise, but at least it opens up a space for a number of ideas.

The positivist view of photography has remained dominant, despite its inadequacies, because no other view is possible unless one comes to terms with the revelational nature of appearances. All the best photographers worked by intuition. In terms of their work, this lack of theory did not matter much. What did matter is that the photographic possibility remained theoretically hidden.

What is this possibility?

The single constitutive choice of a photographer differs from the continuous and more random choices of someone who is looking. Every photographer knows that a photograph simplifies. The simplifications concern focus, tonality, depth, framing, supersession (what is photographed does not change), texture, colour, scale, the other senses (their influence on sight is excluded), the play of light. A photograph quotes from appearances but, in quoting, simplifies them. This simplification can increase their legibility. Everything depends upon the quality of the quotation chosen.

The photograph of the man with the horse quotes very briefly. Kertész's photograph outside Budapest railway station quotes at length.

The 'length' of the quotation has nothing to do with exposure time. It is not a temporal length. Earlier we saw that a photographer, through the choice of the instant photographed, may try to persuade the viewer to lend that instant a past and a future. Looking at the man with the horse, we have no clear idea of what has just happened or what is about to happen. Looking at the Kertész, we can trace a story backwards for years and forwards for at least a few hours. This difference in the narrative range of the two images is important, yet although it may be closely associated with the 'length' of the quotation, it does not in itself represent that length. It is necessary to repeat that the length of the quotation is in no sense a temporal length. It is not time that is prolonged but meaning.

The photograph cuts across time and discloses a cross-section of the event or events which were developing at that instant. We have seen that the instantaneous tends to make meaning ambiguous. But the cross-section, if it is wide enough, and can be studied at leisure, allows us to see the interconnectedness and related coexistence of events. Correspondences, which ultimately derive from the unity of appearances, then compensate for the lack of sequence.

This may become clearer if I express it in a diagrammatic, but necessarily highly schematic, way.

In life it is an event's development in time, its duration, which allows its meaning to be perceived and felt. If one states this actively, one can say that the event moves towards or through meaning. This movement can be represented by an arrow.

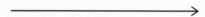

Normally a photograph arrests this movement and cuts across the appearances of the event photographed. Its meaning becomes ambiguous.

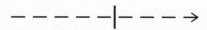

Only by the spectator's lending the frozen appearances a supposed past and future can the arrow's movement be hypothesized.

Above I represented the photographic cut by a vertical line. If, however, one thinks of this cut as a cross-section of the event, one can represent it frontally, as it were, instead of from the side, as a circle. One then has a diagram like this.

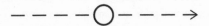

The diameter of the circle depends upon the amount of information to be found in the event's instantaneous appearances. The diameter (the amount of information received) may vary according to the spectator's personal relation to the photographed event. When the man with the horse is a stranger, the diameter remains small, the circle a very reduced one. When the same man is your son, the amount of information gleaned, and the diameter of the circle, increase dramatically.

The exceptional photograph which quotes at length increases the diameter of the circle even when the subject is totally unknown to the spectator.

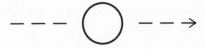

This increase is achieved by the coherence of the appearances – as photographed at that precise conjuncture – extending the event beyond itself. The appearances of the event photographed implicate other events. It is the energy of these simultaneous connections and cross-references which enlarge the circle beyond the dimension of instantaneous information.

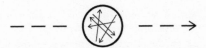

Thus, the discontinuity which is the result of the photographic cut is no longer destructive, for in the photograph of the long quotation another kind of meaning has become possible. The particular event photographed implicates other events by way of an idea born of the appearances of the first event. This idea cannot be merely tautologous. (An image of a person weeping and the idea of suffering would be tautologous.) The idea, confronting the event, extends and joins it to other events, thus widening the diameter.

How is it possible for appearances to 'give birth' to ideas? Through their specific coherence at a given instant, they articulate a set of *correspondences* which provoke in the viewer a recognition of some past experience. This recognition may remain at the level of a tacit agreement with memory, or it may become conscious. When this happens, it is formulated as an idea.

A photograph which achieves expressiveness thus works dialectically: it preserves the particularity of the event recorded, and it chooses an instant when the correspondences of those particular appearances articulate a general idea.

In his *Philosophy of Right*, Hegel defines individuality as follows:

> Every self-consciousness knows itself (1) as universal, as the potentiality of abstracting from everything determinate, and (2) as particular, with a determinate object, content and aim. Still, both these moments are only abstractions; what is concrete and true (and everything true is concrete) is the universality which has the particular as its opposite, but the particular which by its reflection into itself has been equalised with the universal. This unity is individuality.[15]

15 Georg W. F. Hegel, *Philosophy of Right* (London: Oxford University Press, 1975), p. 7.

In every expressive photograph, in every photograph which quotes at length, the particular, by way of a general idea, has been *equalized with the universal*.

A young man is asleep at the table in a public place, perhaps a café (see p. 94). The expression on his face, his character, the way the light and shade dissolve him and his clothes, his open shirt and the newspaper on the table, his health and his fatigue, the time of night: all these are visually present in this event and are particular.

Emanating from the event and confronting it is the general idea. In this photograph the idea concerns legibility. Or, more precisely, the distinction, the stroke, between legibility / illegibility.

Remove the newspapers on the table and on the wall behind the sleeping figure, and the photograph will no longer be expressive – until or unless what replaces them instigates another idea.

The event instigates the idea. And the idea, confronting the event, urges it to go beyond itself and to represent the generalization (what Hegel calls the abstraction) carried within the idea. We see a particular young man asleep. And seeing him, we ponder on sleep in general. Yet this pondering does not take us away from the particular; on the contrary, it has been instigated by it and everything we continue to read is in the interest of the particular. We think or feel or remember *through the appearances* recorded in the photograph, and *with* the idea of legibility / illegibility which was instigated by them.

The print of the newspaper the young man was reading before he fell asleep, the print of the newspapers hanging on the wall, which we can almost read even from this distance – all written news, all written regulations and timetables – have for him become temporarily unreadable. And at the same time, what is going on in his sleeping mind, the way he is recovering from his fatigue, are unreadable for us, or for anybody else who was waiting in the

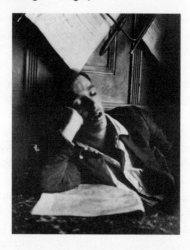

waiting room. Two legibilities. Two illegibilities. The idea of the photo-graph oscillates (like his breathing) between the two poles.

None of this was constructed or planned by Kertész. His task was to be to that degree receptive to the coherence of appearances at that instant from that position in that place. The correspond-ences, which emerge from this coherence, are too extensive and too interwoven to enumerate very satisfactorily in words. (One can-not take photographs with a dictionary.) Paper corresponds with cloth, with folds, with facial features, with print, with darkness, with sleep, with light, with legibility. In the quality of Kertész's *receptivity* here, one sees how a photograph's lack of intentional-ity becomes its strength, its lucidity.

A young boy in 1917 playing in a field with a lamb. He is clearly aware of being photographed. He is both exuberant and inno-cent.

What makes this photograph memorable? Why does it provoke memories in us? We, who are not Hungarian shepherd boys born before the First World War. It is not memorable, as most picture editors might assume, because the boy's expression and gestures are happy and charming. When isolated, photographed gestures and expressions become either mute or caricatural. Here, however, they are not isolated. They contain and are confronted by an idea.

What we see of the lamb – what makes the animal instantly recognizable as a lamb – is the texture of its fleece: that very texture which the boy's hand is stroking and which has attracted him to play with the animal in the way he is. Simultaneously with the texture of the fleece, we notice – or the photograph insists that we notice – the texture of the stubble on which the boy is rolling and which he must feel through his shirt.

The idea within the event, the idea to which Kertész was here receptive, concerns the sense of touch. And how in childhood, everywhere, this sense of touch is especially acute. The photograph is lucid because it speaks, through an idea, to our fingertips, or to our memory of what our fingertips felt.

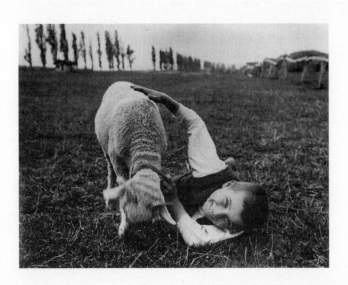

Event and idea are naturally, actively connected. The photograph frames them, excluding everything else. A particular is being equalized with the universal.

In 'A Red Hussar Leaving' the idea concerns stillness. Everything is read as movement: the trees against the sky, the folds of their clothes, the scene of departure, the breeze that ruffles the baby's hair, the shadow of the trees, the woman's hair on her cheek, the angle at which the rifles are being carried. And within this flux, the idea of stillness is instigated by the look passing between the woman and the man. And the lucidity of this idea makes us ponder on the stillness which is born in every departure.

A pair of lovers are embracing on a park bench (or in a garden?). They are an urban middle-class couple. They are probably unaware of being photographed. Or if they are aware, they have now almost forgotten the camera. They are discreet – as the conventions of their class would demand on any public occasion, with or without cameras – and yet, at the same time, desire (or the longing for desire) is making them (might make them) abandoned. Such is the not uncommon event. What makes it an uncommon photograph is that the special coherence of everything we see in it – the concealing screen of the hedge behind them, her gloves, the cuffs of their jackets with the same buttons on them, the movements of their hands, the touching of their noses, the darkness which marries their tailored clothes and the shade of the hedge, the light which illuminates leaves and skin – this coherence instigates the idea of the stroke dividing decorum/desire, clothed/unclothed, occasion/privacy. And such a division is a universal adult experience.

Kertész himself said: 'The camera is my tool. Through it I give reason to everything around me.' It may be possible to construct a theory upon the specific photographic process of 'giving reason'.

Let us summarize. Photographs quote from appearances. The taking-out of the quotation produces a discontinuity, which is reflected in the ambiguity of a photograph's meaning. All photo-

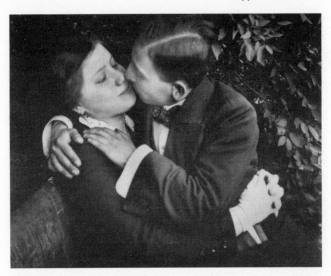

graphed events are ambiguous, except to those whose personal relation to the event is such that their own lives supply the missing continuity. Usually, in public the ambiguity of photographs is hidden by the use of words which explain, less or more truthfully, the pictured events.

The expressive photograph – whose expressiveness can contain its ambiguity of meaning and 'give reason' to it – is a long quotation from appearances: the length here to be measured not by time but by a greater extension of meaning. Such an extension is achieved by turning the photograph's discontinuity to advantage. The narration is broken. (We do not know why the young man asleep is waiting for a train, supposing that that is what he is doing.) Yet the very same discontinuity, by preserving an instantaneous set of appearances, allows us to read across them and to find a synchronic coherence. A coherence which, instead of narrating, instigates ideas. Appearances have this coherent capacity because they constitute something approaching a language. I have referred to this as a half-language.

The half-language of appearances continually arouses an expectation of further meaning. We seek revelation with our eyes. In life this expectation is only rarely met. Photography confirms this expectation and confirms it in a way which can be shared (as we shared the reading of these photographs by Kertész). In the expressive photograph, appearances cease to be oracular and become elucidatory. It is this confirmation which moves us.

Apart from the event photographed, apart from the lucidity of the idea, we are moved by the photograph's fulfilment of an expectation which is intrinsic to the will to look. The camera completes the half-language of appearances and articulates an unmistakable meaning. When this happens we suddenly find ourselves at home among appearances, as we are at home in our mother tongue.

1982

Editor's note

The quotation on pp. 82–3 is Berger's own translation from the French. The passage is translated differently in Roland Barthes, *Camera Lucida*, trans. Richard Howard (New York: Hill and Wang, 1981), p. 8.

Stories

If photographs quote from appearance and if expressiveness is achieved by what we have termed the long quotation, then the possibility suggests itself of composing with numerous quotations, of communicating not with single photographs but with groups or sequences. But how should these sequences be constructed? Can one think in terms of a truly photographic narrative form?

There is already an established photographic practice which uses pictures in sequence: the reportage photo-story. These certainly narrate, but they narrate descriptively from the outsider's point of view. A magazine sends photographer X to city Y to bring back pictures. Many of the finest photographs taken belong to this category. But the story told is finally about what the photographer saw at Y. It is not directly about the experience of those living the event in Y. To speak of their experience with images it would be necessary to introduce pictures of other events and other places, because subjective experience always connects. Yet to introduce such pictures would be to break the journalistic convention.

Reportage photo-stories remain eye-witness accounts rather than stories, and this is why they have to depend on words in order to overcome the inevitable ambiguity of the images. In reports ambiguities are unacceptable; in stories they are inevitable.

If there is a narrative form unique to photography, will it not resemble that of the cinema? Surprisingly, photographs are the opposite of films. Photographs are retrospective and are received as such: films are anticipatory. Before a photograph you search for *what was there*. In a cinema you wait for what is to come next. All film narratives are, in this sense, *adventures*: they advance, they arrive. The term *flashback* is an admission of the inexorable impatience of the film to move forward.

By contrast, if there is a narrative form intrinsic to still photography, it will search for what happened, as memories or reflections do. Memory itself is not made up of flashbacks, each one forever moving inexorably forwards. Memory is a field where different times coexist. The field is continuous in terms of the subjectivity which creates and extends it, but temporarily it is discontinuous.

Among the ancient Greeks, Memory was the mother of all the Muses, and was perhaps most closely associated with the practice of poetry. Poetry at that time, as well as being a form of storytelling, was also an inventory of the visible world; metaphor after metaphor was given to poetry by way of visual correspondences.

Cicero, discussing the poet Simonides who was credited with the invention of the art of memory, wrote:

> It has been sagaciously discerned by Simonides or else discovered by some other person, that the most complete pictures are formed in our minds of the things that have been conveyed to them and imprinted on them by the senses, but that the keenest of all our senses is the sense of sight, and that consequently perceptions received by the ears or by reflection can be most easily retained if they are also conveyed to our minds by the mediation of the eyes.

A photograph is simpler than most memories, its range more limited. Yet with the invention of photography we acquired a new means of expression more closely associated with memory than any other. The Muse of photography is not one of Memory's daughters, but Memory herself. Both the photograph and the remembered depend upon and equally oppose the passing of time. Both preserve moments, and propose their own form of simultaneity, in which all their images can coexist. Both stimulate, and are stimulated by, the interconnectedness of events. Both seek instants of revelation, for it is only such instants which give full reason to their own capacity to withstand the flow of time.

In *Another Way of Telling* we built a sequence of, not four, but a hundred and fifty images. It is entitled 'If Each Time—'. Otherwise there is no text. No words redeem the ambiguity of the images. The sequence begins with certain memories of a childhood, but it does not then follow a chronology. There is no storyline as there is in a *photo-roman*. There is, as it were, no seat supplied for the reader. The reader is free to make his own way *through* these images. The first reading across any two pages may tend to proceed from left to right like European print, but subsequently one can wander in any direction without, we hope, losing a sense of tension or unfolding. Nevertheless we constructed the sequence *as a story*. It is intended to narrate. What can it mean to assert this? If such a thing exists, what is the photographic narrative form?

To try to answer the question, let me first return to the traditional story.

The dog came out of the forest is a simple statement. When that sentence is followed by *The man left the door open*, the possibility of a narrative has begun. If the tense of the second sentence is changed into *The man had left the door open*, the possibility becomes almost a promise. Every narrative proposes an agreement about the unstated but assumed connections existing between events.

One can lie on the ground and look up at the almost infinite number of stars in the night sky, but in order to tell stories about those stars they need to be seen as constellations, the invisible lines which can connect them need to be assumed.

No story is like a wheeled vehicle whose contact with the road is continuous. Stories walk, like animals or men. And their steps are not only between narrated events but between each sentence, sometimes each word. Every step is a stride over something not said.

The suspense story is a modern invention (Poe, 1809–49) and consequently today one may tend to overestimate the role of suspense, the waiting-for-the-end, in storytelling. The essential tension in a story lies elsewhere. Not so much in the mystery of its destination as in the mystery of the spaces between its steps towards that destination.

All stories are discontinuous and are based on a tacit agreement about what is not said, about what connects the discontinuities. The question then arises: who makes this agreement with whom? One is tempted to reply: the teller and the listener. Yet neither teller nor listener is at the centre of the story: they are at its periphery. Those whom the story is about are at the centre. It is between their actions and attributes and reactions that the unstated connections are being made.

One can ask the same question in another way. When the tacit agreement is acceptable to the listener, when a story makes sense of its discontinuities, it acquires authority as a story. But where is this authority? In whom is it invested? In one sense, it is invested in nobody and it is nowhere. Rather, the story invests with authority its characters, its listener's past experience and its teller's words. And it is the authority of all these together that makes the action of the story – what happens in it – worthy of the action of its being told, and vice versa.

The discontinuities of the story and the tacit agreement underlying them fuse teller, listener and protagonists into an amalgam. An amalgam which I would call the story's *reflecting subject*. The story narrates on behalf of this subject, appeals to it and speaks in its voice.

If this sounds unnecessarily complicated, it is worth remembering for a moment the childhood experience of being told a story. Were not the excitement and assurance of that experience precisely the result of the mystery of such a fusion? You were listening. You were in the story. You were in the words of the storyteller. You were no longer your single self; you were, thanks to the story, *everyone it concerned*.

The essence of that childhood experience remains in the power and appeal of any story which has authority. A story is not simply an exercise in empathy. Nor is it merely a meeting-place for the protagonists, the listener and the teller. A story being told is a unique process which fuses these three categories into one. And ultimately what fuses them, within the process, are the discontinuities, the silent connections, agreed upon in common.

Supposing one tries to narrate with photography. The technique of the *photo-roman* offers no solution, for there photography is only a means of reproducing a story constructed according to the conventions of the cinema or theatre. The characters are actors, the world is a decor. Supposing one tries to arrange a number of photographs, chosen from the billions which exist, so that the arrangement speaks of experience. Experience as contained within a life or lives. If this works, it may suggest a narrative form specific to photography.

The discontinuities within the arrangement will be far more evident than those in a verbal story. Each single image will be more or less discontinuous with the next. Continuities of time, place or action may occur, but will be rare. On the face of it there will be no story. And yet in storytelling, as I have tried to show above, it is precisely an agreement about discontinuities which allows the listener to 'enter the narration' and become part of its reflecting subject. The essential relation between teller, listener (spectator) and protagonist(s) may still be possible with an arrangement of photographs. It is, I believe, only their roles, relative to one another, which are modified, not their essential relationship.

The spectator (listener) becomes more active because the assumptions behind the discontinuities (the unspoken which bridges them) are more far-reaching. The teller becomes less present, less insistent, for he no longer employs words of his own; he speaks only through quotations, through his choice and placing of the photographs. The protagonist (at least in our story) becomes omnipresent and therefore invisible; she is manifest in each connection made. One might say that she is defined by *the way she wears the world*, the world about which the photographs supply information. Before she wears it, it is her experience which sews it together.

If, despite these changes of role, there is still the fusion, the amalgam of the *reflecting subject*, one can still talk of a narrative form. Every kind of narrative situates its reflecting subject differently. The epic form placed it before fate, before destiny. The nineteenth-century novel placed it before the individual choices to be made in the area where public and private life overlap. (The novel could not narrate the lives of those who virtually had no choice.) The photographic narrative form places it before the task of memory: the task of continually *resuming* a life being lived in the world. Such a form is not concerned with events as facts – such as is always claimed for photography; it is concerned with their assimilation, their gathering and their transformation into experience.

The precise nature of this as yet experimental narrative form may become still clearer if I very briefly discuss its use of montage. If it does narrate, it does so through its montage.

Eisenstein once spoke of 'a montage of attractions'. By this he meant that what precedes the film-cut should attract what follows it, and vice versa. The energy of this attraction could take the form of a contrast, an equivalence, a conflict, a recurrence. In each case, the cut becomes eloquent and functions like the hinge of a metaphor. The energy of such a montage of attractions could be shown like this:

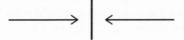

Yet there was in fact an intrinsic difficulty in applying this idea to film. In a film, with its thirty-two frames per second, there is always a third energy in play: that of the reel, that of the film's running through time. And so the two attractions in a film montage are never equal. They are like this:

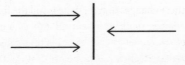

In a sequence of still photographs, however, the energy of attraction, either side of a cut, does remain equal, two-way and *mutual*. Such an energy then closely resembles the stimulus by which one memory triggers another, irrespective of any hierarchy, chronology or duration.

In fact, the energy of the montage of attractions in a sequence of still photographs destroys the very notion of *sequences* – the word which, up to now, I have been using for the sake of convenience. The sequence has become a field of coexistence like the field of memory.

Photographs so placed are restored to a living context: not of course to the original temporal context from which they were taken – that is impossible – but to a context of experience. And there, *their ambiguity at last becomes true*. It allows what they show to be appropriated by reflection. The world they reveal, frozen, becomes tractable. The information they contain becomes permeated by feeling. Appearances become the language of a lived life.

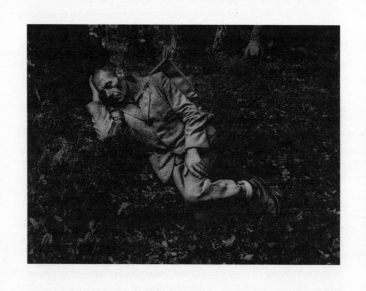

Christ of the Peasants

Markéta Luskačová: *Pilgrims*

I try to imagine how to describe the pilgrim photographs of Markéta Luskačová to somebody who could not see them. An obviously vain exercise in one sense, because appearances and words speak so differently; the visual never allows itself to be translated intact into the verbal. Nothing I could say would enable the reader to imagine a single one of these pictures. Yet what of those who, finding themselves before the photographs, still have difficulty in seeing them? There are good reasons why this might happen. The pictures are of peasants whose experience over the centuries has been very rarely understood by other classes. Worse than that, the pictures are about the experience of religious faith when today most city-dwellers – at least in our continent – have become accustomed to living without any religious belief. Finally, even for the religious minority the pictures may well suggest fanaticism or heresy, because priests and the Church have for so long oppressed peasants, and this oppression has encouraged on both sides the recurring suspicion that principles are being betrayed. The Christ of the peasants has never been the Christ of the papacy. How, then, would I describe the photographs to somebody who could not see them?

I'm inclined to believe that Markéta Luskačová had a secret assignment, such as no photographer had had before. She was summoned by the Dead. How she joined them I don't know. The Dead live, of course, beyond time and are ageless; yet, thanks to the constant arrival of newcomers, they are aware of what happens in history, and sometimes this general, vast awareness of theirs provokes a kind of curiosity so that they want to know more. This curiosity led them to summon a photographer. They told her how they had the impression – and it had been growing for a century or more – that they, the Dead, were being forgotten by the living to an unprecedented degree. Let her understand clearly what they were talking about: the individual Dead had always been quickly or slowly forgotten – it was not this which was new. But now it appeared that the huge, in fact countless, collective of the Dead was being forgotten, as if the living had become – was it ashamed or was it simply negligent? – of their own mortality, of the very consanguinity which joined them to the Dead. Of this, they said they needed no proof, there was ample evidence. What they would like to see – supposing that somewhere in the heart of the continent in which she lived they still existed – were people who still remembered the Dead. Neither the bereaved (for bereavement is temporary) nor the morbid (for they are obsessed by death, not by the Dead), but people living their everyday lives while looking further, beyond, aware of the Dead as neighbours.

'We would like you,' they told her, 'to do a reportage on *us*, in the eyes of the living: can you do that?' She did not reply, for she already knew, although she was only in her early twenties, that the only possible reply could be in the images developed in a darkroom.

Soon after, Markéta Luskačová found herself in the village of Sumiac. Before beginning her assignment proper, she took some pictures to remind the long-departed of the earth on which everything happens. A woman and a horse, with the grass cropped and the footpaths going as far back as living memory. A man sowing, striding slowly through the field he has ploughed, the gesture of his arm like that of a cellist. Three children asleep in a bed.

Then she moved on to the unprecedented challenge of her commission. The people she was photographing trusted her; more than that, they allowed her to become intimate. This was a precondition for her assignment, for she could not photograph the presence of the Dead in the lives of the living from afar: a telescopic lens in this case would have been useless. Nor could she be in a hurry. Intimacy implies having time on one's hands, even a kind of boredom. And further, she could not be in a hurry because the project demanded isolating an instant filled with the timeless, and isolating a set of appearances containing the invisible. These were not impossible demands, since the human eye and the human face are windows on to the soul.

In some pictures she failed – failed for a simple and understandable reason. Sometimes the people being photographed were aware of her being there with her camera, they trusted her completely and so they appealed for recognition. In a flash they imagined how: *Take Us Now = We'll See How We Were at This Moment.*

In other pictures she succeeded; she carried out the assignment and she produced photos such as nobody had ever taken before. We see the photographed in all their intimacy and they are not *there*; they are *elsewhere* with their neighbours: the dead, the unborn, the absent. For instance, her extraordinary photo of the Sleeping Man might be a companion piece to a poem by Rilke:

> . . . You, neighbour God, if sometimes in the night
> I rouse you with loud knocking, I do so
> only because I seldom hear you breathe
> and know: you are alone.
> And should you need a drink, no one is there
> to reach it to you, groping in the dark.
> Always I hearken. Give but a small sign.
> I am quite near.
> Between us there is but a narrow wall,
> and by sheer chance; for it would take

merely a call from your lips or from mine
to break it down,
and that without a sound.

The wall is builded of your images . . .

To stop there would be too resolved, too 'transcendental' for the peasant experience which Markéta Luskačová interprets so faithfully. The peasant, within the secrecy of his own mind, is independent, and he projects this independence on to those he worships. *Nothing is ever quite arranged.*

Italo Calvino has recorded a story from the countryside near Verona; and I think of it when, for instance, I look at the picture of the builders at Sumiac eating a meal:

Once there was a farmer who was devout, but who prayed only to St Joseph. When he died, St Peter refused to let him into heaven. 'No question,' said St Peter, 'you forgot about Christ, God the Father and the Virgin.' 'Since I'm here,' replied the man, 'could I have a word with Joseph?' Joseph appeared, recognized the farmer and said: 'Come in, make yourself at home.' 'I can't,' complained the man, 'Peter here has forbidden me to enter heaven.' Joseph turned to Peter and angrily remonstrated: 'You let him in here, or I'll take my son and my wife and we'll go somewhere else to build paradise!'

1985

W. Eugene Smith

Notes to Help Documentary Film-Maker
Kirk Morris Make a Film about Smith

It's not possible to make a biographical documentary – plus sequences of his own photos – because the true drama of Smith's life and work are not *explicit*. It would be possible, for instance, to use such a method concerning Van Gogh because we have his letters which relate his life with incredible insight. Smith's writings are, by contrast, mostly rantings. Thus the material for a biography is not already there. It has to be written and invented by the film-maker and because the subjective elements in this story are so important – as with the story of any artist – such invention will have to approach fiction. We have the facts of his life but all of them have to be interpreted and ideally these interpretations should lead us to see his work more clearly.

Where did this man come from?

The question is not just geographical but cultural, social, historical. Where did he learn his ideals, his fears, his special kind of pride? He's a man from mid-America. Essentially, he is more like a railroad man, a lumberjack or a folk-singer like Woody Guthrie, than like a New York or European artist of the same epoch. Compare by contrast a man like Arthur Miller or Thornton Wilder. Behind most of Smith's images there is the harshness of a work song: the virtue of virility: the simple destiny of victory or defeat. Such men carry, buried within them, a shyness. And this adds to the image of a typical, Midwest hero. I emphasize this because Smith's physical appearance, especially during the second half of his life, tends to mask this truth and his letters should never be taken as *evidence*. He uses words to make a noise to match the totally inarticulate noise he hears in his head. Smith abuses words and he mistrusted them. This is why he made puns. He wanted to outwit words. One finds the same kind of thing sometimes in bar-room talk.

What drove this man, what demon gave him such energy?

His devotion to photography. His art. But how did he see art? His attitude to words, music, his own art was essentially religious. He saw art as a means of redemption. Music, words, were to him an accompaniment to the drama of looking for goodness. His own photography constituted his way of looking for this, his search.

He was not a cultivated man for this implies belonging to a privileged culture. He was a loner. He sought a truth which, by its nature, was not evident. It was waiting to be revealed by him and him alone. He wanted his images to convert so that the spectator might see beyond the lies, the vanity, the illusions of everyday life. In this profound sense of searching for the immanent truth he was, I believe, the most *religious* photographer in the history of the art. A seer in both the photographic and biblical senses of the term.

His unique use of black and white was intimately tied to his sense of vocation. Through blackness he makes the world his own – turns it into a dark, terrible, moral theatre where souls search for beauty or redemption. (It would be worth looking at some medieval morality plays to find a scene to match this process.) Sometimes the drama which he puts on the stage of his photo is in the subject as given at that moment. The war pictures, for example. But often it is not, often the drama comes from within Smith's vision; then he imposes his vision on what is in front of him with a massive dramatic weight. For example, the evil drama of the three Guardia Civil. For example, the good drama of some of his pictures of Albert Schweitzer in action. His photography uses a biblical language.

Black, for Smith, was the valley of the shadow of death. Light was hope. Compare some of his photos with both icons and certain early Flemish paintings. Not so much from the point of view of light and shade as from that of their expression (the expression of faces) and the relation between figures and background. His most successful pictures look more at home in a church than in a museum. He dreams of speaking to a congregation.

What first formed this man?

How did the moral drama, which is so integral a part of his photography, first begin for him? Unquestionably, profoundly and until the end, it began with his mother. She was, in my opinion, the beginning and end of Gene. All the other women in his life were only planets round her sun (son).

Their relationship was charged with a devotional love, but its language, its form of exchange, was, I suspect, emotional blackmail. Most of Smith's dealings with the world (apart from his photography) were based on the same principle – including, most obviously, all his repeated threats of suicide. He learnt the principle from his mother. She, in her own way, practised it on him. The tools of the blackmail were moralistic and biblical in their scale: sin, the wickedness of the world, the salvation of the soul, future justice, death.

Her son comes to believe that he is only lovable when he is being punished; the punishment comes inextricably mixed with her love and her hopes for him. Like us all, he wanted to be loved and so his life, which more than most men he decided for himself, becomes a story of punishments. To use the term masochist would be a cheap and vulgar simplification. Because from his mother he acquired, not only the habit of punishment, but also the principle of pity and the need to save the world. (Of course his capacity for pity was far greater than hers. In some ways she was perhaps a ruthless woman. Nevertheless I think it was she who taught him the principle of pity.)

What is the genius of his photography?

The authenticity of Smith's photography does not come from his objectivity but from its selectivity. Of the great masters of reportage and of photographic storytelling, Smith is probably the most subjective. For him, appearances only reveal the truth very occasionally. And for him the rest of the time they were lies. For him, Pittsburgh represented the human condition at that time. Far more than a city, it was life on this earth. This is why the project grew so uncontrollably.

Now we can return to our title and to the image of a Pietà – of the man-Christ dead in his mother's lap. An image of tenderness and bereavement. The figure of the victim, suffering or dead, is, by its nature, horizontal. The figure of the healer or the mourner is vertical. The two form a kind of cross and this is where we can notice a simple but quite surprising fact. Among Eugene Smith's fifty most renowned photographs this theme recurs again and again. Sometimes the focus is almost exclusively on the horizontal figure, with only a suggestion of the vertical one. Sometimes the two figures are viewed frontally, sometimes laterally. But again and again we find the same emotional theme of the horizontal sufferer being nursed or mourned or held by somebody, vertical, and moved by pity. Here is a list of some of these outstanding photographs:

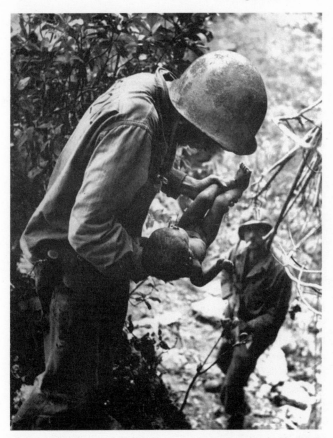

The dying infant found by the GI in Saipan, June 1944; the wounded Marine receiving aid, Saipan, 8 July 1944 (here the vertical figure is symbolized by the water flask being proffered to the victim); the temporary hospital in Leyte, November 1944; the dying man being carried in the battle of Okinawa; the country doctor treating the small baby with a cut on her forehead; many of the images from the story about Maude Callen, the midwife: the wake in the Spanish village; the operation in Schweitzer's hospital; (at the end of his life as a kind of terrible summary of them all) the unforgettable photograph of Tomoko Uemura being bathed by her mother.

Smith identifies with the horizontal figure. This is not to say that he takes himself to be Christ but he identifies with the victim who has suffered unjust punishment. Like his mother, he hated, I think, most of what happened in the world, particularly the metropolitan world, the vicious world of Babylon. He believed profoundly in the Fall of Man. His life's duty was to stalk this world and to lie in wait for its rare moments of nobility, its redemption from the Fall. These were the moments he wished to record. Not only to record but to show in all their terrible glory. The means he had for expressing this glory were black and white. Such moments he then offered back to the world as a form of catharsis. An interesting confirmation of all the above is his very famous picture of the two children walking away from the adult world, their backs towards us, into a glade of light. They are leaving the Fall behind them and Smith himself entitled the picture 'The Walk to Paradise Garden'. It might be possible to deal with this theme by a montage of Renaissance paintings, beginning with Masaccio's *Expulsion* and ending with Grünewald's *Resurrection*.

This view had a lot to do with his running battles with editors. He became a hero of modern photographers because he continually protested against the dishonest or vulgar or over-sentimental use of any of his pictures, and since this is common practice he was entirely justified. Yet Smith's opposition to editorial interference of his intentions had an even deeper basis for he saw, not only certain pictures being misused, but a whole view of the world being substituted for another view. A frivolous one for a sombre, moral one. A magazine cover for a Pietà.

Finally we come to the fulcrum of his genius. He accepted his mother's sombre, condemning view of the world but he judged it far less harshly than she did because he turned the love that he knew through her into a principle to be searched for wherever he went. Love is always, among other things, pity. This is the love of the vertical figure. The love of the mourner and the healer; the love of the survivor for the dead.

Thus we have found an answer to the first and most obvious question, which I didn't pose at the beginning because it would have set up too many prejudices. How is it that a man as patho-logically egocentric as Eugene Smith, and as obsessively selfish as he often was, how is it that he could produce some of the most deeply human photographs of our time? A similar question can be asked about many artists. But in each case the answer has to be specific. There was only one Eugene Smith and he had only one mother.

[written *c.*1988]

Editor's note

When Smith arrived in Pittsburgh in 1955 for a small-scale commission (the project referred to on p. 114), he was expected to stay for a couple of weeks. He ended up spending a year making over ten thousand exposures of every facet of the city and then a further two years trying to print and edit the mass of material into an order that would do justice to 'the tremendous unity of [his] convictions'. By 1959, he had set-tled for publishing a mere thirty-eight pages of photographs. For more on the Pittsburgh project, see Sam Stephenson, *Dream Street: W. Eugene Smith's Pittsburgh Project* (New York: Norton, 2001).

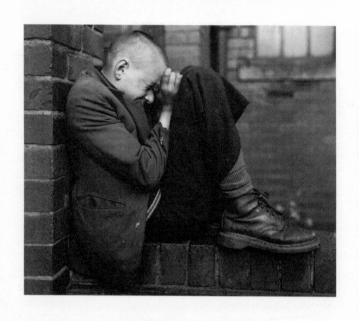

Walking Back Home

Chris Killip: *In Flagrante*

(with Sylvia Grant)

Last Tuesday was the 'Glorious Thirteenth' – the day of the Department of Employment. A place from which we rarely depart for employment. A place where we exchange embarrassment and dependency. It's a journey I make as though I were a little lost girl and my mind never wanders. I catch two buses and I'd prefer to catch them to the dentist's. Our disenchantment exchange. It's a small, long, narrow old building near a fire and railway station. And there we go on our numbered days with our numbered cards and our numbered souls and my mind never wanders. It's painted green; it's long and narrow with grilled windows and long narrow queues. There aren't any green maidenhair ferns or subtle chrome shades. Only fluorescent lights cruelly illuminate our passivity. Posters, detailing all our relevant claims, adorn one wall: UBs, 567s, ABCs. My mind never wanders. The only welfare benefit not advertised is the Death Grant – they rightly assume we've already been there. To sit upon those chairs, upon which you wait only to be called. To rise. To find yourself at a loss, to find yourself a pen and then to make that most sweet and volatile of sounds, a name, silently.

*

To the photographs in his book *In Flagrante* Chris Killip has added two very short texts. His own terse note of explanation ending with the statement, this 'is a fiction about metaphor'. Fiction, I think, because it is a story, not just information. About a human tragedy, not an accident. Metaphor because it is through metaphor that, at first and last, we seek for meaning.

Secondly he has added the searingly apt poem by W. B. Yeats. I say searingly, for it is as if all the photos here have been branded, like a hundred cattle, with the tenderness of those eight lines.

This, our dialogue at the end, is addressed to the reader who is walking back home.

So much that comes from the brightest and best of human instincts is subject to a dry, formal and orderly disintegration. It is happening to this town. There were instincts here as strong, courageous, subtle, supple as anywhere and they were concentrated. Now capital, talent, energy has left, is leaving the place. The town seems sometimes like a black hole that the hills are about to cave in upon.

No new programme of the Labour Party, no new merger of the SDP and the Liberals, not even the Communist Manifesto is going to address the plight of the childhoods, adolescences, virilities, motherhoods and old ages written off here.

There are days, even here where the light is often a strange depleted substance – milk that someone has taken the cream from – there are days when the sun does shine, and somebody with rugged hands shall turn to me on a bus, touch me, give me a smile, and it all becomes an inheritance borne willingly. It was so for my grandfather, my father, my mother.

All but one of the pictures were taken in the North-East of England around Newcastle-upon-Tyne. The coal trade began in this area in the thirteenth century. At the beginning of the nineteenth century George Stephenson started his ironworks in Newcastle. The first locomotives were manufactured there. Ships from Tyneside were famous in ports all over the world. The docks exported coal, iron, steel. Around these activities there developed fine skills, special kinds of courage, prides, struggles, solidarities, which were passed on from generation to generation.

I respect men's brittle strength and feel they are more easily broken. Women are fragile but supple. We don't always break so easy, we crack, we splinter. Ever heard the saying 'She was a china teacup, he was only a mug'? Perhaps incongruous when placed together, but both can hold refreshment. Gifts for each other.

Today the shipyards are silent, many of the mines are closed, the factories shattered, the furnaces cold. The tragedy of this has little to do with new technology as such, or with so-called postindustrialism. It stems, it bleeds, not from the fact that science has discovered electronics, but from the fact that everything which constituted the loves of those living here is now being treated as irrelevant.

Photography has often been used, in a documentary spirit, to record and reveal social conditions. Collected together in exhibitions or books, such work showed to the relatively privileged how the 'other half' lived: sub-proletarians, common soldiers on battlefields, poor farmers, emigrants on ships, the unemployed, the homeless. Whatever the specific subject, the purpose was usually to move the conscientious public to action or protest so that the social conditions might be improved. Look at what is happening! Should this be allowed to continue? Sometimes the future was invoked in a more triumphant sense: look at the richness of the Family of Man, we must do justice to our global heritage!

In Flagrante does not belong to this tradition. Chris Killip is adamantly aware that a better future for the photographed is unlikely.

The debris visible in his photos, the debris which surrounds his protagonists, is already part of a future which has been chosen – and chosen, according to the laws of our particular political system, democratically.

Since Mrs Thatcher was first voted into office the number of people living below even the official poverty lines has doubled. They now number about 12 million. By contrast, during the last four years, the number of millionaires in the country has risen from 7,000 to 20,000. In the North-East it is estimated that there are 1,500 deaths a year due to exposure or starvation. The infamous distinction between the South and North is not one between wealth and poverty but between the safeguarded and the abandoned.

Remember the word 'love'. It was often here. All through childhood, it was here, at the corner shop, on the bus, at the ice-cream van, it was a word preceding others and leading to others, a word of progression, movement, a beginning and an end, a word which was around me all the time. Now it's a word we are sensitive of using; we have heard that to use it often, is to use it lightly. It never felt that way for me. It was a word with substance, surety, certainty. Among lives which bore so much insecurity and social suffering, there was a word which gave security. Yes, Luv.

On page 56 there is a photograph of an old-fashioned ruin, the only picture in the book not taken around the North-East. It is a romantic image – full of a type of grandeur. The new ruins are of a very different character. Thin, torn, worn-out, empty. Circuits which have been liquidated. Spaces which have been abandoned. Zones of the written-off.

In these zones, even the ground is smashed – garden soil, doorsteps, pavements, kerbstones, roads. As if everything, once loved, was now chipped and in pieces.

*

Those men. I'll never forget those men, the ones whose fingers didn't resemble mine, the ones who cried to thank me for staying with them as they smoked a cigarette, the ones who are on the bottom line of 'for each according to his ability'. They'll be there, still in Cedar Ward, they'll be with me all my life, because they're someone's father, and if they aren't then they can be mine. My father would have wished it. Forget 'England Made Me': visits to a hospital helped to make me. And to make me angry.

It's about nature and man. I saw how random and cruel nature can be. I learnt how calculating and cruel man can be. It was the time when the first cut-backs began to take effect. And I knew right from wrong. That it was wrong for the wounded to be the bottom line on a statement of accounts. I could see nature was cruel, but also that those with the swiftest transport, those with houses of strong foundations, escape the harsh effects of floods and earthquakes.

All I know is we require an equal share of protection. The dividends are long overdue.

The abandoned are those born into zones where it is no longer possible to earn a living, and where the idea of any future has been ruptured. The safeguarded are those, elsewhere, who believe that the future belongs only to the profit motive. The profit motive, however, is always clothed in robes which moralize. For example, a secretary to a northern city's Chamber of Commerce declared, 'There are the people who aspire, and the people who can't or won't aspire.'[16] The latter of course live in the zones.

I saw an elderly man with a Tesco carrier and a walking stick. I was on the escalator going down and the one going up was, as usual, broken. If there's a certainty in life, it's that the escalator going up is broken and your shopping bag's full. He was walking up the endless stairs and mildly

16 Quoted by Ian Jack in *Before the Oil Ran Out* (London: Secker & Warburg, 1987).

*struggling. Only struggling mildly. If he had been more obviously disabled
or had been a mother struggling with shopping and a pram, he would
have rightly inspired sympathy. He was just a little, tired, unknown man
struggling mildly. He was just an old man who had maybe paid his taxes,
fought for his country. This beautiful individualism they talk of. By the
time this particular man reaches the top of the stairs, his individual legs
will feel too tired for this particular concept to bloom. Of course if he
had power, money or even just a car, his individualism might flourish.
I don't understand what political people of power mean by that word.
Lots of people I know on estates, in hospitals, in unemployment queues,
now walk on their individual knees and their individual heads are bowed
and they haven't the energy to strengthen their individual spines.*

In the sky, beyond every photograph in this book, is reflected the
blind indifference of the new individualism. Finally history will not
forgive this indifference. Meanwhile in its monstrous light something else becomes visible.

When the first factories and mines were built in the North of
England and Scotland, when the first proletariat ever created,
surged in and out of the iron gates, before barbed wire had been
invented, and, a little later, when Engels and Mayhew made their
pioneer voyages of horrified discovery, the world of 'the labour-
ing classes' was thought of as an underworld, its inhabitants sub-
human, their impulses 'animal', their fates unknowable yet nevertheless the issue of unnameable sins!

Many of the terms used to describe this underworld were borrowed from those which had been used to justify the slave trade,
whose profits had supplied the first capital for launching the new
industries.

Today theoreticians of the New Right denigrate the written-
off in a similar spirit. The epithets may have changed, but not
the principle whereby they explain that the wretchedness they

themselves impose is the consequence of the moral debility of the 'wretched'.

What has become visible and obvious is that this is a lie. This first equality *has* been won. It confers no protection, guarantees no rights. It simply recognizes that those living today in the zones of abandonment differ in no essential way from anybody else.

Not knowing where the dead, the unborn, the skeletons, the embryos live or lie, the dead I see often in the expressions of living eyes, when talking with integrity of other times. Or sometimes in a phrase. I hear a phrase on a bus, full of ambiguity, tenacity and gentility, just a few words spoken to another, and I think to myself: People have been speaking so for centuries. Many places can offer a welcome and sometimes it's all in a phrase, a few words which seem to carry time and life, and each time they're spoken or heard, they restore, re-establish a beauty. And I want to turn round and say 'Did you hear that? Doesn't it make you feel warm, homely, legitimate?'

An elderly man picks over rubbish.

The sea shuts in and, on its beaches, washes up flotsam and jetsam.

Kids sniff glue and find a way out.

Here there will be no more silver-wedding presents.

The travelling people, men and women with saddleless horses who have survived from another century, look across at the ruin of all that once relegated them to the past. They are experts in obsolescence.

*

On these last reaches, people make love, children are born, grand-mothers make pies, families go to the seaside. And they all know what is happening: the boot is being put into the future.

Intently a boy holds a frog in his hand. He's studying it.

Saying what?

I have you. There're my boots on the ground below the sky. In the middle there's you and I only. When I want to, I'll let you go, but I could keep you for days. At home there's a box. If you were under the bed, would you make noises, wet it, move it in the night? I'd be above you, and after the car doors and the bathroom noises and the floorboards, later, I'd hang over to see you down there below, to say hello. We could be together. There could be trouble of course. From the other one, the sister, she might squeal. She's not like Dorothy. Dot and I take the long road home together and if she saw you jump, she'd say 'He's high!' She can howl just like the dogs that come out at night on films I've seen. She's good. Best of all when you're not sure what she'll do. I've had others like you. Once Grandma thought my hedgehog was a brush. She doesn't see very well. They said that with all the crawling things, moving matchboxes, my matchboxes, I was bad for her heart. Grown-ups can be such a long way off, so tall they can't see. But not you. You're all alive and moving. You'll probably move when you're dead.

The first and last pictures show a woman sitting and then lying on a pavement.

She lies on the ground. Perhaps in other places there are those with the privilege of shelter who, in a cautious refined despair, take a bottle to bed, find a hollow in other hills where the eyes of the pavement are easier to bear.
  Not like starlight which is often of beauty, not like the headlight that

slows down in recognition, not like the golden lamps which glow with home through the garden of night trees, not like one who shines in the light of somebody else's eye, alone, you are accommodated by a camera which is held in the arms of a stranger, and you turn away, for you know there are days which die willingly.

It's a tender and vulnerable allegiance we have, I the looker, you the exposed. An association that cannot remain innocent of the crimes of life, of crimes. A love that cannot lie with you but in lying by you cannot lie dormant. There is so much such love cannot do. But it can oppose laws, callous, calculated and protracted which intensify your poverty, castrate your aspirations, compound that fracture of intimacy, from which you will find it hard to rise.

I don't know her name. Asleep, she hears it in her dreams.

Even when empty of most of what you see on closing your eyes, even in those wanton and irreverent things which are dreams, there is a name. A name given only to one when held, plump and proud, to a breast. As close and hot as the space she holds to herself now inside her coat. A name said by another can be sublime. A name said by another can be scathing. And at times a name is a property lost.

On the same pavement a man reads, scrawled in chalk upon the bricks of a wall, the words: TRUE LOVE. Wind blows litter along the pavement. Rain will wash off the chalk. Yet the struggle for meaning which is waged in every soul is immanent in time itself, and in this struggle nothing is repeated. Everything is unique, and, somewhere, is ineradicable. I have no proof of this. It is an article of faith which I think I share with most of the protagonists in this book.

A man walks across a wasteland in biting wind. Behind him is a lorry trailer for hire without a motor. For moving house? How and to where? He advances, driven by his will, head down, carrying what he has gone to fetch.

Once when my aunt was dying, we gathered around her bed. She had ceased to fight. There was and is no possible reason for her to live. To lie in a hospital bed year after year, night after night, to hear others cough and sigh through the dim light.

'Why,' she whispered, 'this time I want to go.'

Perhaps I shouldn't have spoken but I did.

'You're a curious person, Aunty May, you've nowhere to go! Why not stay around out of pure curiosity?'

'Why?' she said.

'Well, Reagan may press the button tomorrow, and you shall have missed it. You will have gone out on a whimper, when you might have gone out on a bang!'

She smiled. 'Trust you!' she said. And she slept.

She's often near death, she's often in despair, but she's remarkable. You wouldn't be aware of courage unless you were aware of her.

The vegetables planted in the soil before the makeshift wind-break on page 32 are, I think, Brussels sprouts. A vegetable which can go on growing when everything else has stopped, in temperatures well below freezing. Sprouts can survive −20°C. Their large, heavily ribbed leaves, like massive hands with fingertips touching, form vaults deep in the snow. These vaults provide air pockets in which small sprouts develop and thrive. Each one has, in addition, its jackets of leaves. The killing cold rarely penetrates more than the first or second layer, beneath which is the green heart. In the winter of this century, children, women and men protect one another with imagination, with violence, with rage, with incomprehension, with ingenuity. The green heart is their capacity to love: their refusal of the principle of indifference.

*

pages to make and little time to spend, of bought packed lunches from Monday to Friday, of a new pair of shoes for Andrew, of 10p off here compared to 15p there, of paracetamol. In Smith's I picked up a book of old photographs. Photos of the North during another recession in the thirties.

Walking Back Home

There was once a Saturday, full of Saturday tension, of people with purchases to make and little time to spend, of bought packed lunches from Monday to Friday, of a new pair of shoes for Andrew, of 10p off here compared to 15p there, of paracetamol. In Smith's I picked up a book of old photographs. Photos of the North during another recession in the thirties.

In the inevitable black-and-white clichés there were the inevitable streets, women in large aprons behind greasy machines, scruffy children pulling up socks, smiling people carrying suitcases with straps around them, they were leaving for their one week's unpaid holiday. There were also men, some only smiling, others, marching, listening, standing. The jackets, the shirts, the clothes they wore, nothing corresponded except in that they were the uniform of the waiting. They were crumpled people, their clothes, socks, faces, like springs that had been compressed for too long. Weary of shrinking, of keeping eyes sharp to avoid the blows. Not in retreat. Just tired.

My mother was looking at the book with me. I glanced at her. In her eyes there were tears. There on that busy Saturday, as people pushed by and said 'Sorry' for your toes, as your hip caught against the metal rim of the counter, tears.

'No,' she said, 'it's all been so rotten, all along they've been treated rotten, all along and it's still going on!'

I was her daughter standing beside her and the resemblance wasn't being taken for granted. I was still learning from her, as I'd learnt to brush my teeth, say 'please' and 'thank you' to others. Some true feelings are like my mother's tears in Smith's, extemporary from the Latin – out of time.

1988

Editor's note

The poem by Yeats mentioned on p. 120 is 'He Wishes for the Cloths of Heaven' from *Collected Poems of W. B. Yeats*, 2nd edition (London: Macmillan 1977), p. 81:

Understanding a Photograph

Had I the heavens' embroidered cloths
Enwrought with golden and silver light,
The blue and the dim and the dark cloths
Of night and light and the half-light,
I would spread the cloths under your feet:
But I, being poor, have only my dreams;
I have spread my dreams under your feet;
Tread softly because you tread on my dreams.

Means to Live

Nick Waplington: *Living Room*

What is remarkable about Nick Waplington's photographs [in *Living Room*] is the special way in which they make the intimate something public, something that we, who do not know personally the two families photographed, can look at without any sense (or thrill) of intrusion. Countless photographs violate the intimate simply by placing it in the public context of a book, a newspaper, a TV slot. Yet others – like most wedding photographs – make the intimate formal and thus empty it of its content.

It is obvious that Nick (the photos make me want to call him by his first name), that Nick knows and loves the friends he has photographed. Obvious because of the way they don't look at him. Sometimes, I guess, they were aware that he was taking a picture (yet another one!), but they were aware of it as they might have been aware that he was smiling, and so he was happy and didn't have to be fussed over.

Other times, they forgot about him altogether. He was just there as naturally as if it were Saturday. No work on Saturday, no looking for work. Day off. Day for having fun. Day for watching football results on the TV. Day for letting the parakeets out of their cages during the halftime break. Day when Nick comes around.

It's not so obvious, but if you look carefully, you can tell that Nick took these photos over quite a long period of time. The reddish wall-to-wall carpet was changed in the living room. To the left of the back door in the kitchen of the other house, there used to be a kind of open cupboard made out of bricks: then Jeff changed it and put up a counter where you can sit, even eat if you want.

When you know them intimately, small houses grow up, acquire habits, create surprises, cause worries, change – not as insistently as the children do, but in their own do-it-yourself fashion. Similarly, Nick's photographs are not about captured moments. They are more experiential, constantly evolving over time, commenting on each other, alive. And always there is that thing he has seen, I think, unlike anybody else.

Pleasure. Not pleasure-seekers. Not luxury. Not ecstasy. Not fashion. Not innocence. But the untidy, crowded, noisy, jokey, sad, persistent, working-class pleasure of being at home on Saturday. It's not a pleasure that idealizes, for it's not a pleasure that looks at itself. It accepts sobbing and tiredness and the bills at the end of the month. It wouldn't exist without pats, slaps, tickles, tears, cuddling up, and what the dictionaries call affection, which is really what body offers body for consolation and confirmation with the knowledge – whatever the doctors and the ministers and the Department of Employment say – that eyes are windows on to a soul.

Taken during those years in Britain (as in the US) when the greed of the ruthless class was impoverishing millions of other people's lives – you can read the signs of the consequent impoverishment in this book – these photos are nevertheless not icons of poverty, but, rather, painted cupolas of play.

Make her hair stand up straight with the vacuum cleaner! Feed the lion! Splash! Eat the slipper! Lovey-Dovey! Fly jet! Ice cream. I scream! Lollapaloosa! Cupolas of games. Shared games, which flare, impertinently and gloriously, against the dark. The sacred canoodling pleasure that grows from the flesh of my flesh.

An artist's vision can never be defined just according to what he or she has seen – how he has seen is equally important. Wap-lington had to discover how to make not records, but images of his chosen subject matter. He had to create images of pleasure to match his subject.

And this is why I think of cupolas. His images are the next-door neighbours to those of baroque ceiling painting – and, in particular, to the work of Peter Paul Rubens. There is an extraordinary affinity of colour, pose, gesture, framing, composition; above all, of the way in which figures relate spatially to one another – look at the three girls and the neighbour in the kitchen, look at the father holding his daughter upside down, or the children on the sofa and the uncle smoking, look at the magic of the vacuum cleaner. I could find bodies of *putti*, men, women, touching, twisting, moving, painted by Peter Paul, to match every one of these. Sometimes they would be almost identical. We could play 'spit' with them all Saturday afternoon.

But it would be only an art-historical game, for the matching is not really important. When Nick took his pictures he wasn't thinking of Peter Paul, and there's little in common between the biographies of the Flemish prince of painting and this kid from Nottingham. The only thing they have in common is a genius for saluting pleasure and a baroque enthusiasm.

I don't know how Nick's notion of using a 6 x 9 camera first came to him. But the baroque was already in this idea. It is a camera designed for panoramic topographical studies. When applied to small interiors and close-up figures, the forms photographed have the space to expand, to become landscapes, or even firmaments. And this is very close to the baroque principle. Baroque wanted to turn the earth-bound into the celestial, and to make human figures appear as at home in the sky as on the ground.

Nick, of course, does not have a sixteenth-century view of the celestial; he has friends in Nottingham. Yet to give expression to the energy of the pleasures of these friends, he needed the visual dynamic of the baroque. And with the help of this camera, he has recycled it.

Any dynamic image begins with what is so dully called composition – how the frame is filled, not just with forms but with movements, and with how these seduce our perception. For example, in the picture of the daughters feeding their father on the kitchen floor: Nick deliberately printed it in reverse (all three appearing left-handed) because like this, the girl on the left takes our hand and leads us with her feet into the picture, as she could never do if she was on the right.

For example, in the flying picture, Nick was lying on the floor because otherwise there would have been no height and the beige ceiling could never have become gold.

For example, in the living room, where the mother is on the sofa and the girl is licking the corner of her mouth; if Nick hadn't put his big feet in it, there'd be no magic circle but just a fragment of a Saturday.

Yet, finally, what is original and moving about Waplington's vision transcends his choice of camera and his skill in composing. I'm talking about his awareness of what is outside the frame. Turning the pages of this book, we also watch the invisible. The paradox of photography is that all great photographers lead us to do this. The invisible has many departments and many moods.

Living Room is in fact a biography of two families in Nottingham. We see them mostly on Saturdays, but we imagine them on every other day of the week; we imagine them in history, which today again tries to treat them like shit; we imagine them all as children; we imagine them all growing old. Each picture holds those whom it shows, as a family name holds for ever the one to whom it has been given. Aunt Elsie is always Aunt Elsie. Dad is always Dad even when he's a granddad. Now we call Mum Mum even when she was a little girl.

The opposite of instant pictures, these photos are as lasting for a lifetime as tattoos, yet all they show are split seconds. This is because, brought there in the concentration of Nick's love, life breathes through every one.

Do you think people'll look at us, Dad? Don't ask me.

Yes, they will. For a very long time. Walt Whitman, who lived before any of us were born, knew why:

> I am the poet of the Body and I am the poet of the Soul,
> The pleasures of heaven are with me and the pains of hell are with me,
> The first I graft and increase upon myself, the latter I translate into a new tongue.
> I am the poet of the woman the same as the man,
> And I say it is as great to be a woman as to be a man,
> And I say there is nothing greater than the mother of men.

Here is what it means to live. As I write in the early weeks of 1991, I know that here is what is reduced to dust when bombs are dropped on cities. Be it Nottingham, Baghdad or New York.

1991

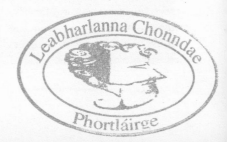

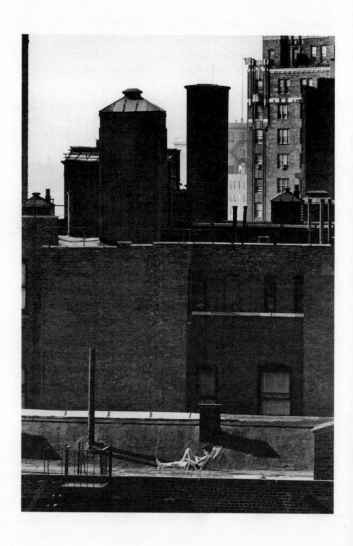

André Kertész: *On Reading*

Each of the sixty photographs in Kertész's book *On Reading* is a particular portrait and an interruption of a particular story which we can never know. Fortunately each image is indescribable in words. Appearances have their own language.

Yet, turning the pages of the book and watching image follow image, I learnt something which I had never noticed before and which I think I can describe.

Usually when we read a newspaper or book, we hold it in our hands. Meanwhile what we are reading, whether it is a news item or a poem or a philosophical thesis, takes our attention and a part of our imagination elsewhere.

The child, who reads, runs panting into the next mystery; the old man remembers. But both of them travel.

Even the reading of a simple word like DANGER or EXIT invokes a displacement: at that moment we foresee danger or imagine following the exit sign.

When the words add up to sentences and the sentences fill whole pages and the pages tell a story, the displacement becomes a journey and the pages become a vehicle, a means of transport. Nevertheless, while reading we hold the pages very still. Thus there is a tension between the manual gesture and the travelling. Long before man could fly, this journey was like flying. Those who first read Homer flew to Troy.

Now Kertész, in photo after photo, reminds us of this. We see readers holding on to pages which are taking off into the air or which have just landed from the air.

The double meaning of the word *missile* (signifying both letter and rocket) is revealing. It is no coincidence that among the sixty photographs in the book, no less than twelve show readers on balconies and the roofs of buildings, which are like launch pads.

The same applies, however, to the old woman reading in her four-poster bed or the wardrobe assistant sprawled on a bench or the kids (of whom we only see the knees) reading in a waiting room.

All of them hold the pages as if those pages were only in momentary contact with the ground, as if they were about to defy gravity or had just done so.

The volatile act of reading!

When we ourselves read, we feel this. What I learnt from Kertész's pictures, and what I didn't realize before, is that this can be seen in the gestures and the body of anybody reading. And for this insight we are once again in the Hungarian photographer's debt.

1996

A Man Begging in the Métro

Henri Cartier-Bresson

It's all a question of time, he says.

I watch him. He is eighty-six and he looks much younger, as if he had a special contract with time passing. His eyes are an intense pale blue, and from time to time they twitch, as a dog's muzzle twitches when investigating a scent. It's hard to watch his eyes without feeling you're being indelicate. They're totally exposed – not through innocence, but through an addiction to observation. If eyes are windows on to the soul, his have neither panes nor curtains, and he stands in the window frame and you can't see past his gaze.

Monet and Renoir, he says, painted the view from this window here. They were friends of Victor Chocquet who lived in the flat below.

Chocquet, the man Cézanne painted a portrait of, with a gentle thin face and a beard? I say.

Yes, he says, Cézanne painted several portraits of Chocquet. Here's a reproduction of the Monet of the Palais Royal. You see how the spire there nicks into the dome, closer than a tangent? Now look out of the window. It's the same. He painted from exactly this spot . . . Photography doesn't interest me any more.

If he was an animal, I think he'd be a hare; all the time he's on the point of bounding away. Not in flight. Not in mockery. But casually, for the hell of it. Instead of ears which bring him the news about everything, he has eyes. Amused eyes.

The only thing about photography that interests me, he says, is the aim, the taking aim.

Like a marksman?

Do you know the Zen Buddhist treatise on archery? Georges Braque gave it to me in '43.

I'm afraid not.

It's a state of being, a question of openness, of forgetting yourself.

You don't aim blind?

No, there's the geometry. Change your position by a millimetre and the geometry changes.

What you call geometry is aesthetics?

Not at all. It's like what mathematicians and physicists call elegance, when they're discussing a theory. If an approach is elegant it may be getting near to what's true.

And the geometry?

The geometry comes in because of the Golden Section. But calculation is useless. Like Cézanne said: 'When I start thinking, everything's lost.' What counts in a photo is its plenitude and its simplicity.

I notice the small camera on the table beside him, within easy reach.

I gave up photography twenty years ago, he says, to go back to painting and above all to drawing. Yet people keep on asking me about photography. A while back I was offered an award for my 'creative career as a photographer'. I told them I didn't believe in such a career. Photography is pressing a trigger, bringing your finger down at the right moment.

He imitates the gesture comically in front of his nose. And, as I laugh, I remember the Zen Buddhist tradition of teaching by jokes, of refusing anything ponderous.

Nothing is lost, he says, all that you have ever seen is always with you.

Did you ever want to be a pilot?

Now it's his turn to laugh because I've guessed right.

I was doing my military service in the Air Force, stationed at Le Bourget. Not far away, towards Paris, was the family factory. The well-known Cartier-Bresson reels of cotton! So they knew I was the kid son of a bourgeois. I was put to sweeping out the hangars with a broom. Then I had to fill out a form. Did I want to be an officer? No. Academic achievements? None, I wrote, because I hadn't passed my *baccalauréat*. What were my first impressions of military service? I replied by quoting two lines from Jean Cocteau:

> don't go to so much trouble
> the sky belongs to us all . . .

This, I thought, expressed how I wanted to be a pilot.

I was called before the commanding officer who asked me what the hell I meant. I said I was quoting the poet Jean Cocteau. Cocteau what? he shouted. He went on to warn me that, if I wasn't pretty careful, I'd be drafted to Africa in a disciplinary battalion. As it was, I was put into a punishment squad in Le Bourget.

He has picked up the camera and is looking at me – or, rather, around me, as if I had an aura, as he speaks.

When I was demobilized, I went to the Ivory Coast and earned my living there hunting game. I used to shoot at night with a lamp on my head like a coal miner. There were two of us, and my companion was an African. Then I fell ill with blackwater fever. I'd have certainly died but I was saved by my brother hunter who was skilled, like a medicine man, in the use of herbs. He had already poisoned a white woman because she was too arrogant. Me, he saved. He nursed me back to life . . .

As he tells me this story, it reminds me of other stories I've heard and read about lost travellers being brought back to life by nomads and hunters. When they're brought back, they're not the same. Their sign has been changed by an initiation. The following year, Cartier-Bresson bought his first Leica. Within a decade he was famous.

The geometry, he is now saying, comes from what's there, it's given to one, if one is in a position to see it.

He puts down the camera he was pointing at me without using it.

I want to ask you something, I say, please be patient.

Me? I can't help it. I'm impatient.

The instant of taking a picture, I persist, 'the decisive moment' as you've called it, can't be calculated or predicted or thought about. OK. But it can easily be lost, can't it?

Of course, for ever. He smiles.

So what indicates the decisive split second?

I prefer to talk about drawing. Drawing is a form of meditation. In a drawing you add line to line, bit to bit, but you're never quite sure what the whole is going to be. A drawing is an always unfinished journey towards a whole . . .

All right, I reply, but taking a photograph is the opposite. You feel the moment of a whole when it comes, without even knowing what all the parts are! The question I want to ask is: does this 'feeling' come from a hyper-alertness of all your senses, a kind of sixth sense –

The third eye! He puts in.

– or is it a message from what is in front of you?

He chuckles – like hares do in folk tales – and leaps away to look for something. He comes back holding a photocopy.

Here's my answer – by Einstein.

The quotation has been copied out in his own handwriting. I read the words. They are taken from a letter of Einstein's addressed to the wife of the physicist Max Born in October '44. 'I have such a feeling of solidarity with everything alive that it doesn't seem to me important to know where the individual ends or begins . . .'

That's an answer! I say. Yet I'm thinking about something different. I'm thinking about his handwriting. It's large, easy to read, open, rounded, continuous and surprising.

When you look through the view-finder, he says, whatever you see, you see naked.

His handwriting is surprising because it's maternal, it couldn't be more maternal. Somewhere this virile man who was a hunter, who was co-founder of the most prestigious photo-agency in the world, who escaped three times from a prisoner-of-war camp in Germany, who is a maverick anarchist and Buddhist, somewhere this man's heart is that of a mother.

Check it with his photos, I tell myself. Check it against the men in bowler hats, the abattoir workers, the lovers, the drunks, the refugees, the tarts, the judges, the picnickers, the animals and, on every continent, the kids, above all the kids.

Only a mother can be that unsentimental and love without illusion, I conclude. Maybe his instinct for the decisive moment is like a mother's instinct for her offspring, visceral and immediate. And who really knows whether this is instinct or message?

Of course the heart, maternal or otherwise, doesn't explain everything. There's also the discipline, the persistent training of the eye. He shows me a painting by Louis, his favourite uncle, a professional artist who was killed in Flanders during the First World War, aged twenty-five. We examine other drawings by his father and grandfather. Topographical landscapes of places they found themselves in. A family tradition, passed from generation to generation, of minutely observing branches and patiently drawing leaves. Like embroidery, but with a male, lead pencil.

When he was nineteen, Henri went to study with André Lhote, the Cubist master. And there he learnt about angles, walls and the way things tilt.

Some of the drawings, I say to him, some of your still lifes and Paris street-scenes make me think of Alberto Giacometti. It's not an influence so much as the two of you sharing something. You both share, in your drawings, a way of squeezing between a table and a chair, or between a wall and a car. It's not you physically, of course. It's your vision that slips through to the other side, to the back—

Alberto! he interrupts. Despite all the hell of this life, a man like him makes you realize it's worth being alive. Yes, we slip through . . .

He has picked up his camera and is looking at what is around me again. This time he clicks.

Slipping through, he says. Take coincidences, there's no end to them. Maybe it's thanks to them we glimpse an underlying order . . . The world has become intolerable today, worse than the nineteenth century. The nineteenth century ended in about 1955, I think. Before, there was hope . . .

He has bounded away again to the edge of the field.

We look together at a photo he has just taken of the Abbé Pierre. It's an image which shows the compassion, the fury and the godliness of that remarkable man who fights for the homeless and is the most loved public figure in France. Photographer and priest must be about the same age. A picture of one tireless old man taken by another. And if the Abbé's mother could see Pierre today, she'd see him, I think, as he is at this instant in this photo.

Finally I say I must leave.

People ask me about my new projects, he says, smiling. What shall I say to them? To make love tonight. To do another drawing this afternoon. To be surprised!

I take the lift down from the apartment on the fifth floor and I think he may do another drawing.

In the Métro I find a seat in a coach which is more than half full. At the end of the coach, a man in his early forties makes a short speech about his handicapped wife whom he is leading by the hand and who follows him with her eyes shut. They've been turned out of their lodgings, he says, and they risk being separated if they apply to any institution.

You don't know, the man tells the coach, what it's like loving a handicapped woman – I love her most of the time, I love her at least as much as you love your wives and husbands.

Some passengers give him money. To each one the man says: *Merci pour votre sensibilité.*

At a certain moment during this scene I suddenly glanced towards the door, expecting him to be there with his Leica. This gesture of mine was instantaneous and without reflection.

Photography, he once wrote in his maternal handwriting, is a spontaneous impulse which comes from *perpetually* looking, and which seizes the instant and its eternity.

1996

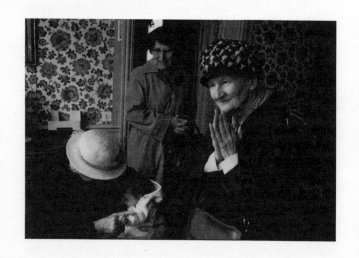

Martine Franck

Fax Foreword to *One Day to the Next*

Fax: 16.43

03/03/98

Martine,

Why don't we begin at the end? A story becomes a story when its end is known. Adam and Eve in the Garden of Eden became a story after the Expulsion, not really before. Cinderella has to lose her glass slipper.

Your book – which is haunting because the pages turn as if they made a single story (although in reality you were making many separate reportages) – your book ends with eight photographs taken on Tory Island, out in the Atlantic off the west coast of Donegal in Ireland.

The place is so bare it has no trees. Its extremity is to do with the fact that you can't go any further on land and in this it's like other places along the western coast of Europe – the Hebrides. Land's End. Finistère in Brittany. Finisterre in Galicia. Literally, the end of the earth. Now I want to ask you about landscape. What are the first ones or the most striking ones you remember as a child? Or the most reassuring ones? Where would you like to be buried?

John

Fax: 11.10

05/03/98

John,

I am in the Channel tunnel, precisely in a no man's land: it's like closing my eyes and letting images, words, come up to the surface.

You ask about landscapes. My earliest memories are of the desert: huge fierce cacti erect, rocks, sand, dried-up river beds – almost monochrome apart from the occasional tiny flower that surprises by the intensity of its colour. We had gone to live in Arizona for a few months on account of my brother's asthma. I became acutely aware of this landscape clutching on to a runaway horse. If I had fallen off, it would have been on to rocks or prickly plants. I was lost; I didn't know where I was going; I was prisoner to a bolted horse that wanted to get rid of its mount and go back to its stable. Curiously enough, I associate this terrifying episode with my first lie. The day-school I attended was on the edge of the desert, and every afternoon we would rest on a large wooden balcony overlooking the desert and a plump matron would hand us out a book for our *siesta*. I demanded a book in French; she looked most surprised and asked, 'Can you read French?' 'Yes,' said I haughtily. A little later she caught me out gazing at the book upside down!

I have never really wanted to think about where I am going to be buried, but now you ask me. I think I want to be cremated and my ashes spread under a beautiful tree. I like the idea of being recycled into the earth – but not right away, please!

Martine

Fax: 16.47

06/03/98

Martine,

The runaway horse and the first lie – as you call it. Aren't both of them to do with a jump or a leap ahead? (Later you would read

French, and often kids' fibs are like that – little prophecies, no?)
For some reason, the two stories together make me think of your
photograph of the little girl in the Pushkin Museum, reading the
title of a painting. Another runaway animal in the painting! And
this goes further than an anecdotal coincidence, for many, many of
your pictures are to do with anticipation or a leap ahead. The old
woman in Ivry, joking with you about the picture you are about to
take, is using the right tense. *Future immediate*. Can you see what I
mean? Of course there are exceptions. But often there's the 'leap'
– either physical, like the kids on the wall in Donegal or the juggler
in Paris, or else psychic, like the *petits rats* at the opera *waiting* to
go on and dance, or like the Tulkus learning to *become* wise.

Not all photos are like this. There's your portrait of Paul Strand.
I didn't know you knew him. He was a great tree of a man, wasn't
he? His pictures were of the *historic present*, don't you think? Sometimes they were almost like dams to keep the water still. Yours dart
forward. Did you always want to be a photographer? Never an
acrobat (of some kind)? I keep on coming back to the term anticipation. What children and actors play with continually.

John

Fax: 11.40

07/03/98

John,
No. I never wanted to be an acrobat, but I did enjoy ski racing as
an adolescent and, as a child, leaping into the water. My father,
among other things, was a distinguished yachtsman and raced in
two Olympic Games as captain in the six-metre class. We would
spend many a summer and Easter holiday sailing, but I have never
conquered my fear of the sea or, should I say, respect for the 'elements' that are so unpredictable. The most recent picture I took
for this book, the huge wave crashing on the rocks at Tory, scared

the wits out of me; I kept trying to get closer and yet was fearful of the unexpected wave or of slipping on the rocks and breaking a leg or being stranded where no one would have found me. I kept saying to myself, what a stupid way of dying!

My grandfather killed himself falling off the dike in Ostend while photographing my two cousins. This can happen so easily when looking through a lens; for a split second nothing else exists outside the frame, and to get the right frame one is constantly moving forwards, backwards, to the side. A movie-cameraman is often guided, held, when filming; a photographer rarely. This year I am the same age as when my grandfather died.

Photography came as a substitute. I was painfully shy and found talking to people difficult; a camera in hand gave me a function, a reason to be somewhere, a witness but not an actor.

A photograph is not necessarily a lie, but it isn't the truth either. It's more like a fleeting, subjective impression. What I like so much about photography is precisely the moment that cannot be anticipated; one must be constantly on the alert, ready to acclaim the unexpected.

Martine

P.S. I am back in Paris.

Fax: 16.45

07/03/98

Martine,
We're saying the same thing. You: 'One must be constantly on the alert, ready to acclaim the unexpected.' And me with my *future tense* and anticipation. This is something very specific to you. Of many photographers it's not necessarily true. For example, Markéta Luskačová, Edward Weston, Sebastião Salgado, Walker Evans. And Henri Cartier-Bresson is different again. His 'decisive moment' is

chosen or seen, as if from the sky, where all time is laid out. But you are waiting for what is going to happen unpredictably. There's something of Tom Sawyer or Huck in you! Look at the Carnival picture in Cologne! Look at the first twelve pictures in the book. Or look – because it's not a question of kids being the subject – look at that marvellous picture of the old women in Cabourg. Look at all three of the women in it considering the baby – an expectancy which is close to devilry. The girl on Tory with the doll is a self-portrait! Admit it. (Have you ever taken a self-portrait? Fax me one, if you have.) Lili Brik is planning mischief. And the fabulous composition shows her already halfway there!

Does one get less shy with age? Shyness is a strange thing. It's not quite the same as being timid. Because there's an element of curiosity in shyness, no? It's to do with *daring*. That's the paradox. It's the adventurous who are shy.

Perhaps fear is never conquered. But an antidote to fear (contrary to what people imagine) is speed. You sailing. You on your skis. Me on my motorbike. Maybe it's an atavism of the nervous system. Fear meant running! What allows an image to suggest speed is pretty mysterious. For instance, for me your very still picture of two gulls on a cliff face on Tory; and, equally, the following photograph of the nude couple on the beach. What speed!

And with speed we're again talking about anticipation and readiness.

How did the theme of the monks come about? Was it like any other project for you, or was it special?

John

Fax: 10.05

08/03/98

John,

Yet another coincidence: you ask me about the little monks and today I shall be photographing the demonstration to commemorate the Tibetan uprising against the Chinese (10 March 1959). I remember, years ago, you mentioned Susan Meiselas as being a Shakespearian messenger for the resistance in Latin America and now for the Kurds. I would like to think of myself as adding a grain of sand in favour of the Tibetan cause. How can you show the Tibetans' plight without referring to Buddhism – their whole culture is linked, and these young lamas I have been photographing over the past few years will one day become the spiritual leaders of the Tibetans (hopefully, not only those in exile). Like our Middle Ages, it is in the monasteries that their culture is preserved and transmitted. Their life is somewhat similar to an English boarding school, without the competitive emphasis on sports; it is Spartan, disciplined, they wear a 'uniform' and are educated to become an elite, but with a lot more affection bestowed upon them than in England. Monks can be very motherly. My mother gave me Mark Twain to read as a child, also Conan Doyle; Sherlock Holmes and Hitchcock are still a passion of mine. And that brings us back to the mystery of life, the unexpected side of reality that is constantly taking us by surprise, off our guard. I think, basically, that is why I never get bored photographing.

You have been asking all the questions. May I ask one? Are you happy?

Martine

Fax: 15.34

11/03/98

Martine,

Am I happy? I don't really believe that happiness is a *state*. Unhappiness can be but happiness is, by its nature, a moment. The moment may last a few seconds, a minute, an hour, a day and a night, but I don't think it can ever last *as such* for as long as a week. Unhappiness is often like a long novel. Happiness is far more like a photo! And it's closely connected with what you say: the sense of marvelling.

I think the second half of my life has been happier than the first – there have been more such moments. Maybe when they were rarer, they were more intense. (Memory plays as many tricks as photography.) I'm not sure. I have the impression that, when I was young, the moments of happiness were pushed close to the point of pain, whereas now they are like a place of shelter.

Is this old age, or the times we live in? Happiness changes its character, too, in the Dark Ages. In our Dark Age. I'm happy to be able, at certain moments, to marvel. Like at your tree in Djibouti!

I want to quote (another way of answering your question) some lines from the Argentinian poet – ah! you should make a portrait of him! He lives in Mexico – Juan Gelman.

The Deluded

hope fails us often
grief, never.
that's why some think
that known grief is better
than unknown grief.
they believe that hope is illusion.
they are deluded by grief.

It's snowing this afternoon. I see you with snow on your shoulders. Where are you?

John

Fax: 21.58

14/03/98

John,

I was in Barcelona participating in an exhibition organized by 'les petits frères des Pauvres' [the Little Brothers of the Poor]. I did a book many years ago on their relationship to old people; some of my photos were on show and there was also a group exhibition on the theme of 'poverty and exclusion'. The setting was surreal – a magnificent medieval palace next to the Cathedral with Gothic paintings of saints and martyrs on the walls, sculptures of *Mater Dolorosas* and, mingled in between, photographs of the 'martyrs' of today: the poor, the excluded, the junkies, the Aids victims. I wonder if the public will see the irony of it all.

Barcelona is a photographer's paradise; the streets are so lively and you can get lost in the old city, which hasn't been restored or spoilt by the tourists. The Catalan museum of Romanesque frescoes is mind-boggling. These painters were such great portraitists, earlier than Giotto, and we don't even know their names.

Martine

Fax: 11.20

16/03/98

Martine,

Last night, while thinking about what makes a picture by you visibly *yours*, I had a little vision.

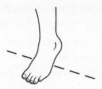

Does this drawing make any sense to you? Do you see what it refers to?

John

Fax: 13.56

16/03/98

John,

Your drawing makes me think of someone tripping gently along the path – tiptoeing so as not to be seen or heard.

In fact, I am always fearful of stubbing my toes, even in summer. I rarely walk barefoot or wear sandals, especially when photographing. 'Sensible shoes' are what allows a photographer to be agile.

Martine

Fax: 16.31

16/03/98

Martine,

The drawing was not meant to show someone gently tripping along a path, though this is surely what it looks like – bad drawing! It was meant to show a foot crossing a line – a broken line, maybe – crossing a kind of frontier.

In picture after picture by you I have this sense of a frontier – the frontier of a moment – as in the photo of the Tulku with the pigeon on the monk's head; a frontier of experience, as in the portrait of Chagall; a frontier of comprehension, as in the study of Mnouchkine imagining a midsummer night's dream; the frontier of a continent, as in several of the pictures of Donegal. Always this stepping over, or this about-to-be-stepping over, a line of demarcation . . .

On the other side it's not the same. Yes, I think it's with that sentence that I would sum up the intimation I have before this collection of your work.

John

Fax: 19.14

16/03/98

John,

Your words evoke so many images to me, but I am not sure they are the same for us both. You say: 'On the other side it's not the same.' On the other side of what? The camera?

The camera is in itself a frontier, a barrier of sorts that one is constantly breaking down so as to get closer to the subject. In doing so, you step over limits; there is a sense of daring, of going beyond, of being rude, of wanting to be invisible.

To cross on to the other side, you can only get there by momentarily forgetting yourself, by being receptive to others: hence, as a photographer, I am in two different worlds at once. That is all I can really say about what I feel when photographing – the rest remains in the domain of the unconscious.

Transgression is the word I have been searching for all along.

Martine

Fax: 22.15

16/03/98

Martine,
Yes, *transgression.*

Its first meaning, of passing a legal limit, is important. There's a subversive tendency in most of the photography you and I admire. (Although, God knows, photographs are also used a million times a week across the world today to pander to the new world order, which at the moment is that of the Free Market and Neo-liberalism.)

There is also the other, geological, meaning of the word transgression. This refers to the way one geological stratum uncomfortably overlaps another – particularly when the movement of the sea is involved. So we are back at Land's End, at Finistère, at a demarcation line which offers *perches* from which one can dive into the unknown!

John

1998

Editor's note

Juan Gelman's 'The Deluded', quoted on p. 153, is taken from *Unthinkable Tenderness: Selected Poems*, ed. and trans. Joan Lindgren (Berkeley: University of California Press, 1997), p. 167.

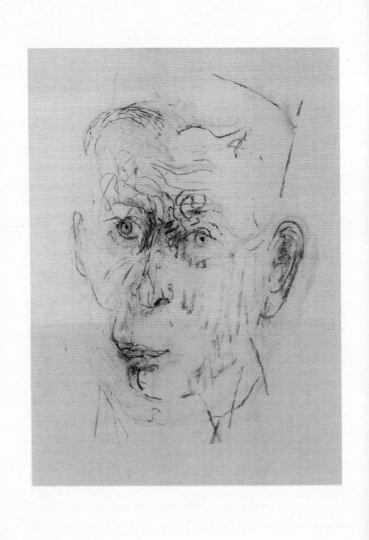

Jean Mohr: A Sketch
for a Portrait

Over the thirty-five years of our friendship, Jean has taken many photographs of me. Sometimes people who don't know me well propose that I write an autobiography. It's hard to explain to somebody who doesn't see it, why storytellers, as distinct from novelists, aren't very interested in autobiography. And anyway the story exists, written in the laughs, the gestures, the wrinkles, the lines, the fatigue, the smiles, the grimaces, the fury, to be found in the countless pictures which Jean has taken of me and which now fill how many yellow boxes? Many of course were taken without my realizing it, for I have become so used to seeing Jean holding up a camera before his broken nose that I no longer ask what he's looking at.

A few weeks ago, I decided to turn the tables on him. Will you pose for me? I asked. Can I bring my camera? Of course, I said.

And so Jean came and posed for several hours while I tried to draw him. I had drawn him once before – about five years ago – but I had forgotten that drawing and I didn't want to look at it again for the moment.

In the studio we listened to music (Jean shared with his father a love of Mahler, Schubert, Berg) and when the music stopped, we talked about how it felt to be seventy years old, and we remembered old friends, some of them lost, and we named old loves, and all the time, throughout the music or the talk or the silences, I was trying to read the face of this man, with whom I had learnt so much, and with whom I had been to many places for the first time.

I was drawing with charcoal on large sheets of Ingres paper, about life-size. I did three drawings, all of them bad, but becoming perhaps a little less bad. At the beginning all you can do is to make a clumsy map of the face. Three and a half maps.

Finally it was time for him to leave. He settled into his driving seat, raised two fingers of his left hand like a pilot before taxiing to the runway, and said: It was good to be together. Then he drove off.

I went back, took another sheet of paper and sat there, huddled over the drawing board. Naturally I was no longer looking at Jean, for he was no longer there. I was studying the maps on the floor and trying to forget.

When you're trying to make a portrait of somebody you know well, you have to forget and forget until what you see astonishes you. Indeed, at the heart of any portrait which is alive, there is registered an absolute surprise surrounded by close intimacy. I'll certainly be misunderstood but I'll take the risk and say: to make a portrait is like fucking.

After many re-beginnings, a drawing emerged. In it I see a dog and a boy, and both are contained in the face of a man of my age. In the look of neither of them is there anything in the least naïve. (If it's naïveté you're after, you should concentrate on Successful Men.) What is here which might be mistaken for naïveté by the naïve – is the habit of being startled, for to both dog and boy the world is startling. Often alarmingly, and occasionally miraculously, the world is continually startling. The photos Jean has taken all his life are the product of an alertness which comes from being startled.

I have often seen Jean with dogs, but rarely in the role of the dog's master. If he raises his voice and says words curtly, the dog obeys him, no doubt. But this is unusual. More often he is making dog noises with the dog and, far from being masterly and upright, is somehow doubled up and as close to the ground as the animal. One of his books is entitled *A Dog and His Photographer*. The dog in question was called Amir and was a Persian Saluki.

I have other memories of Jean sitting with guests at a formal dinner table, or drinking coffee in a drawing room, and, without warning, because he has spotted a cat or maybe a stranger's dog through the window – he starts, without the slightest warning, to make animal or bird noises himself. His face absolutely impassive, his mouth slightly pursed yet quite still, the focus of his very pale blue eyes very far away, almost at the world's end. If there are children present, they are delighted and adopt him immediately. The adults look uncomfortable.

In the rest of his life Jean is more than usually formal. You feel the example of his father, a highly cultivated German scholar who, because he was uncompromisingly anti-Nazi, left Germany to settle in Switzerland in the late 1930s.

I knew Jean's mother and I've seen some of his father's library, but his father had already died when Jean and I first met. Nevertheless I have a vivid image of his father. Perhaps because Jean admired him very much. I see the way he holds himself very upright and a little stooped. I see his blue eyes half shut against the light, and I hear his modulated, calm voice.

I guess that of the six children it is Jean who resembles his father the most. Jean, however, has lived more precariously than his father did. Precariously, in this context, refers to time: his father thought and felt in terms of decades or half-centuries. Jean thinks and feels in minutes or split seconds. This historical difference was encapsulated in Jean's eventual decision to become a photographer.

He might also have been a pilot. If I had to name a writer to accompany Jean in a double portrait of two men, it would be Antoine de Saint-Exupéry. (I say this, although I'm not sure that we have ever discussed the writer, and I can guess that Jean would be sceptical about the myth surrounding the man.) Yet I see both of them as discreet, eccentric travellers, loving people and loving distances even more.

Every large family in the Alpine village where I live has its own collection of Mohr photos. Sometimes there's one framed on the mantelpiece; others are in a box which is brought out when people start to reminisce. Frequently they are photos which they have asked him to take at a wedding, a village gathering, a dance.

Today, all the young in the village have colour films and cameras and videos. But when Jean first started coming to visit, pictures were still rare and a photographer was thought of as some kind of inspector, or obscure state spy.

If they quickly accepted Jean, and then invited him to take pictures (in exchange for bottles of illicit *eau de vie*), it was because this man who came from the ends of the world, this man with a black bag always slung over his shoulder and a slightly foreign accent and a curious love of mountains (shepherds can understand such a love better than peasants), this man, unlike an inspector, was clearly and startlingly observant all the while, as they themselves had to be because they lived unprotected lives and it is therefore necessary to observe everything. And then, later, they found that the photos he took and gave them were a kind of company – like the melodies of tunes they knew and might sing when together. The photos became in black and white the incarnations of certain names: Théophile, Marius, Jeanne, César, Angeline, Marie, Basil.

The other night I had a dream about Jean. We were in a car together and he was driving. As one might expect of an airline pilot, he drives decisively and very well. At a certain moment he braked and we stopped on a deserted road, a mountain landscape around us.

'Il faut tirer les photos,' he said. In French *tirer les photos* means develop the photos, but, literally, it can also mean pull out the photos. We opened both doors of the car and he, having stepped outside, pulled out from under the bonnet three large photographs which were masked with adhesive paper. All three were rectangular and one of them was long and narrow. As soon as I saw them, I realized that the long one had the same dimensions as the windscreen, and the other two were the size of the side windows of the car.

Carefully and slowly, I pulled off their adhesive covering. Underneath were three landscapes. I cannot really describe them, but they were beautiful and, although the photos were black and white, I knew that they would change colour when the sun went down – in the same way as the white mountain snow does. In each picture one could see something which was partly hidden under a kind of geological cornice, like somebody sheltering under the eaves of a roof.

I fixed the three photos to the windscreen and the two windows. As I had foreseen, they fitted perfectly. We shut the doors, and Jean drove off. He drove with the same decisiveness as before. I did not know whether he was driving blind or with a kind of clairvoyance. But I was filled with a sense of well-being and assurance. Then I woke up.

Even among his confrères, Jean is a widely travelled photographer. He has been to many countries in the five continents, many corners of the world. Not, first of all, to take photographs but to notice. His pictures never suggest that he was searching, rather they suggest that he happened to be passing by. There is something strangely casual, offhand, about his images. A kind of nonchalance. Yet a caring nonchalance. And this is precisely why one believes in the special authenticity of his photos.

Both Jean and I have a considerable admiration for Eugene Smith. He, however, when he set out on a reportage, was intent on finding what he was looking for, and in one way or another, he was usually looking for the same thing – a Pietà. Edward Weston was looking for a manifestation of harmony; Walker Evans for qualities of endurance. Jean, I believe, looks for nothing. What he finds is what he happens to come upon. And not infrequently this involves somebody else looking at him!

This casualness, however, has nothing whatsoever to do with indifference; it is a simple precondition for being open to surprise. In principle nothing surprises Jean Mohr – he has seen and observed so much; in practice almost everything he notices surprises him because, in its minute or overwhelming way, it is unique.

Here we are at the secret of the best travellers' tales: a whispering between the familiar and the outlandish, between the banal and the unknowable, between routine and fatality. Jean's tales spare nothing and nobody and they never judge: they often make the heart bleed and they don't exaggerate.

I'm of course generalizing about a life's work. Jean has more than half a million photographs in his archives and I'm trying to define the quality which makes them unmistakably his. I'm not claiming that if I was shown any one of these images I would immediately recognize it as his. But if I was shown a dozen, I think I would immediately say: Jean! and I would recognize them by their specific quality of surprise, a spontaneous surprise, never one which has been sought for.

The way Jean became a photographer may help to explain this. Like Cartier-Bresson and like Salgado, Jean became a photographer by default. He did not set out to spend his life taking pictures with a camera.

At the University of Geneva he studied economics and fantasized about becoming a painter. He then volunteered, in 1949, to be sent as a delegate for the International Red Cross to take care of Palestinian refugees on the West Bank and in Jordan. (Thirty years later he would make a whole book about the Palestinian struggle and tragedy with Edward Said, *After the Last Sky*.) While there on the Red Cross mission, he had the chance of buying an East German camera. He bought it to give as a present to one of his brothers. Then, unexpectedly, he started using it himself. He began to take pictures so as not to forget the unpredictable and incongruous details – often painful, sometimes desperate, occasionally illuminated – concerning the lives he was witnessing.

He returned to Europe in 1951 and settled in Paris to study painting. There he showed his Palestinian photographs to painter friends, and they told him that they were surprising!

He decided to try portraits. First, however, before taking out his camera, he would sit down to draw his sitters and they for their part were a little nonplussed. They glanced at the drawings and asked: What on earth are you doing? You are meant to be a photographer, aren't you?

Consequently, bit by bit, Jean's eyes became accustomed to black and white, to split seconds, to the darkroom. A habit of looking-around-all-the-while, an habitual alertness, started to develop. And a demon was born.

In 1955, to earn money, he agreed to work with a couple of acquaintances who had thought up a scheme of taking aerial photographs in the countryside and then selling prints to the farmers and proprietors of the land photographed. Black and white, later hand-coloured by a girlfriend. Jean in the little monoplane worked fast and under cramped conditions, but the business never got going and the money ran out. Instead of being paid for the work he had done, he was given an enlarger and two Leicas. This is how he set up as a professional.

He began working from Geneva for different branches of the United Nations – and in particular for the World Health Organization and the High Commission for Refugees. His job was to make pictures about their ongoing international projects and programmes. He was never a press or war photographer, although often his pictures, supplied by the UN, were used in newspapers.

This special freelance status – and it continued for over twenty-five years – allowed him to work in his own way. He was continually going to faraway places and his travelling was paid for. Further, when he was on a mission, he was not under the time pressure which most press photographers have to work with; his trips were relatively unhurried.

Consequently, apart from the reportage he delivered to the organization which had sent him, he was able to take tens of thousands of pictures for himself. These pictures were purposeless – in the sense that they were not taken to prove or demonstrate a preconceived idea. They were offhand, casual, maverick, personal records of moments which astonished or startled him.

Jean's work is deeply committed to what happens, and at the same time it shows an *elsewhere*. Even when the subject is familiar to a spectator, the image will still communicate a kind of surprise. And this is the more striking because his photographs refuse formal tricks.

Finally, their surprise derives from the quality of their observation: the startled observation of a boy and dog who have accompanied a highly experienced and intrepid traveller.

With Jean – as with most true artists – the relationship between modesty and pride is a complex one. Or maybe it's simpler than I think. He is modesty itself with those who are modest. And he is as recalcitrant as hell with those who are arrogant. What he and I both share is nevertheless a sense of measure. This helps to explain how we have been able to collaborate over many years – and why our collaboration has been productive. Less modest than he, I will say that with the example of three books, *A Fortunate Man*, *A Seventh Man* and *Another Way of Telling*, we have considerably extended the narrative dialogues possible in book form between text and images.

We started from what Walker Evans and James Agee achieved

in their magnificent *Let Us Now Praise Famous Men*. Exactly where we ended, it is for others to judge, but we covered a lot of ground and have already had a considerable influence on the way other photographers and writers across the world have made books.

So we share a sense of measure. Where mine comes from, I don't know. Perhaps Jean does. Maybe it comes from the process of correcting and correcting again the exaggerations with which I usually begin a project or a vision. It's what comes after a kind of recklessness.

Jean's sense of measure comes from something different. His acquired stance towards life – coming perhaps from his father – is classical. He is clearly aware of the dangers of excess. And yet, inside him, are the dog and the boy. Maybe it's exactly for this contradiction that I love him. In any case it's from the pain of this contradiction that his stoicism is born and it's from his stoicism that comes his sense of measure.

We have needed a shared sense of measure in order to create pages which flow. A book has to advance on two legs, one being the images, the second the text. Both have to adapt to the pace of the other. Both have to refrain from repeating what the other has already done. What so often checks any flow, when images and text are used together, is tautology, the deadening repetition of the same thing being said twice, once with words and once with a picture.

To avoid this and to walk together in step with the story, a sense of measure is essential. Perhaps this is true – at another level – for all long-standing (long-walking?) friendships.

The Edge of the World. I've tried to suggest why such a location, such an *elsewhere*, is intrinsic to Jean's vision and *oeuvre*. I could put it differently: Jean is always on foreign soil, or Jean is always the stranger. Yet, like all nomads, he knows how the guest behaves and how the host receives. And the paradox is that it's there on the Edge of the World that he is at home, as both host and guest. And it is there that I had the privilege and luck of his offering me his friendship.

1999

Editor's note

'The Edge of the World' is what the mountains near Geneva are known as locally, and it was here that Mohr was recovering from a serious operation in 1996.

A Tragedy the Size of the Planet

Conversation with Sebastião Salgado

Sebastião Salgado. Nationality: Brazilian. His look suggests that if he had been born in another century he would have been a navigator, an explorer. Profession today: photographer. He was trained as an economist, and one day he asked himself whether pictures might not reveal as much or more than statistics.

John Berger. Nationality: British. Profession: writer. Trained as a painter. I try to put into words what I see.

It was in my kitchen that the two of us met to talk about Salgado's latest book *Migrations*. He travelled for six years, visiting forty-three countries. Everywhere he went he found people on the move, looking for somewhere, some way, to earn their living and feed their children. During those six years, the economist – who became a photographer – took pictures of the face of globalization.

After talking we went for a walk and an alpinist coming down the local mountain noticed that Salgado was carrying a camera. 'Would you like me to take a picture of you both?' he asked us.

What follows are passages, unlaundered, from this conversation.

*

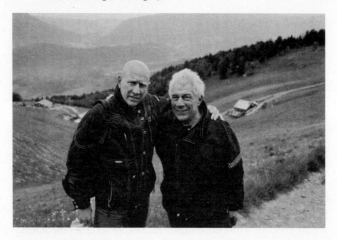

SEBASTIÃO SALGADO:

I saw sometimes die per day 10,000 people. It's very hard, it's very hard to see 10,000 people die, and 10,000 people with good health, they were not starving, they were dying because we had not any way to save them.

This happens in many different places today, and I ask myself the question if there is not a correlation between the number of televisions produced in some factories, the number of cars produced, the number of profits the banks make, with the number of people who die in this moment like this . . . This story, this book, these pictures is a globalization picture, these are the globalized people.

JOHN BERGER:

Globalization means many things. At one level, it talks of trade, which since the sixteenth century has exchanged goods and now, increasingly, ideas and information across the globe. But also globalization is a view of the world, it is an opinion about man and why men are in the world.

One in five of all the people on the globe benefit from this system. Four in five suffer in different degrees from the new unnecessary poverty.

Part of the fanaticism of the economic system which we now call globalization, part of its bigotry, as always occurs with bigotry, is that it pretends – and it is a lie – it pretends that no alternative is possible. And it's simply not true, and it is said in the face of the whole of human history.

SEBASTIÃO SALGADO:

This phenomenon in Africa to have more and more refugees, more and more disintegration of countries, has to do with this new economic system and what they receive against their production, the goods that they produce. The price of these products is not fixed in the Ivory Coast, is not fixed in Liberia, is not fixed in Brazil, *is* fixed in London, *is* fixed in New York by trading companies, and they don't take into consideration the needs of the life of this population. And what happens? The cake is each time smaller for a population that is each time bigger.

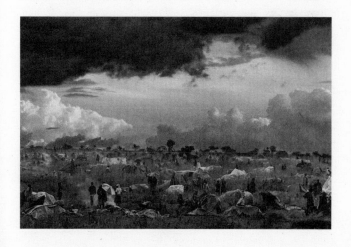

The problem is an economical problem in the start of all these stories.

I know these people from Rwanda from long ago. I came to Rwanda the first time, 1971, as an economist. I came to work in the tea plantations, and the tea plantations had a very equilibrated way of life. Rwanda was not an underdeveloped country, was not a poor country, was a developing country. When I came back to this tea plantation recently, all was burnt, all was destroyed. All the effort that all these people made was lost. These people were in the road, in the death. And up to this moment, until the days I took these pictures, I was sure that evolution was positive. After this I ask myself the question: what is evolution? Evolution can be towards anything, it can be in any direction, we can evolve negatively, going to the death, going to the final point, going to the most brutal end, and we adapt to it also.

JOHN BERGER:

In a strange way, in all these pictures, one feels in your vision the word 'Yes', not that you approve of what you see, but that you say 'Yes' because it exists. Of course you hope that this 'Yes' will provoke in people who look at the pictures a 'No', but this 'No' can only come after one has said, 'I have to live with this.' And to live with this world is first of all to take it in. The opposite of living with this world is indifference, is a turning away.

The point about hope is that hope is something which occurs in very dark moments, it is like a flame in the darkness, it isn't like a confidence and a promise.

SEBASTIÃO SALGADO:

As you say, there is for me a lot of hope here. All the migrants I photographed once lived in a stable way. Now they suffer transition, and what they have with them is just a small slice of hope. And it is with this hope that they are trying to get another stable position in life.

If the person looking at these pictures only feels compassion, I will believe that I have failed completely. I want people to understand that we can have a solution. Very few of the persons photographed are responsible for the situation that they are now in. Most of them don't understand why they are in the road with thousands of others. They lost their house at the end of the last brick, because they were bombed, fired, destroyed, and they are in the road and they don't understand why. They are not the reason for their being there; it is other things. And about these other things we have to choose.

JOHN BERGER:

If you added up all the time of the instants in this book . . .

SEBASTIÃO SALGADO:

Probably here we have altogether one second! And this for me is the magic of this kind of photography because in this one second I believe you can understand very well what is going on in the planet today.

JOHN BERGER:

This photo?

SEBASTIÃO SALGADO:

This man, he was a teacher and he was completely, completely in despair, and nobody else was there to understand him. Only his community was there to understand what they had lost.

JOHN BERGER:

Which makes me think of the French philosopher Simone Weil and something she wrote in the forties. It's a kind of a summing up, I think, of what you were saying: 'There are only two services which images can offer the afflicted. One is to find the story which expresses the truth of their affliction. The second is to find the words which can give resonance, through the crust of external circumstances, to the cry which is always inaudible: "Why am I being hurt?"'

SEBASTIÃO SALGADO:

We speak a lot about statistics; we don't speak about real feeling. I came one year ago to Kosovo and I was reminded exactly of this. During this war we were given a lot of statistical information, information about the number of bombers that had been bombing Kosovo, the number of pilots that were used to attack Serbia, but nobody spoke about real people, about the suffering of those living it.

Crossing the border from Kosovo to Albania, the refugees were expecting people to receive them with open arms, to bring them to their countries, to bring them to France, to bring them to Germany, to the United States. And they were wrong, nobody was waiting for them. We made a big war, we expended billions of dollars in their name and we made nothing for them.

JOHN BERGER:

If we accept what is happening in pictures like these, we are face to face with the tragic. And what happens in face of the tragic is that people have to accept it and cry out against it. Although it won't change anything. And they cry out, very frequently, to the sky. In many of your pictures the sky is very important. Spectators who have lost any sense of tragedy look at these skies and say, 'Ha. What a beautiful set, what a beautiful decor, what a well-chosen moment.' But it isn't a question of aesthetics. The sky is the only thing that can be appealed to in certain circumstances. Who listens to them in the sky? Perhaps God. Perhaps the dead. Perhaps even history.

SEBASTIÃO SALGADO:

They are living their lives inside a tragedy the size of the planet.

People come to you, to your lens, as they would come to speak in a microphone. You assume a big responsibility then, you have to tell their stories; this means you must show their pictures. I don't want to create a bad conscience in those who look at them, because the majority of the people who look at them have a proper house, they have work, they have health. And it is correct that they have these things. What needs to be different is that all the planet has these things.

JOHN BERGER:

How did these portraits of children come about?

SEBASTIÃO SALGADO:

I was working in Mozambique, in a camp, a big camp of displaced population. Most of them were children because in Mozambique there were about 350,000 children who had lost their families. These children were making a big fuss to be in the pictures, because that is the way of children to be in the picture, it's natural, it's normal. And I had an idea. I said, 'Guys, I do a picture of each one of you, and after that you behave normally, and let me work.'

The moment these children stepped out of their group to sit in front of the lens, they become individuals. Individuals. They were innocent, they were pure, but from their eyes it was possible to see what they had lived, what was their life.

JOHN BERGER:

They stood there presenting themselves: 'I, I'm here, this is me.'

SEBASTIÃO SALGADO:

'I exist.'

JOHN BERGER:

Something else is happening, isn't it? Because they are looking at the camera, they know that they are looking at the world. And so they address a question to the world: 'What are you, you out there?' Or: 'Is there anything else out there?'

Following their questions, we could ask ourselves three questions.

1. The priorities according to which we perceive and react to the world might be changeable?

2. Those kids, the true spectres of hope, look at us from the five continents – embodying whose hope?

3. Who needs who the most, they us or we them?

SEBASTIÃO SALGADO:

Probably to do a film is a wrong way. Probably to do a show of posters is not correct. But I sincerely want to know what is correct. Because, if it is correct, I believe that I must go and do it. I believe we have a responsibility in the time we are living to provoke a discussion, to provoke a debate, to ask questions. A debate everybody should participate in and have a responsibility for. If we want to survive as a species we must find a proper direction to go, we must choose another way. Because what I saw in these pictures is not the proper way. This is not the correct way the one we have chosen.

2001

Recognition

Moyra Peralta: *Nearly Invisible*

To know a person you have to be known by that person. Between people there is no such thing as unilateral one-way knowledge. Moyra Peralta knows the people she photographs. We, who look at her photographs, are witnessing an exchange. We overhear, with our eyes, two or more voices talking to one another. And the voices have allowed us to be there. Make yourself at home, the voices suggest. And this is startling, even disturbing, because the photographs are of the homeless.

The photographs are close-ups not in the photographic but in the human sense of the term. Yet the men and women who are their subjects are normally in everyday life ignored, or passed over, as if they were not visible, not there. When we encounter one of them in the street, we tend to look away. In certain cities the authorities of so-called law and order forbid the homeless access to the most frequented parts of the city. Turning the pages of *Nearly Invisible* we come upon close-ups of the excluded, of those who suffer from being treated as if they ought to be invisible.

A few years ago I was writing a story about the homeless. In it a sixty-year-old man talks to his dog about one of the reasons for this aspect of their exclusion: the need of the rest of society not to see them.

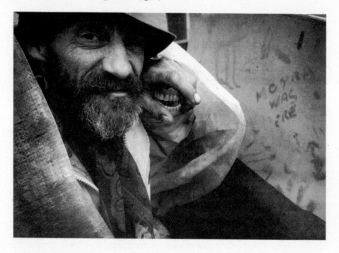

We are being wiped off the earth, not the face of the earth, the face we lost long ago, the arse of the earth. Because we are their mistake, King. And a mistake is hated more than an enemy. Mistakes don't surrender as enemies do. There's no such thing as a defeated mistake. Mistakes either exist or they don't, and if they do exist, they have to be covered over, they have to be made invisible. We are their mistake, King.

The poverty recorded in this book is a new poverty, such as did not exist before. Dying from the cold at night, having hunger pains in the guts, drinking anything alcoholic to numb the mind – this is the same whatever the kind of poverty. Nevertheless, the context in which the poverty occurs is important and may contribute to the pain involved.

Until the middle of the twentieth century poverty, on a world scale, was linked with scarcity; today the new poverty's linked with overproduction and ever-increasing consumerism. Four-fifths of the world's population's growing poorer every year, and the gap between rich and poor is wider than it has ever been in history. The marginalized men and women in the close-ups of this book represent, in this comparative sense, the global majority. Once fallen into – or born into – the new poverty is limitless.

Why? The new economic order, based upon the free market and the pursuit of ever-increasing profits (for otherwise the system collapses), is maintained, managed and directed by an international elite who have untiring energy (until they are burnt out) and no vision of the future at all. They live from hour to hour, day to day. Their absolute maximum future projection – always tentative – might be five years.

The barbarism we have entered – and maybe in this it resembles all barbarisms – takes account of only the short term, only the immediate gain (or loss), only the present advantage here and now. (Never have the generations to come been less considered.) Nothing else and nothing more counts than the immediate.

The homeless have been turned out and are obliged to live as best they can in the streets, because the single world economy – with its unsurpassed productivity and turnover – is, for the moment, being operated by marketeers who calculate (and speculate) with the time perspective of a destitute: a destitute desperately asking her- or himself: how will I get by until the day after tomorrow?

This brutal and monstrous paradox requires thinking about.

Return to Moyra Peralta's photographs, taken over a decade, of some of the people she knows. None of them can be reduced to an argument – even a passionate argument – against the new world economic order. Each person she photographs is unique, each one has her or his own world, which they struggle every hour to somehow preserve.

The close-up is the opposite of a statistic. The love which the photographer has for her subjects is the opposite of philanthropy.

There are impulses deeper than generosity. What first matters is recognition. Recognition. The word appears to make no claim and to sound poor. Yet that perhaps is how it should be.

I know of nobody who has understood half as much about recognition as the philosopher Simone Weil (1909–43). What she wrote could only have been written in the twentieth century with its climax of intolerable human contrasts.

> There is a natural alliance between truth and affliction, because both of them are mute suppliants, eternally condemned to stand speechless in our presence.
>
> Just as a vagrant accused of stealing a carrot from a field stands before a comfortably seated judge who keeps up an elegant flow of queries, comments and witticisms while the accused is unable to stammer a word, so truth stands before an intelligence which is concerned with the elegant manipulation of opinions.
>
> To love one's neighbour is a question of being able to ask simply: what is your torment? Of knowing that affliction exists, not as a statistic, not as an example from a social category labelled 'underprivileged', but as something which happens to a human being, exactly comparable with us, who one day was struck and marked down with a mark that is like no other, by affliction. And to know this it is sufficient – but indispensable – to be able to look at this person with recognition and attention.

Following the example of Moyra Peralta, let us look at the close-ups to come with attention. They will then surprise us with their resilience, their wit, their indomitability and their despair.

2001

Editor's note

The first quotation on p. 180 is from 'Human Personality' in *Simone Weil: An Anthology* (London: Virago, 1986); the second is from 'Reflections on the Right Use of School Studies with a View to the Love of God' in Simone Weil, *Waiting on God* (London: Fontana, 1983).

Tribute to Cartier-Bresson

At every railway crossing in France there is a solid notice, a panel with writing on it which reads: 'Attention! Un train peut en cacher un autre.' Cartier-Bresson, whatever the event he was photographing, saw the second train and was usually able to include it within his frame. I don't think he did this consciously, it was a gift which came to him, and he felt in the depths of his being that gifts should continually be passed on. He photographed the apparently unseen. And when it was there in his photos it was *more than visible*.

Yesterday he joined the second train. At the age of ninety-five – with all his agility – he jumped it. He has joined his inspiration. Six years ago he wrote something about inspiration: 'In a world collapsing under the weight of the search for profit, invaded by the insatiable sirens of Techno-science and the greed of Power, by globalization and the new forms of slavery – beyond all of this, friendship and love exist.' He wrote this in his own handwriting, which was open like a lens which has no shutter.

Bullshit! I now hear him saying. Look at my drawings, there is no second train in them!

So I look at some reproductions of some of his drawings. How drawings change – even twenty-four hours after a death; their tentativeness disappears, they become final. He said repeatedly in his later years that photography no longer interested him as much as drawing. Drawing – or anyway drawing as he drew – has less to do with the sense of sight than with the sense of touch, with touching the substance and energy of things, with touching the enigma of life without thinking about eternity or the second train. Drawing is a private act. Yet Cartier-Bresson returned to it, knowing very well that it was an act of solidarity with both those who see the second train and those who don't.

That's better, he says.

An epitaph for him? Yes, a photo he took in Mexico in 1963. It shows a small girl in a deserted street carrying a framed daguerreo-type portrait of a beautiful and serene woman which is almost as large as the child. Both are about to disappear behind a tall fence. The last second of visibility, but not of the woman's serenity or the girl's eagerness.

2004

Between Here and Then

Marc Trivier

My son, Yves, made a drawing of a clock when he was thirteen.
The clock was manufactured in Ansonia, Connecticut, towards
the end of the nineteenth century. The manufacturing company
– according to the label found inside the clock, when you open the
door to wind it up – specialized in 'time pieces for ships, steam-
boats, locomotives and dwellings'. On the glass of the clock's little door is engraved an image of an ancient hive with bees flying
around it. A beehive is a traditional, originally Greek, symbol for
the natural passing of time. Beverly inherited the clock from her
father, Howe Bancroft.

When Howe died in 1985, I wrote these lines about him.

> I know you
> by my ignorance
> and its space
> which shyly
> you filled with quotations
>
> I know you
> by the half smile of your reticence
> and the space

of a pride
you hid in patched sleeves

I know you by the moment before death
and the space
of God
you found in the lament of words

I know you
by your daughter
and the space
of the words
between here and then

The clock stands on the mantelpiece of the high chimney in our kitchen. I can only reach it, my hands above my head, standing on tiptoe beside the stove. It needs winding up about every two and a half days, every sixty hours. Once it used to chime but the mechanism is broken. It keeps good time when the weight on the brass pendulum is properly adjusted.

Sometimes I forget to wind it up. When it stops, however, the inhabitual silence in the kitchen – which is the room we live in most of the time – attracts my attention and, standing on tiptoe, I open its door and rewind the mechanism with the key, kept on the mantelpiece to the right of the clock. Then with my forefinger I tap the pendulum gently to the left (never to the right), the ticking re-begins, and I invariably have the sensation that the kitchen, which was holding its breath during the silence, is breathing normally again.

A room needs an awareness of the passing of human time. Otherwise it risks becoming inanimate. Or, to be more accurate, its silence risks becoming inanimate. My ritual, of reaching up to the clock high above my head, is like putting a bowl of water down on the floor for a silence to drink. Thirsty silences devastate.

One day when I was inattentive while winding it, the foreseeable happened. The clock toppled, and fell between my arms. I was able to break its fall but it landed on the asphalt floor. Asphalt because around the chimney wooden planks would be too dangerous.

The door had come off its hinges, and the mechanism was damaged. It had to go to a clock-maker to be repaired. I knew of one in the next village.

A dark shop with an old woman peeling vegetables behind the counter. A very limited choice of engagement rings. A few silver necklaces with crosses. Some quartz alarm clocks. And at the end of the counter a door that opened on to a clock-maker's deserted workshop. On the workbench I could see tiny, fastidious tools and a couple of eyepieces.

My brother will look at it, says the woman. My husband is now past it; he can't see any more – it's a trade that ruins the eyes. Come back in a month.

Perhaps, I suggest, I could phone in a few days to see whether or not he can fix it?

We never answer the telephone, she replies, but I won't forget – come back in a month.

The kitchen was changed by the absence of the clock. (We could tell the time by the electric digital clock above the oven on the gas stove.) The kitchen breathed less deeply; nevertheless it survived. It was a hard winter, and all day every day finches, some blue tits and a robin came to the windowsill to peck at sunflower seeds. A kind of ticking of bird time, much faster than our time.

When I was next in the clock-maker's village I couldn't believe my eyes. The shop had disappeared! No shop sign, no shop window, no engagement rings. Every window of the building shuttered. I rang the doorbell. Total silence on the other side of the door.

I went to inquire in a neighbouring shop, which was a pharmacy, and the chemist, a very precise man in a white coat, informed me that the clock-maker's family had moved out the week before, taking everything with them in a lorry.

To where?

He had no idea.

You could ask the midwife, he suggested. She might know because she's a cousin; on the other hand, she might pretend she doesn't.

I felt a kind of resignation rising in me, somewhat like the expression on the faces of clocks that no longer tell the time.

Your photos, Marc, propose that an unphotographed world would be like a house without time! They propose that cameras and timepieces are, in some way, complementary.

Ever since its beginning photography has provoked speculations about time. The nostalgia implicit in any photograph. Time stopped in its tracks. The decisive moment. The trace left behind. The photo-finish. Such notions have been much thought about and discussed.

Yet what you propose – or rather the proposal of your black-and-white untampered-with photos – is, I think, somewhat different. Photography and empiricism grew up together – both of them materialist, secular, pragmatic. Whereas you argue for a metaphysical approach. You don't exactly argue. You infiltrate with a metaphysical question.

Your concern is not with the moment, but with the past and future. And you ask a strange question: what happens if (or when) the past and future stop? Does this change the *now*, and if so, how?

Roland Barthes wrote poignantly about the connivance between a photograph and death; both of them stop time, both inflict a *coup de grâce*. Your question is about something other. What happens if past and future stop and the present is extended indefinitely? What happens in the silence of a kitchen without a clock?

The sitters in nearly all of your portraits are looking for an answer to this question. Continuous, normal human time has just left and they, eyes fixed on the doorway through which it departed, are either celebrating or waiting for its return.

I see two exceptions – one is Jean Genet, who's listening to bird time, and the other is Bram van Velde, to whom the same thing has happened many times before, so that when it happens again, he thinks about Spinoza.

Each of the other sitters is distinctly her- or himself. Each *now* in each life is unique. But the way the past and future have been arrested is the same for all of them, and they are all listening to the silence which follows this arrest.

Sometimes you juxtapose one of these portraits with an image taken in an abattoir. This is shocking but not arbitrary. For the photographed animals past and future are about to be felled in a single blow; their arrest will not be a speculative one, but physical and final. No questions are being asked. The abattoir images, however, force us to think about sacrifice, and as soon as we start speculating about the past and future, the notion of sacrifice is inseparable from the notion of survival. (One of the surprising things about abattoirs is the sense of continuity they exude.)

The way you place your abattoir photos reminds me of the way certain Renaissance painters sometimes placed a skull on a table or shelf, with the consent of the sitter, when painting a portrait.

As I write these words I'm listening to the ticking of the clock made in Ansonia. Two months had passed and one day the clock-maker's wife phoned. Your clock is repaired, she said, it took so long because there was a small piece we couldn't find a replacement for. If you fix a time, my brother will deliver it to you.

He came, and naturally I invited him in for a coffee. Together we installed the clock on the mantelpiece and set it in motion. Its ticking made the silence of the kitchen sigh. I settled the bill. It cost a lot.

I've never in my life seen another timepiece quite like it, the brother said. Would you mind if I took a photo of it up there?

Of course not, I replied.

He went out to his car to fetch his camera. And I sat at the table listening again to time passing.

Your last book you called *Paradise Lost*. The title was accompanied by an image like that of a reflection in a driver's rear mirror – an image that is being left behind. An orchard and the long shadows of two people. Paradise was before any past or future existed. There was no question of stopping them because they hadn't started.

Understanding this, I see that your vision as a photographer begins with the notion of an impossible return. What has made us human, what makes us what we are, is our awareness of past and future. Consequently we are no longer fit for paradise. In fact there'll be nobody there. And as the Arab saying puts it: a paradise without people is not worth stepping into.

Arresting past and future may, though, be a way of momentarily entering eternity. The opposite of the eternal is not the ephemeral but the forgotten.

The repaired clock, for the first time in my hearing, has just chimed.

[written *c*.2005]

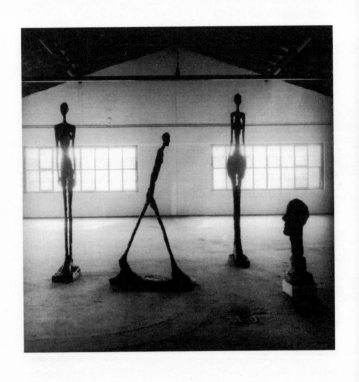

Marc Trivier: *My Beautiful*

Marc Trivier's photographs of Giacometti's sculptures are not what they first appear to be. They are not 'reproductions' of the sculptures, as in a good art catalogue. They do not record, they collaborate. Instead of facing the sculptures, the photographer put himself, and his talent for waiting with the camera, beside them. Then they all turn and advance in an Indian file. The sculptures leading and the photographs following behind, often stepping into the same footprints.

Maybe these words can join the file.

I remember two stories. The first about Trivier, the second about Giacometti. Marc was taking his photos and shifting the sculptures around a lot in order to find the place and light each one needed. Each time he carried *Annette* (see p. 194), who is only 60cm high, he found himself holding her tight against his chest. He couldn't keep her at arm's length, and this he found surprising.

One day somebody asked Alberto: When your sculptures finally have to leave the studio, where should they go? To a museum? And he replied: No, bury them in the earth, like that they may be a bridge between the living and the dead.

The light in the photograph of a single leg is like the light in an indoor swimming pool. I learnt to swim in such a pool in

Eastbourne with my father. There was a lifebelt hanging on the wall of white tiles and on it was printed Eastbourne Town Council. I think I learnt to read easily and to swim in the same year – 1931.

After 1945 Giacometti's sculptures of people (and a cat and a dog) became thinner and thinner and so it was concluded that they were on the point of disappearing. Trivier doesn't see them like that; for him they are at the point of arrival, they have just appeared. *Annette* arrives at the same instant as he considers her. *Annette is* the attention she is attracting. The truth of this has something to do with desire but it is too soon to speak of it.

Annette is persistent. She does not allow us to leave easily. She does not look at us. We have to imagine her doing so. It is partly for this that we stay.

In the Indian file I spot Katrin. Here is a photo of her. I pinned it to the wall above my working table after she died.

Katrin Cartlidge, actress. We often discussed the parts she was playing or was about to play in a film or on the stage. Each time she performed a role I had the impression she was playing one of her hundred previous lives. Her hundred very distinct lives, which meant she was familiar with a hundred very distinct wounds. When she sent me an SMS she signed off with the name – Wing. It had something to do with a joke between us.

About two months after her entirely unexpected death, I had the impression, when I pictured her in my mind, that she was withdrawing or had withdrawn. (I'm not sure whether this happened gradually or in a quantum leap; I suspect the latter.) She was no less present but her way of being present was altered. Previously she would be there in a particular place or context, which changed from day to day. A street market or a path through a wood, or she was asleep on a train, or she was reading out loud in a café something I'd written, or she was laughing fit to kill herself on a staircase. Now she seemed to be in several places at the same moment. No, more than that: she was at the same moment in a multitude of places or lives such as I couldn't envisage. Couldn't, not through a lack of imagination on my part, but through a lack of magnanimity. Her presence was as precise as before but it had become unlimited. Her *here* had become everywhere.

Now she's interrupting:

Sweetheart! That sounds good but it's not accurate. You're not in a position to say *here* about where I am!

I should say *there*?

It would be better, Sweetheart, or you could say *here* and *here* and *here* and *here* and *here* and *here* – and never stop!

Like a frog!

Laughter. Then words spoken quietly. (Her frequent laughter often led to a quiet.)

The word *or* implies a choice and I no longer have to choose, John. I've replaced the word *or* with the word *and* and I love it. Isn't *and* the word both *Annette* and I make you think of?

> *And* is neither a relation nor really a conjunction, it subtends all relations, is their flow, is what allows them to overspill beyond their boundaries, beyond what can be thought of as Being, beyond One or All.

Those words are not mine but Gilles Deleuze's. He loved collaborations and a multitude of voices.

The resemblance between *Annette* and Katrin is striking. The holding of their heads, the pits of their two necks where they join their chests, the swivel of their chins, the direct current, the charge, running between their faces and bodies – all this is similar. But their resemblance comes from something deeper. In the bronze statue and in the black-and-white snapshot, each of them has left behind everything; each of them has brought nothing but herself. This irreducibility is what they have in common.

The irreducible was Giacometti's ideal. His figures are there,

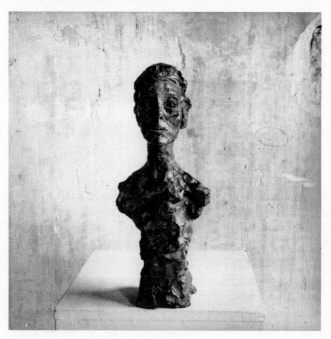

with what is left after air and light and usage have dispersed with the rest. They are like skeletons? The opposite. They concern what anatomy can never categorize or identify. They show how, in the depths of a body, there is an interface, a shared skin between the physical and metaphysical.

Most portraits in the history of art refer first to the gender and class and milieu to which their sitters belonged, and secondly to what was particular and unique about the particular person posing. Doña Cobos de Porcel in Goya's portrait of her is first a woman, an aristocrat, a desperado of the First Spanish Civil War, and then she is Isabel with her fateful, special attraction towards what may harm her. Each of Giacometti's sculptured portraits seems to present an irreducible self, who only then happens to be woman or man, old or young, philosopher or gangster's moll. Each of his portraits is like a first name cast in bronze.

Annette.

When discussing the Stoic philosophers, Gilles Deleuze wrote:

> Between physical things in depth and the surfaces of metaphysical events, there is a strict complementarity.

Jump from the Stoic philosophers, referred to by Gilles, into the municipal swimming pool. Not the one in Eastbourne but another in the Parisian suburb of Fresnes, where the notorious Maison d'Arrêt is.

People of all ages go to the pool. Fathers take their sons. Quite a number of regulars go alone. They may nod to one another. Sometimes there are seven swimmers, sometimes seventy. It depends upon the day of the week, the hour and the season. The kids address their fathers. Otherwise words are deemed superfluous.

Most of the swimmers wear dark goggles to protect their eyes from the chlorine. Bonnets are obligatory – even for the bald. Everybody is concentrated on the act of swimming. Some dive in. Others step slowly down a ladder. They swim in order to keep healthy, to lose weight, to exercise their hearts, for the pleasure of being in the water, or for the odd and deep pleasure of carrying out something private and alone in company! Occasionally there's a swimmer who is dreaming of becoming a local champion. Everyone swims side by side, length after length, each following her or his own unmarked, narrow channel.

When you climb out, you notice, if you've been swimming like me without goggles, a slight haze around those still swimming or those leaving the pool to have a shower before dressing and drying their hair. The haze comes from your sore eyes, yet I like to believe it may also have something to do with thought. I've never accepted that thinking only clarifies; it fills an emptiness too. Thought has its own opacity.

The standing or striding figures in the swimming pool at Fresnes when I watch them are as blurred as are Giacometti's standing and striding figures in one of Marc's photos.

A tall young man under a shower soaping his long legs. A middle-aged woman holding on to the pool's edge, looking concentratedly at the water, which reaches her collarbones, as if it's a book she's reading. A man of my age swimming the crawl slowly towards his past. An eleven-year-old walking along the side of the pool savouring the treasure of her hips.

There's no place for sexiness here, the location doesn't allow it. It's a place where there's a lot of Desire – and many desires – but sexiness is elsewhere.

I imagine the young man, the portly woman, the septuagenarian, the eleven-year-old, whom I have just described, returning to their private lives and being recognized and welcomed by someone with whom they are intimate.

My beautiful.

Sexual desire, when reciprocal, is a plot, hatched by two, in the face of, or in defiance of, all the other plots which determine the world. It is a conspiracy of two.

The plan is to offer to the other a reprieve from the pain of the world. Not happiness but a physical reprieve from the body's huge liability towards pain.

Within all desire there is pity as well as appetite; the two, whatever their relative proportion, are threaded together. Desire is inconceivable without a wound.

If there were any unwounded in this world, they would live without desire.

The human body has prowess, grace, playfulness, dignity and countless other capacities, but it is also intrinsically tragic – as is no animal's body. (No animal is naked.) Desire longs to shield the desired body from the tragic it embodies, and what is more it believes it can.

The conspiracy is to create together a place, a locus, of exemption, and the exemption, necessarily temporary, is from the unmitigated hurt which flesh is heir to.

The *locus* is the inside of the other's body. The conspiracy consists of passing into the other, wherein each will be unfindable. Desire is a movement of hiding-places being exchanged. (To reduce this to a 'desire to return to the womb' is a trivialization.)

Touch a leg with a lover's hand. Whether to arouse or calm makes no difference. The touch seeks to reach further than femur, tibia or fibula, to the leg's very core, and the entire lover hopes to follow that touch and to reside there. Giacometti's leg of the Eastbourne baths is about (among other things) Desire.

There is no altruism in desire. From the start, two bodies are involved, and so the exemption, when and if achieved, covers both. The exemption is bound to be brief and yet it promises all. The exemption abolishes brevity – and along with it the hurts associated with the threat of the brief.

Observed by a third person, desire is a short parenthesis; experienced from within, it is an immanence and an entrance into a plenitude. Plenitude is usually thought of as an amassing. Desire reveals that it is a stripping away: the plenitude of a silence, a darkness.

I think of the legend of the Golden Fleece. (It granted an exemption from a sacrifice.) It lies hanging in its hiding-place, curly, inviolate, complete, worn by nobody. When Marc held *Annette* against his chest, she became a Golden Fleece. See her silhouette in the photo.

*

I once did a drawing of Andrei Platonov from a picture in a newspaper. Maybe the drawing came from some of his words too. Words which, for me, had to be translated since he wrote in Russian. A muttered Russian of the small hours. He was born in Voronezh in 1899 and he died in Moscow in 1951. At the bottom of the drawing I stuck a train ticket and wrote a sentence from one of his stories: 'He went far away for a long while – perhaps for ever.'

Andrei has now joined the Indian file and Katrin is listening to him talking as he follows her.

In a book entitled *Djann* he tells the story of a group of nomads who have ended up in a salt desert (desolate) somewhere near the Sea of Aral in Uzbekistan. They have lost everything – means of survival, possessions, cattle, any notion of the future and all illusions.

He wrote the book in 1935 and it was first published after his death in the 1960s. Andrei Platonov was an errant poet of sharing and penury. To share, he once said, gives you back a sense of the real. I can't hear what he's saying to Katrin. He believed that ultimate losers are loved yet don't know it, and that in this ignorance of theirs, there is something more sacred than anything else on earth.

In the middle of the story, one night before the onset of the merciless winter, the principal protagonist overhears a man and woman whispering in their bare hut.

We are both good for nothing, says the woman, you are thin and useless, as for me my breasts are withered and there's a pain in the marrow of my bones.

I won't stop loving what's left of you, says the man.

They say nothing else. Doubtless they are lying together so as to hold in their hands their one happiness.

I won't stop loving what's left of you.

The extremity of these eight words is close to the extremity of *Annette*'s stance.

Not long ago I was in Firenze. Snow was falling on the Duomo, and the Arno running under the bridges was the colour of an old skull. The city was as cold as a garrison town in winter. Usually the weather and all the produce from the Tuscan hills mask the fact that Firenze was (is) the sharpest, the least indulgent of the great Italian cities.

At a certain moment I took refuge from the icy streets in the Museo del Bargelo and there I came upon a coloured porcelain head of a young saint – or is she an angel? – by Luca della Robbia. He made it when he was in his sixties. It has only three colours. A flaxen ochre for her or his hair, a sorrel green for the collar of the tunic, and the inimitable della Robbia blue for the tunic itself and his or her cap. The flesh is porcelain white. How to describe the della Robbia blue? It combines an Aegean Sea with the Madonna's robe, it promises Memory; it is the blue of music. The colours have nothing to do with life but the angel is lifelike.

When Luca was younger, before the family business of making coloured busts and reliefs and medallions to make the city seem more innocent than it was had got under way, he was Donatello's equal as a sculptor in bronze. His *Singing Gallery*, a sequence of high reliefs about musicians, singers and dancers making music, is amazing. I know of no other work which shows so precisely in its depiction of bodies the power of music to carry away players and listeners. When you look at it, you think that Elvis, Jim Morrison, Miles, Bird, Ferré or Piotr were already announced in bronze at the beginning of the Quattrocento.

Luca has joined the file and Andrei is explaining to him that his father worked on the railways as an engine-driver and that he himself, before he became an engineer, studied at the Railway Polytechnic.

Luca della Robbia was an exact contemporary of the painter Masaccio. The latter died at the age of twenty-nine and the former lived to the age of eighty-two. Masaccio's fresco of Adam and Eve in the church of Santa Maria del Carmine, which is ten minutes' walk away from the Museo del Bargelo, is one of the most eloquent evocations ever of how the human body is intrinsically tragic.

Luca is now talking to Katrin. She has green eyes.

The angel was beautiful. I'm thinking of her presence, not about the outcome of some struggle to make art. I did a drawing to try to understand better the expression of her face. And while I was drawing her expression, I understood something quite different.

Her face assures you that you're being looked at by her. Beauty here is not what you enjoy looking at but what you want to be looked at by! Beauty is the hope of being recognized by, and included within, the existence of what you're looking at.

This hope of being looked at and recognized doesn't only occur before portraits of sexy Florentines. A lion drawn in the dark on a rock face thirty thousand years ago offers, apart from the elegance of his profile, an inclusion in the world in which he exists. And the same is perhaps true when the beautiful is not man-made, when it is found in a sunset, a plant, an animal, a mountain. Any of these is beautiful when they answer the same hope as the angel's face seemed to do.

We are waiting for *Annette* to look.

Stop reading. Find the photo. Her body is looking straight at us.

Giacometti and Trivier in *My Beautiful* search for a zone of experience where a coming-into-view is the equivalent of a meeting. Or, to put it another way: both testify, not to a state of being, but to a shared movement of becoming. Both leave behind them a gesture of stepping, not forwards but towards. Stepping towards, with legs and a looking and a tongue and a listening and a solitude.

Last week, Mélina, my granddaughter, learnt to walk.

Such a zone of experience is entered innumerable times every day. In Fresnes and in Firenze. Everywhere. Yet each entry bears a different first name, and the zone itself remains nameless.

My beautiful.

2004

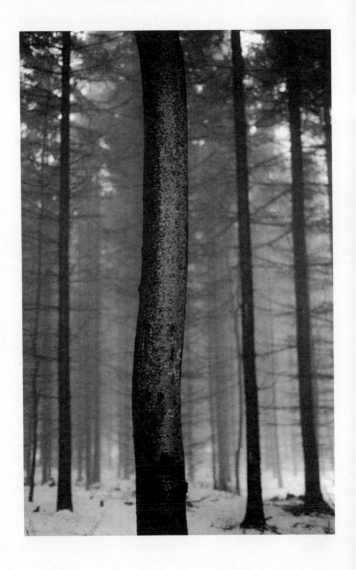

Jitka Hanzlová: *Forest*

The way I go is the way back to see the future.

Jitka Hanzlová

The forest in question is far away, near the Carpathian mountains, beside the Czech village where she lived as a child. The images could be of another forest, but not for Jitka. Over the years she has returned to hers. She goes into it alone, and if not alone does not take pictures.

Many nature photographs are like fashion photos. This is not to dismiss them; they record and admit pleasure. Mountaintops, waterfalls, meadows, lakes, beech trees in autumn, are asked to stand there, wearing themselves and giving the camera a moody look. And why not? They are reminders of the pleasure of at last arriving after hours in airports. Nature as hostess.

In Jitka's pictures there is no welcome. They have been taken from the inside. The deep inside of a forest, perceived like the inside of a glove by a hand within it.

She speaks of the between-forest. This is because, in the same valley as her village, there are two forests which join. Yet the preposition *between* belongs to forests in general. It's what they are about. A forest is what exists between its trees, between its dense undergrowth and its clearings, between all its life cycles and their different time scales, ranging from solar energy to insects that live for a day. A forest is also a meeting-place between those who enter it

203

and something unnameable and attendant, waiting behind a tree or in the undergrowth. Something intangible and within touching distance. Neither silent nor audible. It is not only visitors who feel this attendant something; hunters and foresters who can read unwritten signs are even more keenly aware of it.

> I went to the forest-hills early in the morning when the forest awakes. Standing there I breathed in the wind, the unruffled voices of the birds and the silence which I love. And then when I was concentrating on a picture, I stopped hearing the silence around me. It was as if I was somewhere else, like in a film. The forest started to move and, as I looked through the camera, I experienced fear. Maybe it was just the framing and the stillness of the evening. As if the birds and the crickets had stopped their singing, as if the wind had come to a stop in the valley. Nothing, but nothing to hear. No birds, no wind, no people, no crickets. The darkness of the light and this other silence made my hair stand on end . . . I could not exactly place the fear, but it was coming from the inside. It was the first time I felt this so intensely, but not the last. I escaped! What's the basis of this fear of mine? Why? I'm not afraid of animals or of the forest. The place is safe.

Throughout history and prehistory forests have offered shelter, a hiding-place, while also being places in which a wanderer can be ultimately lost. They oblige us to recognize how much is hidden.

It's a commonplace to say that photographs interrupt or arrest the flow of time. They do it, however, in thousands of different ways. Cartier-Bresson's 'decisive moment' is different from Atget's slowing down to a standstill, or from Thomas Struth's ceremonial stopping of time. What is strange about some of Jitka's forest photos – not her photos of other subjects – is that they appear to have stopped nothing!

In a space without gravity there is no weight, and these pictures of hers are, as it were, weightless in terms of time. It is as if they have been taken *between* times, where there is none.

What is intangible and within touching distance in a forest may be the presence of a kind of timelessness. Not the abstract timelessness of metaphysical speculation, nor the metaphorical timelessness of cyclic, seasonal repetition. Forests exist in time, they are, God knows, subject to history; and today many are catastrophically being obliterated for the quick pursuit of profit.

Yet in a forest there are 'events' which have not found their place in any of the forest's numberless time scales, and which exist between those scales. What events? you ask. Some are in Jitka's photographs. They are what remains unnameable in the photographs after we have made an inventory of everything that is recognizable.

The ancient Greeks named events like these *dryads*. My lumberjack friends from Bergamo refer to the forest as a separate kingdom, a 'realm' on its own. Wilfredo Lam painted equivalent events in his imagined jungle. Yet let's be clear. We are not talking about fantasies. Jitka spoke of the forest's silence. The diametric opposite of such a silence is music. In music every event that occurs is accommodated within the single seamless time scale of that music. In the silence of the forest, certain events are unaccommodated and cannot be placed in time. Being like this they both disconcert and entice the observer's imagination: for they are like another creature's experience of duration. We feel them occurring, we feel their presence, yet we cannot confront them, for they are occurring for us, somewhere between past, present and future.

The philosopher Heidegger, for whom a forest was a metaphor for all reality – and the task of the philosopher was to find the *Weg*, the woodcutters' path, through it – spoke of 'coming into the nearness of distance' and I believe this was his way of approaching the forest phenomenon I am trying to define. Just as Jitka's formulation is another. 'The way I go is the way back to see the future.' Both reverse the hourglass.

To make sense of what I'm suggesting it is necessary to reject the notion of time that began in Europe during the eighteenth century and is closely linked with the positivism and linear accountability of modern capitalism: the notion that a single time, which is unilinear, regular, abstract and irreversible, carries everything. All other cultures have proposed a coexistence of various times surrounded in some way by the timeless.

Return to the forests that belong to history. In Jitka's one there is often a sense of waiting, yet what is it that is waiting? And is waiting the right word? A patience. A patience practised by what? A forest incident. An incident we can neither name, describe nor place. And yet is there.

The intricacy of the crossing paths and crossing energies in a forest – the paths of birds, insects, mammals, spores, seeds, reptiles, ferns, lichens, worms, trees, etc., etc. – is unique; perhaps in certain areas on the seabed there exists a comparable intricacy, but there man is a recent intruder, whereas, with all his sense perceptions, he came from the forest. Man is the only creature who lives within at least two time scales: the biological one of his body and the one of his consciousness. (This is perhaps what grants him his sixth sense.) Every one of the crossing energies operating in a forest has its own time scale. From the ant to the oak tree. From the process of photosynthesis to the process of fermentation. In this intricate conglomeration of times, energies and exchanges there occur 'incidents' that are recalcitrant incidents, unaccommodated in any time scale and therefore (temporarily?) waiting *between*. These are what Jitka photographs.

The longer one looks at Jitka Hanzlová's pictures of a forest, the clearer it becomes that a breakout from the prison of modern time is possible. The dryads beckon. You may slip between – but unaccompanied.

2005

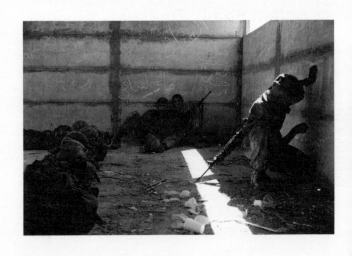

Ahlam Shibli: *Trackers*

First, a distinction between being simple and simplifying. The former has something to do with reducing or being reduced to the essential. And the latter – simplification – is usually part of a manoeuvre in some struggle for power. Simplifications are self-serving. Most political leaders simplify, while the powerless react simply to what is happening. There is often an abyss between the two.

Now let's look at Ahlam Shibli's photographs without making simplifications. They offer, among other things, a political lesson and are, in this sense, exemplary. But we'll come to that later. She calls the sequence of pictures *Trackers*, and this requires an explanation.

There are one million Palestinians today living with official papers, as underclass citizens, in the state of Israel. In the media they are described as Israeli-Arabs. They are never referred to as Palestinians. Among the Israeli-Arabs are Bedouin families.

From these families a small number of men – less than a hundred a year – volunteer to join the Israeli army, where they will be trained and used as military scouts, who are known as trackers. The trackers, who are exclusively 'Israeli-Arabs', do much of the army's dangerous field-reconnaissance work. It is they who are sent ahead, whenever the Command reckons there may be resistance, to clear a terrain of land-mines, snipers, possible ambushes. The trackers are initially trained together in groups of about twenty or thirty.

Once trained, they are separated out and allotted alone to units of the Israeli Defence Force, or the IDF as the army calls itself.

After three years' service, a tracker may volunteer again to become a professional soldier, whereby he will be very much better paid. The IDF Command accept only a small number of such volunteers. The professional trackers have an advantage over Israeli soldiers because of their familiarity with local customs, habits and ways of calculation.

Ahlam Shibli's pictures are discreet, elusive and persistent. They contain the minimum of general information and they never report about incidents or events. One has the impression that each one has been taken just after something has happened. Not because Shibli was too slow, but because what interests her is *affect*. Events, as such, do not (at least in this project) concern her; the impact of an event on a life does. And so she is prepared to wait.

She watches the military training of the trackers, trackers going on leave, a cemetery with soldiers' graves, the taking of an oath of allegiance to the IDF sworn on the Koran, the interior of a house with family pictures on the wall, new houses being slowly built thanks to the professional army pay the trackers are earning. Each different location leads slyly to a query. For these men what constitutes a home? Or, more slyly: to where and what do they have a sense of belonging?

There is never anybody there in the picture to tell us what happened just before it was taken. All we can do is to look at the participants who remain and then guess for ourselves and, like Shibli, wait. The effect of the whole series (eighty-five photos) is cumulative. They fit together to make a whole. Yet what does the whole add up to?

For Bedouin the issue of home and what constitutes a home is as entwined as a rope. Traditionally they are a nomadic people. Two or three generations ago, particularly in the Sinai, many Bedouin families became sedentary, yet the land they settled on belonged to somebody else, and on it they had minimal rights. A confused situation in which atavistic memories perhaps play a part. For nomads, home is not an address, home is what they carry with them.

What do the trackers carry?

Ahlam Shibli is soul-searching. Yet she avoids soulfulness and never seeks a confession. She watches patiently from the side. One might say she was a storyteller, yet this would be to simplify her chosen role. (There are great photographic storytellers – André Kertész, for example.) Ahlam Shibli, I would say, is a fortune-teller. She observes intensely, reads the signs, guesses and proffers her prophecy which, like a soothsayer's, is both sharp and unclear; it lays out the chances like playing cards, yet doesn't select one.

Select three. In the first, three trackers, sheltering, take a rest, and one of them is writing something on a public wall. In the second, a man asleep in the daytime, has pulled a cover over his face. In the third are the photos a tracker has framed of himself as an IDF warrior, on a wall in his house, beside an old map of Palestine.

In each one, differently expressed, is the same dilemma concerning identity and whereabouts.

What are they carrying?

Traditionally, and over the centuries, nomadic Bedouin clans have offered their services to any invading force – be it Egyptian, Turkish, British – whenever they recognized that they themselves, with all their guerrilla skills, were nevertheless outflanked. They did this, however, to avoid being disbanded and in order to remain independent, unchallengeable on their own, almost impenetrable territories. It was a cunning strategy for continuity, which often succeeded.

Today the circumstances for Israeli Bedouins have become very different. They have been hounded off their land and stripped of their economic means of survival. In their own Negev Desert they are treated as criminal trespassers, and their crops are sprayed with herbicide from IDF helicopters.

To grasp finally what this means we have to take account of the extremity of the Palestinian situation in general. The Palestinian–Israeli conflict has lasted nearly sixty years. The military occupation of Palestine – the longest in history – has lasted nearly forty years. Scarcely necessary to repeat all the facts that this occupation entails, for they have been internationally recognized and condemned. The Palestinian economy and everyday life have been reduced to rubble. The illegal Israeli settlements encroach upon and devour Palestinian land each week. The illegal Wall, implacably advancing, is dividing up what remains of that land into future 'Bantustans'. East Jerusalem, occupied and transformed into an Arab ghetto, is being dismantled piecemeal.

What is sometimes forgotten about this continuing conflict – for the Palestinians continue to resist – is the disparity, the inequality of means, whether in terms of firepower or defence. The IDF are armed with everything that modern technology can supply, from helicopters and guided missiles to surveillance cameras and computerized tracking methods, whereas the Palestinians have recourse to small arms, home-made explosives, a few mortars, occasional suicide martyrs, and stones. Their single advantage is their enduring faith in the justice of what they are defending. Against this, the state of Israel, besides enlisting a few Bedouin trackers, enjoys the unconditional support of the world's first megapower, the USA.

Such a disparity of resources and arms recalls the mid-twentieth-century colonial wars of liberation, and if we want to understand the trackers' dilemma we could not do better than consult the writings of Frantz Fanon, who was a visionary prophet of those struggles. At the end of *Black Skin, White Masks*, he writes: 'At the conclusion of this study, I want the world to recognise, with me, the open door of every consciousness.' (Ahlam Shibli, writing about her *Trackers*, refers often to Frantz Fanon.)

As a doctor and psychiatrist from Martinique working in Algeria, Fanon explained how colonial domination, how the disparity of means between the invader and the indigenous, how the contempt inwritten into every encounter between the armed and the unarmed, besides producing revolt, can also lead to a gash in those allegiances which maintain a person's sense of self. And that this happens most frequently and woundingly among the poorest and the most underprivileged of the trampled-on.

An image may help to make this more clear. Consider the opposite syndrome, which is that of the megalomaniac. Every encounter with another person works for the megalomaniac like a held-up mirror in which he sees himself reflected and decked out in his own glory. For the colonized, who has lost his sense of self, every encounter is a mirror in which he sees nothing but a soiled djellaba. Both held-up mirrors hide the other as she or he really is. And so it happens that the colonized, in order to disassociate himself from the soiled djellaba, dreams of wearing the uniform or carrying the flag of his oppressor. Not his enemy, his oppressor.

The Bedouin are among the most underprivileged of Palestinians and they have lost, for the most part, their nomadic liberty and the pride that went with it. So it can happen, as Fanon foresaw, that they split themselves in two, and tearing themselves apart, wear the mask of their oppressors. Many change their names from Ahmed to José, from Mohammed to Moshe. Yet, in doing this, the trackers do not refind their own bodies, their noble bodies that are calumnied by the false image of the soiled djellaba.

The man with the bedcover pulled over his head is dreaming of what? One can never guess at what somebody else is dreaming. *Yet he can probably not guess at his own dream.*

Something like this is what the trackers carry.

*

This work of Ahlam Shibli makes no direct political comment on the Israeli–Palestinian conflict, it refrains from slogans. Yet I believe that in today's global context it is politically important – or, as I said, exemplary. And I will try to explain why.

Ahlam Shibli herself comes from a Bedouin family. As a young girl she was herding goats in Galilee. Later, after studying at university, she became a photographer of international renown.

Long ago she made the opposite existential choice to the trackers whom she shows in these photos. She believes in the justice of the Palestinian cause and has protested as a patriot and a photographer against the illegal Israeli occupation. For her, as for most Palestinians, the trackers can be considered traitors. They have joined an army which is oppressing the Palestinian people and they stalk to kill and capture those who actively resist that army. Traitors . . . In certain circumstances, they must be treated as such.

Nevertheless Ahlam Shibli feels a need to go beyond, and search behind, the simplifying label. Because she is a Bedouin herself? Maybe, but the question is naïve. What counts is the result. Because she is Bedouin, she was able to search behind the label and discover what she had to discover. With these photographs she posed the question: what price are they paying for their decision to become trackers? Then she waited for the enigmatic answers which she found in her darkroom. And these she makes public.

How is this political? In the mid-twentieth century Walter Benjamin wrote: 'The state of emergency in which we live is not the exception but the rule. We must attain to a concept of history that is in keeping with this insight.'

Within such a concept of history we have to come to see that every simplification, every label, serves only the interests of those who wield power; the more extensive their power, the greater their need for simplifications. And, by contrast, the interests of those who suffer under or struggle against this blind power are served

now and for the long, long future by the recognition and acceptance of diversity, differences and complexities.

These photographs are a contribution to such an acceptance
and recognition.

I will end by quoting Frantz Fanon once more:

No, we do not want to catch up with anyone. What we want to do
is to go forward all the time, night and day, in the company of Man,
in the company of all men. The caravan should not be stretched
out, for in that case each line will hardly see those who precede it;
and men who no longer recognise each other meet less and less
together, and talk to each other less and less . . .

2007

Editor's note

The closing quotation from Frantz Fanon is taken from *The
Wretched of the Earth* (New York: Grove Press, 1963), p. 314,
while the quotation on p. 212 is from *Black Skin, White Masks*
(London: Pluto, 1986), p. 181.

Sources

'Image of Imperialism': from John Berger, *The Moment of Cubism* (London: Weidenfeld & Nicolson, 1969). First published in *New Society*, 26 October 1967 and 18 January 1968; reprinted in John Berger, *Selected Essays and Articles: The Look of Things* (Harmondsworth: Penguin, 1972) and *Selected Essays* (London: Bloomsbury, 2001).

'Understanding a Photograph' and 'Political Uses of Photo-Montage': from *The Look of Things*. First published in *New Society*, 17 October 1968 and 23 October 1969 respectively; reprinted in *Selected Essays*.

'Photographs of Agony', 'The Suit and the Photograph', 'Paul Strand' and 'Uses of Photography': from John Berger, *About Looking* (London: Writers and Readers, 1980). First published in *New Society*, 27 July 1972, 22 March 1979, 30 March 1972 and 17 and 24 August 1978 (in two parts, in slightly different form) respectively; reprinted in *Selected Essays*.

'Appearances' and 'Stories': from John Berger, *Another Way of Telling* (London: Writers and Readers, 1982).

'Christ of the Peasants': from John Berger, *Keeping a Rendezvous* (London: Granta, 1992). First published as text for Markéta Luskačová, *Pilgrims* (London: Arts Council, 1985).

'W. Eugene Smith': written around 1988 and previously unpublished.

Sources

'Walking Back Home': afterword to Chris Killip, *In Flagrante* (London: Secker & Warburg, 1988).

'Means to Live': from Nick Waplington, *Living Room* (New York: Aperture, 1991).

'André Kertész: *On Reading*': first published in German translation in *Die Weltwoche* in 1996. Previously unpublished in English.

'A Man Begging in the Métro': from John Berger, *Photocopies* (London: Bloomsbury, 1996).

'Martine Franck': foreword to Martine Franck, *One Day to the Next* (London: Thames & Hudson, 1998).

'Jean Mohr: A Sketch for a Portrait': from Jean Mohr, *At the Edge of the World* (London: Reaktion, 1999).

'A Tragedy the Size of the Planet': from the film *The Spectre of Hope*, directed by Paul Carlin (Icarus Films, 2001). Part of the text was published in the *Guardian*, 18 May 2001.

'Recognition': from Moyra Peralta, *Nearly Invisible* (London: Inside Eye, 2001).

'Tribute to Cartier-Bresson': from the *Observer*, 8 August 2004, published under the title 'John Berger pays tribute to his good friend'.

'Between Here and Then': written to accompany a planned exhibition of photographs by Marc Trivier in 2005. Previously unpublished.

'Marc Trivier: *My Beautiful*': from Marc Trivier, *My Beautiful* (Nord-Pas-de-Calais: Centre Régional de la Photographie, 2004).

Sources

'Jitka Hanzlová: *Forest*' and 'Ahlam Shibli: *Trackers*': from John Berger, *Hold Everything Dear* (London: Verso, 2007). 'Jitka Hanzlová: *Forest*' first published as text for Jitka Hanzlová, *Forest* (Göttingen: Steidl, 2005), and 'Ahlam Shibli: *Trackers*' first published as text for Ahlam Shibli, *Trackers*, ed. Adam Szymczyk (Cologne: Verlag der Buchhandlung Walther König, 2007).